AF307906

D. Pickuth • Essentials of Ultrasonography: A Practical Guide

Springer
*Berlin
Heidelberg
New York
Barcelona
Budapest
Hong Kong
London
Milan
Paris
Tokyo*

Dirk Pickuth

Essentials of Ultrasonography
A Practical Guide

In Collaboration with
Christella A. Grover, M. Chiara Bossi, Rajendra P. Kedar

With Forewords by
V. R. McCready, G. van Kaick, U. Veronesi

With 256 Figures, 1 Chapter in Colour

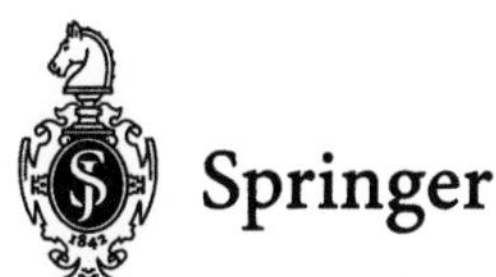 Springer

Dr. Dirk Pickuth, MD
Department of Radiology
German Cancer Research Centre
Im Neuenheimer Feld 280
D-69120 Heidelberg

Title of the German Edition:
D. Pickuth: Sonographie – systematisch
© 1993 by UNI-MED Verlag AG, Lorch, Germany

ISBN-13:978-3-642-79581-7   e-ISBN-13:978-3-642-79579-4
DOI: 10.1007/978-3-642-79579-4

Library of Congress Cataloging-in-Publication Data

Pickuth, Dirk, 1966– [Sonographie–systematisch. English] Essentials of ultrasonography: a practical guide/Dirk Pickuth, in collaboration with Christella A. Grover, M. Chiara Bossi, Rajendra P. Kedar; with forewords by V.R. McCready, G. van Kaick, U. Veronesi. p. cm. Includes bibliographycal references and index. ISBN-13:978-3-642-79581-7(hardcover:alk. paper)1.Diagnosis, Ultrasonic. I. Grover, Christella A., 1922- . II. Bossi, M. Chiara, 1954- . III. Kedar, Rajendra P., 1961- . RC78.7.U4P5313 1995 616.07'543 – dc20 95-31138 CIP

© Springer-Verlag Berlin Heidelberg 1995
Softcover reprint of the hardcover 1st edition 1995

The use of general descriptive names, registered names, trademarks, etc. in this publication does not imply, even in the absence of a specific statement, that such names are exempt from the relevant protective laws and regulations and therefore free for general use.

Product liability: The publishers cannot guarantee the accuracy of any information about the application of operative techniques and medications contained in this book. In every individual case the user must check such information by consulting the relevant literature.

Typesetting: Data conversion by Springer-Verlag

SPIN: 10134013   21/3135 – 5 4 3 2 1 0
Printed on acid-free paper

To my parents,
a wellspring of love and support
without bounds

D. Pickuth

Authors

Dr. D. Pickuth, MD
Department of Radiology, German Cancer Research Centre, Heidelberg, Germany; formerly Clinical Research Fellow, Diagnostic Imaging Department, The Royal Marsden Hospital, London, United Kingdom; formerly Clinical Research Fellow, Diagnostic Imaging Department, The Royal Infirmary, Edinburgh, United Kingdom

Dr. C. A. Grover, BSc, MB, ChB, MRCGP
Diagnostic Imaging Department, The Royal Marsden Hospital, London, United Kingdom

Dr. M. C. Bossi, MD
Department of Radiology, European Institute of Oncology, Milan, Italy; formerly Locum Consultant, Diagnostic Imaging Department, The Royal Marsden Hospital, London, United Kingdom

Dr. R. P. Kedar, MD
Department of Radiology, Bridgeport Hospital, Affiliate of Yale University School of Medicine, Bridgeport, United States of America; formerly Clinical Research Fellow, Diagnostic Imaging Department, The Royal Marsden Hospital, London, United Kingdom; formerly Associate Professor, Department of Radiology, King Edward Memorial Hospital, Bombay, India

For Sect.1.1:
Dipl.-Ing. S. Longstaff
Dipl.-Ing. P. Ziebart
Picker International, Espelkamp, Germany

For Sect.1.2:
Dr. R. Schlief, MD
Schering, Berlin, Germany

Foreword I

This textbook is designed for physicians, students, and radiographers who wish to learn ultrasonography concisely and comprehensively. All general aspects of diagnostic ultrasound are covered. The text encompasses principally those disorders that are encountered in the daily routine of scanning, but mention is also made of rarer conditions which must be considered in differential diagnosis.

The authors present the subject systematically and practically, and with the facility of quick reference in mind. For didactic purposes they use many flow-charts, tables and teaching points. The book will be invaluable for learning and for scanning, as well as for reporting.

Dr. Dirk Pickuth, who has been Clinical Research Fellow in our Diagnostic Imaging Department, conceived the idea of this international publication. As the main author he was supported by his British, Italian, and Indian colleagues, and the four physicians collaborated in this Department most amicably, which has resulted in this highly commendable book. I wish it every success.

Prof. V. R. McCready
Chief, Diagnostic Imaging Department
The Royal Marsden Hospital
London, United Kingdom

Foreword II

Ultrasound still continues to develop, with the clinical spectrum of its application becoming ever wider. Accordingly, the number of ultrasound textbooks has increased considerably in recent years.

The question of which is the right ultrasound textbook for the beginner or for the more experienced sonographer is very difficult to answer, because many of these books are impractical by virtue of their complexity and size.

These difficulties have been overcome by the production of this book. It systematically presents the principles of ultrasound. Each chapter has the same format, making cross-references easy for the reader. This concept is unique and differs from the traditional organization of an ultrasound textbook. The main advantages of the book are its conciseness, preciseness, and comprehensiveness, making it a select choice for all who are interested in ultrasound.

I have no doubt that the efforts of the authors will be rewarded by a successful contribution to sonographical education.

Prof. G. van Kaick
Chief, Department of Radiology
German Cancer Research Centre
Heidelberg, Germany

Foreword III

This book provides an excellent comprehensive and practical text encompassing all major aspects of ultrasound that are routinely in clinical use. It is beautifully illustrated, using clear diagrams and high-quality images. The lists of diagnostic criteria found in each chapter is a particularly attractive feature.

I welcome this book, which was conceived at The Royal Marsden Hospital, London, known internationally as a centre of oncology research. Ultrasound is employed daily to detect or to exclude cancerous conditions and to assess their diffusion; the recognition of its features is vital in differentiating many benign diseases which may simulate malignancy.

The book has achieved a commendable logic in the complex process of reaching a diagnosis; it is easy to consult, both by the learner and by the more experienced, and should prove to be a valuable companion to all who are involved in ultrasound.

Prof. U. Veronesi
Scientific Director
European Institute of Oncology
Milan, Italy

Preface

With the vast number of publications on the subject of ultrasound, yet another based on teaching and use seemed un-called-for; however, we realized there was an absence of a concise but comprehensive manual available for ready reference, to those engaged in daily scanning and interpretation, or to those who desire knowledge of ultrasound in the scheme of diagnostic medicine. Therefore one may say that it was a fortuitous coincidence that four of the authors, each from a different country but sharing enthusiasm, found themselves working together at The Royal Marsden Hospital, London. Realizing that the material, experience, and expertise were available, they conceived the idea of the production of this book.

To our knowledge, the subject has not previously been presented in this format, and our aim was to encompass the principles of ultrasound with a methodical approach in practice towards the diagnosis of disease, in a manual which is readily at hand to facilitate reference and reporting. The book will be invaluable to the beginner, from whatever discipline, first starting to work in medical ultrasound, but it should also contain useful hints for even the most experienced practitioner.

In conclusion, acknowledgement should be made to Dr. David O. Cosgrove whose teaching and scanning skill provided the invaluable basis which inspired the production of this book.

D. Pickuth
C. A. Grover
M. C. Bossi
R. P. Kedar

Contents

Explanatory Notes

The first chapters of the book are on physical principles and technical considerations, including how to adjust equipment for best images, and on ultrasound contrast media and artefacts.

The book then details the sonoanatomy and the sonopathology of each organ. All chapters have the same format:

x.1   Imaging Modalities
x.2   Ultrasonography
x.2.1   Examination Technique
x.2.2   Sonoanatomy
x.2.2.1 Normal Dimensions
x.2.3   Sonopathology
          – Clinical Data
          – Sonographic Diagnosis
          – Sonographic Differential Diagnosis
x.2.4   Checklist for Reporting

The book provides many images, flow-charts, tables, and teaching points to add clarity to the explanations given in the text.

Part I

Chapter **1** Introduction

1.1 Basics

What Is Ultrasound?

Sound waves with a frequency above that which can be heard (>16 kHz) are referred to as ultrasound. At the present time frequencies of between 3 and 10 MHz are the most commonly used in medical diagnostic ultrasound. The speed of sound through a medium depends upon the density and the elastic modulus of the medium.

What Happens When an Ultrasound Wave Passes from One Medium to Another?

When an ultrasound wave meets a boundary between two media, the energy is reflected, refracted, scattered, and absorbed in the medium.

Reflection. Reflection takes place at the boundary between two media of differing acoustic impedance. The greater the difference between the acoustic impedances of the individual media the greater the reflection. In the case of a boundary between air and tissue approximately 99% of the wave is reflected. For this reason an ultrasound contact gel is used to reduce the reflection at the boundary between the transducer and the skin surface. The intensity of the reflected wave also depends upon the angle of the incident wave. As the incident angle increases, so the reflected intensity decreases. What this means for the operator is that a reflector parallel to the transducer is displayed brighter than one which is at an angle to the transducer.

Table 1. Speed of ultrasound, acoustic impedance, and density

	Speed (m s^{-1})	Density (g cm^{-3})	Impedance (g cm^{-2} s^{-1})
Air	331	0.0013	$0.00043 \cdot 10^5$
Bone	3600	1.7	$6.12 \cdot 10^5$
Muscle	1568	1.04	$1.63 \cdot 10^5$
Water	1492	0.9982	$1.489 \cdot 10^5$
Fat	1450–1470	0.97	$1.38\text{–}1.42 \cdot 10^5$

Refraction. Sound behaves as light in that, when a sound wave meets at an angle other than a right angle the boundary between two media, it is refracted. The angle of refraction depends upon the difference in the speed at which sound travels in the two media. This effect is usually of little importance. It should however be taken into account when performing a biopsy on a fluid-filled organ.

Scatter. When a sound wave meets a rough surface where the size of the irregularities are of a size similar to or smaller than the wave length of the sound wave, the wave is randomly reflected, that is, scattered. At the present time medical diagnostic ultrasound depends mainly upon the effect of reflection, and scatter is an unwanted side effect. Only in Doppler is the scatter effect of importance.

Absorption. As a sound wave passes through tissue its intensity is reduced as the distance that it passes through the tissue increases. This effect, known as attenuation, is a result of various factors. The main factor affecting the attenuation of ultrasound in tissue is absorption. The rate of absorption increases as the frequency of the ultrasound wave increases. For practical purposes, attenuation is taken to be 1 dB/MHz for each centimetre depth of the reflector. For example, a 5-MHz transducer receiving an echo from a reflector at depth 6 cm records a reduction of 30 dB in intensity (or attenuation of 30 dB). To counteract attenuation the operator selects transducer frequencies according to the depth of the structure being examined and compensates for attenuation by adjusting the gain control.

How Is Ultrasound Power Defined?

Normally ultrasound power is stated as a spatial peak temporal average (SPTA) value in mW/cm^2. The SPTA value means the peak power of the pulse at the focus point averaged over the time between pulses. Often the SPTA value is given as an in vitro value. The effect of attenuation requires that the value must be corrected to provide an in vivo value. At the present time the accepted maximum SPTA value for diagnostic purposes is 100 mW/cm^2 (recommendation of the World Health Organization).

How Is a Transducer Constructed?

The transducer consists of a crystal (PZT), a backing layer, various matching layers, and a silicon lens. After the crystal has been excited with a short electrical pulse, the crystal continues to vibrate. This ringing reduces the axial resolution. To reduce the ringing a material with a similar acoustic impedance is attached to the rear of the crystal but this also reduces the reception sensitivity. The transmitted sound wave passes through the matching layers to the skin surface. The matching layers are so selected that the acoustic impedance between the crystal and the skin surface is reduced as much as possible. The silicon lens used on the linear, convex, and phased array probes focuses the ultrasound beam in the slice plane to a fixed point to reduce and thereby improve the slice thickness.

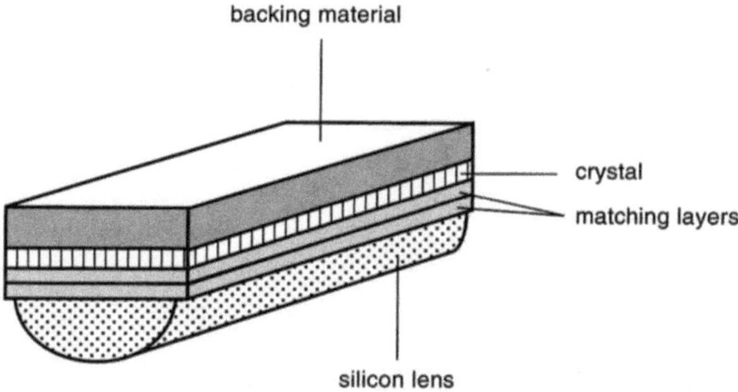

Types of Transducer: Advantages and Disadvantages

Single Element Transducer. The single crystal is usually internally focused, the resulting concave form is filled with a material to form a flat surface. Its use is now only found in the A- and M-modes. When the crystal is separated into two halves then one half can be used as a transmitter while at the same time the other half can be used as a receiver. This type of transducer is used as a pencil probe for continuous-wave Doppler.

- ◆ Advantages
  - – Small coupling area
  - – Cheap
- ◆ Disadvantage
  - – Cannot be used in real-time B-mode

Mechanical Sector Transducer. This transducer consists of a crystal which is mechanically oscillated through an arc. The position of the crystal is detected by an encoder and the resultant information passed to the ultrasound unit. After one display line has been processed, the motor positions the crystal for the firing of the next beam. This is repeated until a sector image is produced.

- ◆ Advantages
  - – Small coupling area
  - – Cheap
- ◆ Disadvantages
  - – Static focus
  - – Mechanical wear
  - – Small near field
  - – Unlinear line density

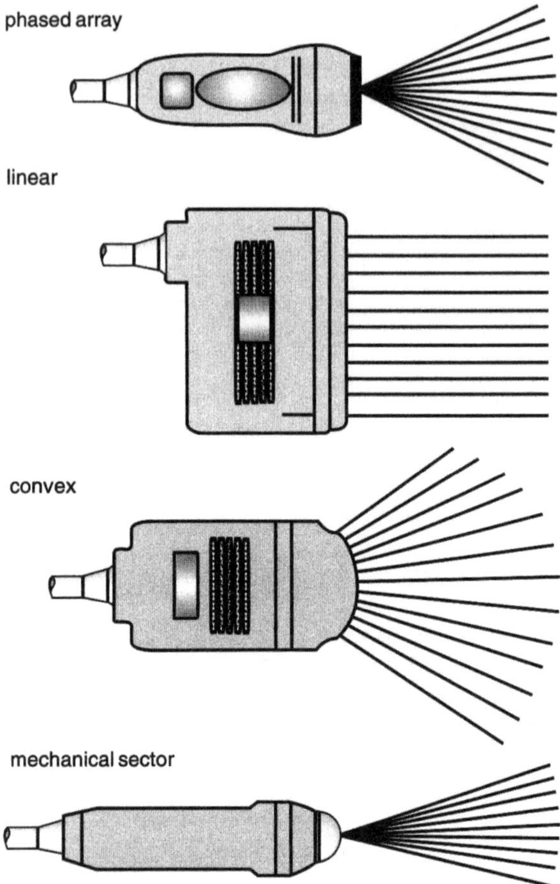

Fig. 1.2. Important types of transducer

Annular Array Transducer. This is used in the mechanical sector transducer to overcome the problem of static focus by enabling electronic focusing. The crystal is constructed of annular elements which are activated at different time intervals. The image is achieved as in the mechanical sector transducer by oscillating the array.

- ◆ Advantages
  - – Small coupling area
  - – Variable focus
- ◆ Disadvantages
  - – Mechanical wear
  - – Small near field
  - – Unlinear line density

Linear Transducer. The linear transducer consists of a row of rectangular elements. Groups of elements are used in such a manner that the effect of moving a single transducer backwards and forwards produces a rectangular image.

◆ Advantages
- Large near field
- Linear line density
- Electronic focusing
◆ Disadvantage
- Large coupling area

Convex Transducer. The convex transducer is a curved linear transducer. Electronically it is controlled as a linear transducer whereby the convex form of the image is dictated by the form of the transducer.

◆ Advantages
- Small coupling area
- Large near and far field
- Electronic focusing
◆ Disadvantage
- Unlinear line density

Mini Convex Transducer. The mini convex transducer is a miniaturized form of the convex transducer. It finds its application in such transducers as finger tip or top transducers, endoscope or vaginal transducers. Despite the small contact area its convex form makes possible a wide far field.

◆ Advantage
- Small coupling area
◆ Disadvantage
- Unlinear line density

Phased Array Transducer. This transducer is similar in form to the linear in having a row of rectangular elements, but fewer and smaller. Typical for this kind of probe all the elements are used to provide an ultrasound beam. A phased delay between the activation of the elements produces a sector image. The phased array probe is used mainly in cardiology.

◆ Advantages
- Small coupling area
- No mechanical wear
- Electronic focusing
◆ Disadvantages
- Expensive
- Unlinear line density
- Small near field

What Is Electronic Focusing?

To achieve a focused ultrasound beam from a group of elements they are electronically aligned. The focus point is physically closer to the middle elements than to the outer elements of the group. To compensate for the longer times necessary for a sound wave to travel to and from the outer elements, the signals from the middle of the group are delayed. By varying this delay time the focus depth can be selected. During the receive period the focus point can be continuously changed (dynamic focus) producing a more uniform receive beam form.

What Happens When More Than One Focus Is Selected?

One transmit focus only can be selected for each transmit cycle. If, however, it is necessary for a larger area to be focused then the transmit cycle is repeated with a different focus. The information from the new focus area is then substituted (accordingly) in the previously obtained line. This procedure is repeated until the required number of focus areas have been captured. More sophisticated units are equipped with dynamic receive focusing so that an almost constant lateral resolution can be achieved over the total depth. The disadvantage of selecting more than one focus is that the transmit firing sequence must be repeated according to the number of focuses selected. This reduces the speed with which the image is produced and accordingly decreases the frame rate.

How Is an Ultrasound Image Produced?

An ultrasound unit comprises a transducer, a transmitter, a receiver, a scan converter, and a monitor.

- Ultrasound units use a method known as pulse echo.
- A sound wave is produced by exploiting the piezoelectric property of the crystal contained in the transducer. The transmitter in the unit provides a voltage pulse which, by exciting the transducer elements, produces a burst of acoustic energy. This burst is transmitted through the contact gel to the body. When the burst meets an acoustic boundary part of the energy is reflected, this echo is detected by the transducer. The unreflected energy proceeds further into the body to be reflected at an acoustic boundary deeper in the body. At a velocity of 1540 m/s a sound wave requires 13 μs/cm travelled. Thus, if an image is to be displayed showing a depth of 20 cm, the receiver waits 260 μs before the echoes from 20 cm depth are received.
- By means of the reversed piezoelectric effect the reflected sound waves are transformed by the crystals in the transducer into an electrical signal. The amplitude of the electrical signal is proportional to the acoustic properties of the tissue interface. The time interval between transmit and receive is proportional to the position of the tissue interface in the body. The signal energy is very low and decreases as the depth of the tissue interface increases. The signal must therefore be amplified in the receiver. The operator is able to compensate for the attenuation effect by means of a variable depth gain control (TGC).

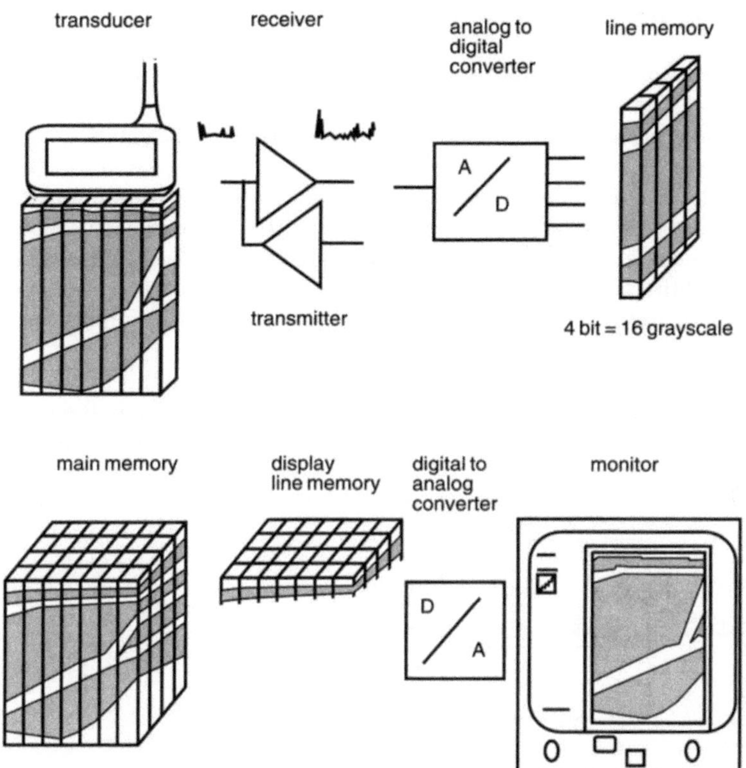

Fig. 1.3. Ultrasound unit

- In the scan converter the amplified signal is converted into a digital signal enabling it to be easily processed and stored.
- A system using a digital signal size of 4 bits produces an image of 16 different shades of grey.
- The resultant pixels (picture elements) are then stored vertically in the image memory.
- The transmit and receive process is repeated for each line of the image and the resulting line stored next to the previous line. This process is repeated until a complete image is stored in the memory.
- To enable the use of standard video systems the memory is read out horizontally and processed via a digital to analog converter into the CCIR video format.
- The scan converter not only stores the ultrasound image, it also provides a graphic overlay displaying such information as caliper markers, operating parameters, text, and various other kinds of information.
- The video signal is finally converted into an image on the monitor screen.

Ways of Displaying the Echo Information

A-Mode. A-mode denotes the method of displaying the received echo information as an amplitude signal. The amplitude is proportional to the reflection coefficient of the tissue interface and is projected in the x-axis. Depth is displayed in the y-axis.

M-Mode. M-mode denotes motion mode in which the trace displays motion with respect to time. The y-axis displays the depth in the body while the x-axis is a constant speed sweep. The z-axis is controlled by the A-mode signal so that the echo intensity is converted into brightness, the higher the amplitude the brighter the trace. This mode displays the change in position of tissue interfaces with respect to time. It is mostly used in cardiology.

B-Mode. The brightness mode uses the A-mode information for the z-axis, the x- and y-axes produce the positional information and place the brightness information of the

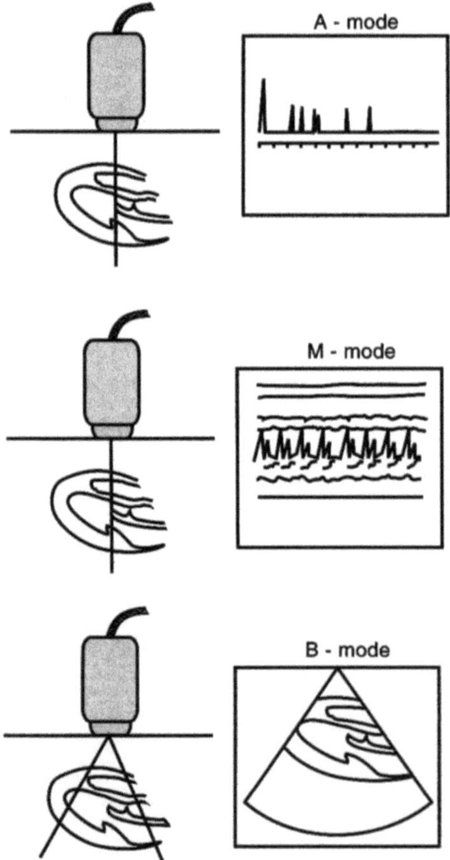

Fig. 1.4. A-mode, M-mode, B-mode

tissue interface at the appropriate point in the image. An image of a body slice is produced. The form of the image depends upon the type of transducer used.

Factors Influencing Image Quality

The image quality is influenced by:
- Resolution
  - Axial resolution
  - Lateral resolution
  - Slice thickness resolution
- System sensitivity
- Dynamic
- Line density
- Frame rate
- Patient

Resolution. Resolution may be defined as the degree to which two objects in proximity to one another are displayed as distinctly separate objects. This often referred to property has practical value only when the dB value is also stated. Normally the 6 dB value is given (half amplitude).

The axial resolution is the resolution achieved in the direction of the ultrasound beam and depends basically upon the frequency of the transmit pulse. The higher the transmit frequency the better the axial resolution. Because the attenuation of sound is proportional to the frequency of the sound wave it is not possible simply to increase the frequency and unfortunately a compromise between display depth and resolution must be accepted.

The lateral resolution is the resolution achieved at right angles to the ultrasound beam and depends upon the form of the beam. The form of the beam is determined by the number and size of the elements as well as by the electronic and mechanical focusing. The lateral resolution is normally much worse than the axial resolution.

The slice thickness is at right angles to the lateral and axial resolution planes. It depends upon the acoustic lens of the transducer. In the case of linear convex and phased array the lens is optimized for the individual transducer type by the manufacturer.

System Sensitivity. The sensitivity of the system depends upon the quality of the transducer and the receiver. The transducer quality of performance depends upon bandwidth, the beam form, and the efficiency of the elements. The determinant of receiver performance is its signal to noise ratio. To improve the ratio the bandwidth is moved from a higher frequency for the near field to a lower frequency for the far field. Because higher frequencies are attenuated more at greater tissue depth, echo information of higher frequency received from these regions can be presumed to be noise.

Dynamic. The dynamic is the difference between the smallest and the largest received echoes. Most systems allow the dynamic to be appropriately preset by the operator according to the type of examination.

Line Density. The line density is proportional to the number of transducer elements per centimetre. By using a half pitch stepping technique it is possible to double the number of lines produced. It is also possible to interpolate between adjacent lines to improve further the line density.

Frame Rate. The frame rate is important when viewing moving parts. If the frame rate is slower than the moving part then the movement within the image becomes erratic. For abdominal examinations a frame rate of 15 frames/s, and for cardiac examinations a frame rate of 30 frames/s, are sufficient to produce a stable image.

Patient. However effectively the operator sets up and uses the ultrasound unit the image quality varies from patient to patient.

A Simple Setting-Up Procedure

1. Switch on the unit and allow it to warm up for a few minutes.
2. Adjust the monitor by selecting maximum contrast and then reducing the contrast until the characters are clear and sharp while still maintaining the maximum possible brightness.
3. Adjust the brightness level so that the first grey level can just be seen against the background.
4. If the ultrasound power is too low then the echo intensity of structures in the far field is insufficient. If one tries to compensate by increasing the gain then the image becomes too noisy. Set the power at as low a level as is possible without adversely affecting image quality (as low as reasonably achievable, ALARA). This is especially important in M-mode, Doppler mode, and colour mode since a much higher ultrasound power is produced in these modes than in normal B-mode.
5. With the depth selective gain control set at the centre position, adjust the main gain so that the centre of the ultrasound image has the correct intensity. Then the depth selective gain control should be adjusted so that an homogeneous image is achieved.
6. Select the dynamic value. For abdominal and near field (thyroid, breast) studies the highest value should be selected to enable the diagnosis of even small tissue differences. For cardiac examinations a better differentiation of the heart valves is achieved by selecting a low dynamic value (30 or 40 dB).
7. Select the focus area so that it lies within the region of interest. The number of focuses should be reduced until a sufficiently high frame rate is achieved.
8. The linear gamma curve should be used as a standard grey scale curve. Post processing should be used only when it is necessary to enhance small changes in the grey scale. Most sophisticated units allow the parameters to be stored in a preset menu.
9. If the image movement appears to be erratic then the following parameters should be adjusted:
   - Frame rate
   - Depth
   - Image width
   - Number of focuses
   - Scan correlation

1.2 Ultrasound Contrast Media

1.2.1 General

Ultrasound contrast media are an innovation in ultrasound diagnosis. Because of their special physical nature, the pharmacokinetics of these acoustic media differ from those of contrast media for radiology or magnetic resonance imaging in that they do not diffuse in the body fluids, but remain in the vascular bed or in the cavity of the body into which they were administered. The main fields of use resulting from this are:

◆ Amplification of the echo signals of the blood flow in the chambers of the heart and the vessels
◆ Demonstration of body cavities and communications

Quantitative examination techniques which allow clinical information about cardiac and circulatory function to be obtained from the arrival and run-off kinetics of an echocontrast medium, are still in the early stage of research.

1.2.2 Principles and Characterization

All currently known industrial developments of echocontrast media are based on microbubbles. Because of their special acoustic properties, microbubbles play a role in the production of ultrasound contrast media of similar importance to that of iodine in radiology and of gadolinium in magnetic resonance imaging. The short life span of these microbubbles in vivo constitutes a basic problem. The microbubbles need to be highly stable to survive passage through the capillaries of the lungs. As far as is known from the world literature, there are as yet only two preparations undergoing clinical development which offer the required degree of microbubble stability and with which – as described further below – echo signal enhancement can also be achieved in the left heart and the arterial vascular bed after intravenous injection.

The currently known echogenic contrast media can be divided into three physically different types, each of which represents different principles of microbubble stability:

◆ Microbubble-containing solutions
◆ Gas-filled microspheres
◆ Microbubble-containing suspensions

Microbubble-Containing Solutions. The use of agitated or foamed-up injection solutions to produce echogenic effects in the blood during echocardiographic examinations has been known since 1968. In the following years, various injection solutions were investigated as vehicles in an attempt to increase the reproducibility of the contrast effect and the in vivo life span. Different preparation techniques were also compared (shaking, foaming). Although the superiority of the sonication method in respect of microbubble size and intensity of the contrast medium effect has been reported in several papers, no one has yet succeeded in producing microbubbles in a purely liquid vehicle so reproducibly and in stabilizing them to such an extent, that a dosable contrast medium could be claimed. Moreover, the in vivo stability so far attained is still not good enough for the production of diagnostic contrast effects after passage through the pulmonary capillaries. The use of contrast media of this type therefore remains confined to venous vessels, the right heart, and body cavities (right-heart contrast media).

Gas-Filled Microspheres. Using a special sonication method and human albumin as the carrier solution, researchers have succeeded in producing air-filled microspheres which survive passage through the pulmonary capillaries and which produce contrast effects in the left heart after intravenous injection. Apart from published self-produced preparations, this type of echogenic contrast media is represented by the industrial development Albunex. The preparation is undergoing clinical trials in the United States (Molecular Biosystems, Mallinckrodt), Europe (Nycomed), and Japan (Shionogi) as an echographic contrast medium for B-mode scanning.

Microbubble-Containing Suspensions. Microbubble-containing suspensions of specially produced galactose microparticles form the basis of the first industrial development of echocontrast media, which began around 10 years ago and was successfully concluded with the marketing of the first ultrasound contrast medium (Echovist, Schering). Galactose microparticle granules produced in a special manufacturing process are suspended by shaking either in galactose solution (Echovist) or in sterile water (Levovist) shortly before use. After intravenous injection of the microbubble-containing milky white suspension, the blood becomes temporarily echogenic during passage of the bolus until the acoustic microstructures dissolve in the blood stream.

After leaving the right heart, Echovist dissolves as a result of mixing with and becoming distributed in the blood serum before the left heart is reached. Consequently, it is suitable for contrast echocardiographic examinations of the right heart by B-mode scan and Doppler and of the venous circulation (right-heart contrast medium). It is also employed as an echogenic indicator solution for the sonographic demonstration of Fallopian tube patency.

A derivative of Echovist with an extended in vivo life span bears the development code name SH U 508 A. This preparation (Levovist) leads, after intravenous injection, to an increase of the echogenicity in the blood which survives pulmonary passage and, therefore, reaches the arterial vascular bed. The flow of echogenic blood produced by a suitably dosed bolus leads to echogenic contrasting of the right and left heart chambers in the sector image or to an increase of the Doppler signal intensity in the heart and the entire arterial vascular bed further to the periphery.

After the acoustically active microstructures have dissolved in the bloodstream, the galactose is broken down physiologically – mainly in the liver – independently of insulin. Galactose is a non-toxic monosaccharide and has no known allergenic potential. The small total amount of air in the microbubbles (approximately 100 μl) is eliminated in exhalation.

While the acoustically active microstructures of type I (microfoam) and III (microparticle suspension) contrast media dissolve in the blood stream after injection, little has been published about the break-down of microspheres. They are most probably eliminated by the reticulo-endothelial system by means of phagocytosis.

1.2.3 Diagnostic Fields of Use

Right-Heart Contrast Media

Contrast Echocardiography of the Right Heart. Contrast echocardiography of the right heart is particularly suitable for the diagnosis of shunts at the atrial or ventricular level and for the demonstration of valvular incompetence. Also, demarcation of the endocardium is improved by the echogenic contrasting of the chambers of the right heart. The very fact that the right-heart contrast medium is not normally expected to survive pulmonary passage is an advantage in the diagnosis of small shunts as well as, in particular, an open foramen ovale, since leakage of even minimal amounts of contrast medium from the right to the left ventricle is recognizable.

The use of echocontrast media in colour Doppler echocardiography increases the sensitivity of blood flow detection, allowing questionable shunts or valvular incompetence to be clearly visualized particularly in patients with poor Doppler signal to noise ratios. Figure 1.5 shows a shunt flow from left to right in the presence of an atrial septum defect which was demonstrable only after injection of Echovist.

Phlebocontrast Sonography. The peripheral and central venous injection of echocontrast material permits observation of the haemodynamics in B-mode or increases the intensity of Doppler sonographic flow signals. This offers diagnostic advantages in the exclusion of thrombosis and vascular occlusion in cases which were questionable at plain sonography, in the follow-up of thrombolysis, in the demonstration of venous insufficiency, and in the functional evaluation of dialysis shunts and vena cava filters.

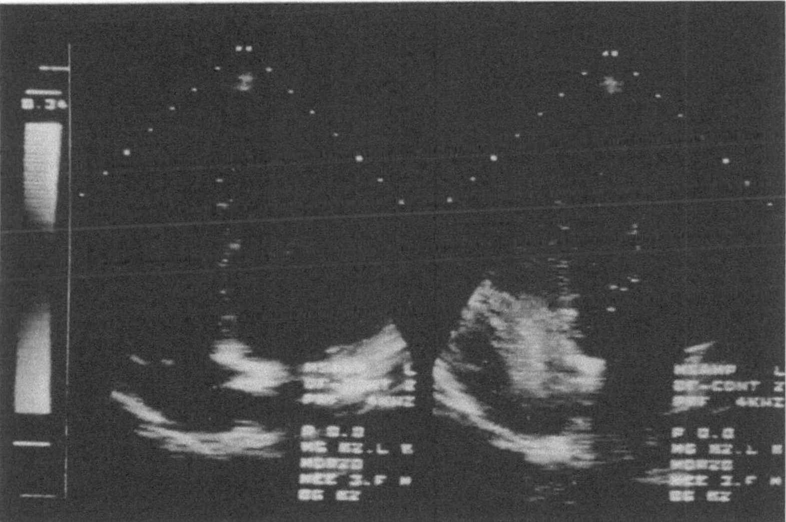

Fig. 1.5. Apical four-chamber view in colour Doppler echocardiography. Atrial septum defect with left-right shunt before (*left*) and after (*right*) injection of Echovist

Hystero-Salpingo Contrast Sonography. The use of the first echogenic contrast medium combined with a transvaginal examination technique made it possible to develop a sonographic method as an alternative to X-ray hystero-salpingography. Transcervical administration and pertubation of Echovist led to the sonographic demonstration not only of uterine anomalies, but also of patency of the Fallopian tubes. The advantages of this method over conventional procedures are the elimination of radiation exposure and the absence of allergoid contrast medium reactions or surgical risks. On-line observation of the examination and display of the results are also possible. Clinical studies have shown a specificity of 100% and a sensitivity of 88% for the demonstration of patent tubes in hystero-salpingo contrast sonography compared to conventional diagnostic procedures (laparoscopy, X-ray hystero-salpingography). The method therefore seems ideal as a future, virtually non-invasive screening procedure in the diagnosis of sterility. Figure 1.6 shows an example of echogenic demarcation of bilaterally patent tubes by transvaginal sonography.

Preliminary experience with pulsed-wave and colour Doppler vaginal transducers suggests that the diagnostic reliability particularly in suspected tubal occlusion, as well as the documentation of the findings, can be further improved by additional Doppler recording.

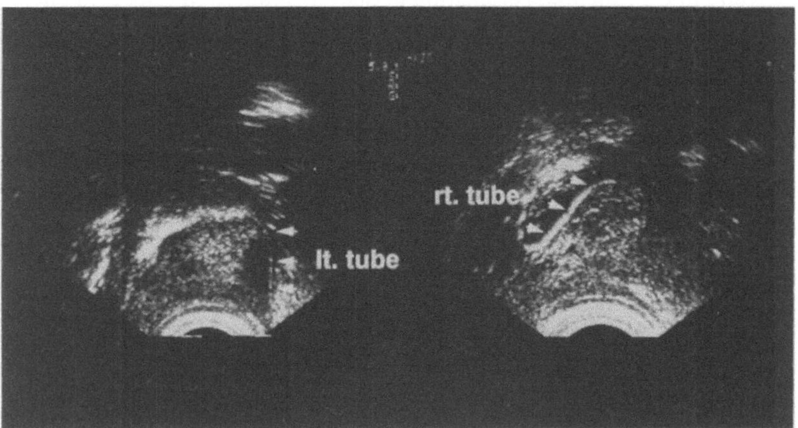

Fig. 1.6. Transvaginal hystero-salpingo contrast sonography of the left tube (*left image, arrows*) and right tube (*right image, arrows*). The recognizable flow patterns during pertubation of the contrast medium in real-time scanning facilitate demonstration of tubal flow as confirmation of patency

Stable Transpulmonary Contrast Media

Contrast Echocardiography of the Left Heart. In line with the properties of B-mode echocardiography, the basic fields of use of echocontrast media in the left heart concern all questions of the anatomical demarcation of blood-filled cavities and myocardial structures and of the identification of haemodynamic phenomena. Thus, the indications for the use of contrast media include the clarification of pathological changes such as tumours, intracardiac thrombi and septum defects, and disturbances of movement as part of coronary heart disease. In addition, valvular incompetence can be recognized by means of contrast medium regurgitation, although this problem is nowadays mainly investigated by means of colour Doppler techniques. Figure 1.7 shows a sequence of echocardiographic apical four-chamber views before and in three time phases after contrast medium injection.

In colour Doppler echocardiography, the injection of contrast medium makes a diagnosis possible in those cases in which the intensities of the Doppler signals are too low for a diagnosis without contrast material. The increase of the Doppler signals in the left heart and in the arteries after intravenous injection of SH U 508 A amounts to between approximately 15 and 25 dB and, in the great majority of cases, leads to qualitatively good demonstration of the Doppler signals. Figure 1.8 shows an example of echocardiography of mitral incompetence, clearly demonstrable only after contrast medium injection.

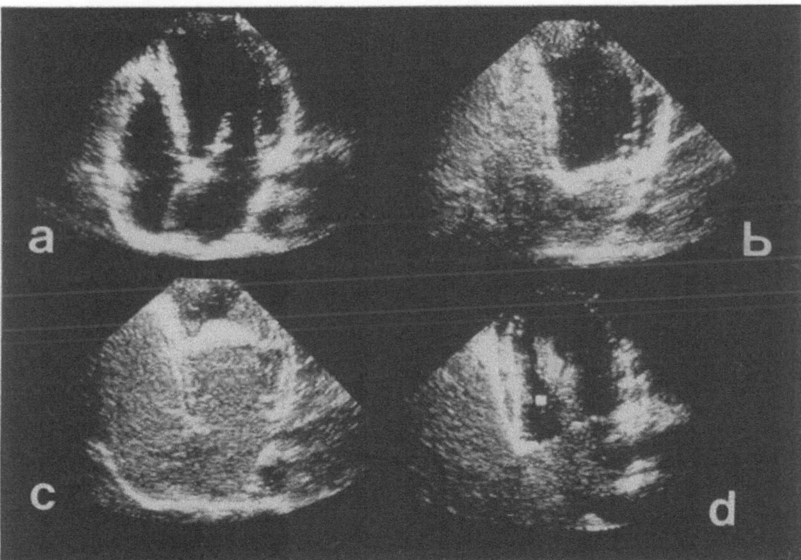

Fig. 1.7. Echocardiographic apical four-chamber view before (**a**) and after (**b–d**) injection of SH U 508 A. **b** The echogenically labelled blood flow in the right heart chambers and the influx into the left atrium after pulmonary passage. **c** First diastolic influx into the left ventricle. **d** Corresponding end-systolic phase with contrasted residual blood

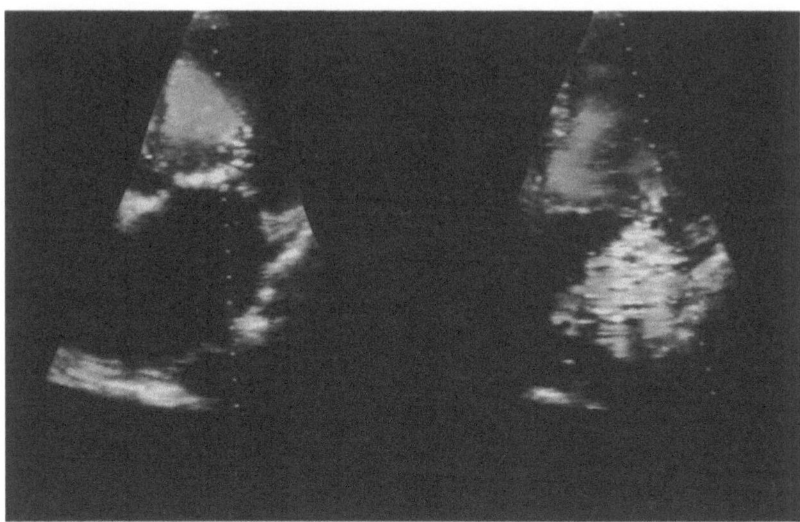

Fig. 1.8. Echocardiographic colour Doppler sonography of the left heart before (*left*) and after (*right*) injection of SH U 508 A. The systolic reflux through the mitral valve into the atrium is visible only after contrast medium enhancement of the Doppler signals (demonstration of mitral incompetence)

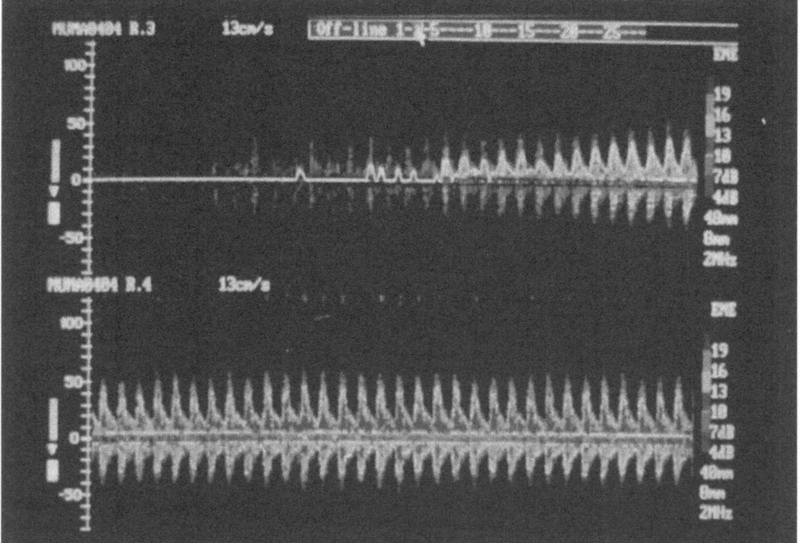

Fig. 1.9. Transcranial Doppler examination of the middle cerebral artery before and after intravenous injection of an ultrasound contrast medium

Figure 1.9 shows a Doppler pulse curve of the middle cerebral artery (transcranial Doppler recording) which was adequately demonstrable only after administration of contrast medium (SH U 508 A).

A new field of use particularly for the colour Doppler technique is the comparative evaluation of vascularization especially of tumour regions. Since such examination techniques are performed at the limits of equipment technology because of the small size of the vessels being examined, contrast enhancement is expected to make a major contribution to the reliability of the findings.

1.3 Standardized Examination

Display of sections on the monitor:
- All sections
  - Upper part of the screen: near to the transducer
  - Lower part of the screen: away from the transducer
- Longitudinal section
  - Left side of the screen: cranial side of the patient
  - Right side of the screen: caudal side of the patient
- Transverse section
  - Left side of the screen: right side of the patient
  - Right side of the screen: left side of the patient

In ultrasonography it is essential to have a systematic and standardized scanning technique. Only in this way can one ensure that:
- The findings are comprehensible.
- No pathology is overlooked.
- The findings are reproducible.

Standard section levels include:
- Lateral longitudinal section on the right side
- Paramedian section on the right side
- Paramedian section on the left side
- Lateral longitudinal section on the left side
- Upper transverse section
- Middle transverse section
- Lower transverse section
- Subcostal section on the right side
- Oblique section on the right side
- Intercostal section on the right side
- Suprapubic longitudinal section
- Suprapubic transverse section

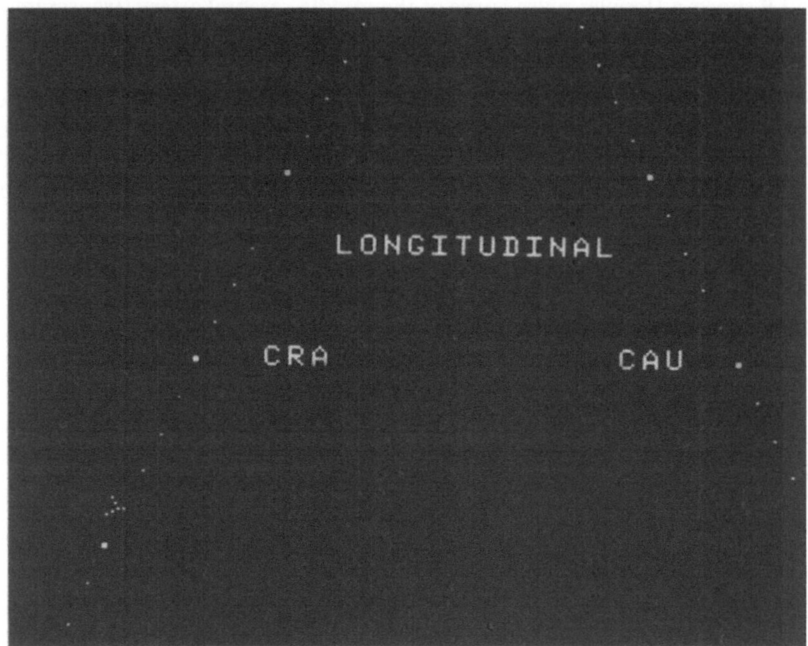

Fig. 1.10. Longitudinal scan. *CRA*, cranial; *CAU*, caudal

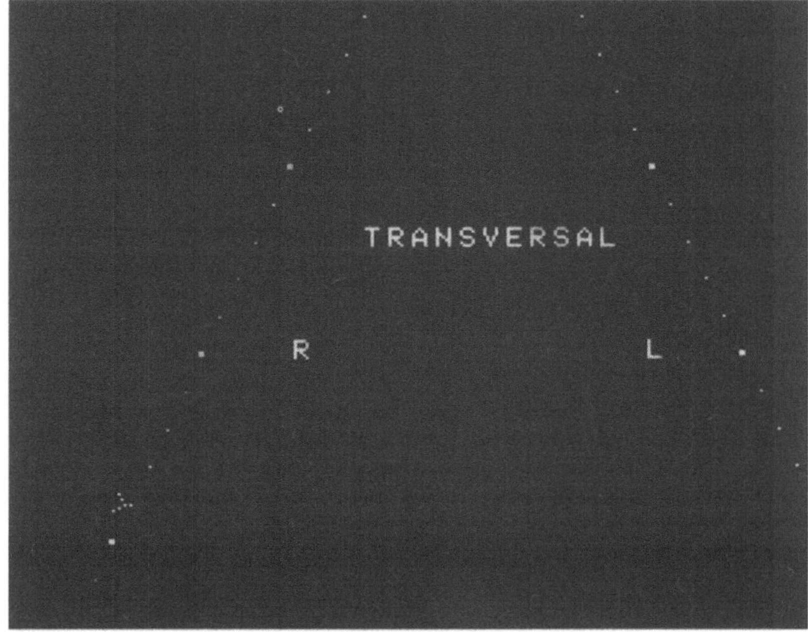

Fig. 1.11. Transverse scan. *R*, right side; *L*, left side

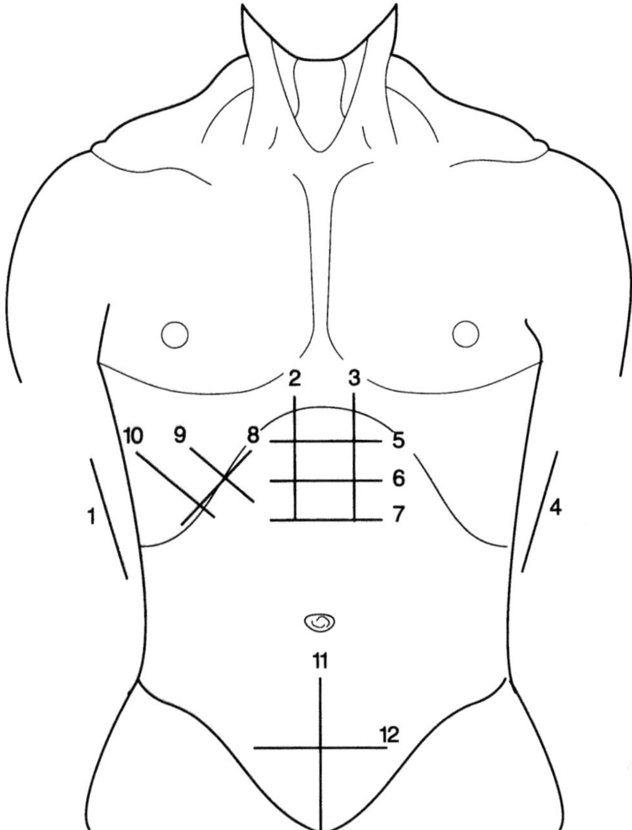

Fig. 1.12. Standard section levels. *1*, Lateral longitudinal section on the right side; *2*, paramedian section on the right side; *3*, paramedian section on the left side; *4*, lateral longitudinal section on the left side; *5*, upper transverse section; *6*, middle transverse section; *7*, lower transverse section; *8*, subcostal section on the right side; *9*, oblique section on the right side; *10*, intercostal section on the right side; *11*, suprapubic longitudinal section; *12*, suprapubic transverse section

Lateral Longitudinal Section on the Right Side

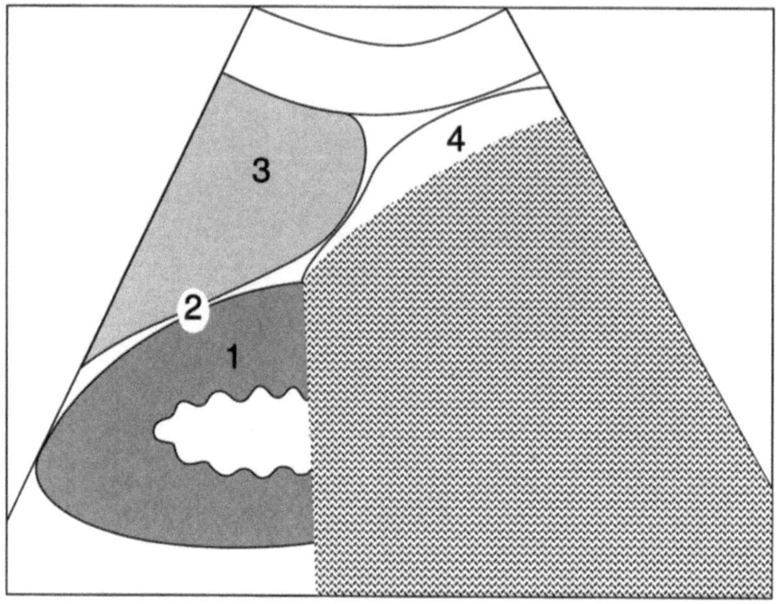

Fig. 1.13. Lateral longitudinal section on the right side. *1*, Kidney; *2*, Morrison's pouch; *3*, liver; *4*, colonic flexure

Paramedian Section on the Right Side

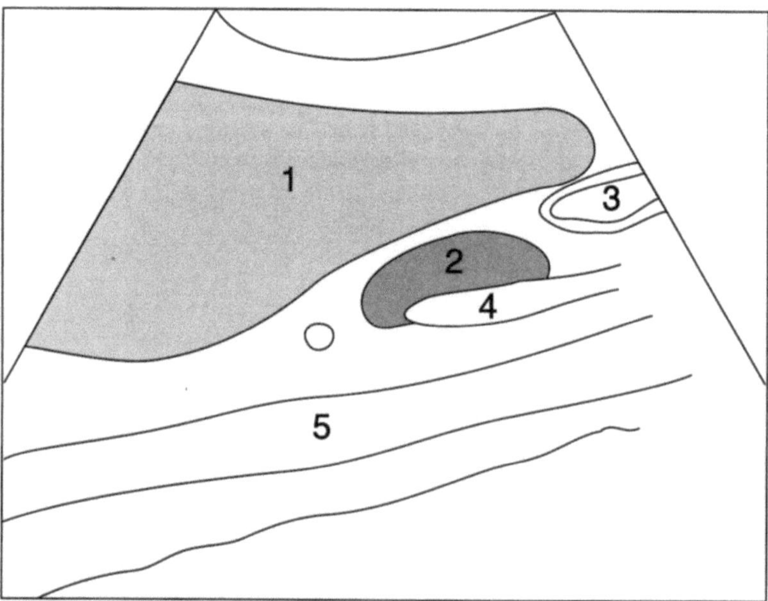

Fig. 1.14. Paramedian section on the right side. *1*, Liver; *2*, head of pancreas; *3*, antrum of stomach; *4*, superior mesenteric vein; *5*, inferior vena cava

Paramedian Section on the Left Side

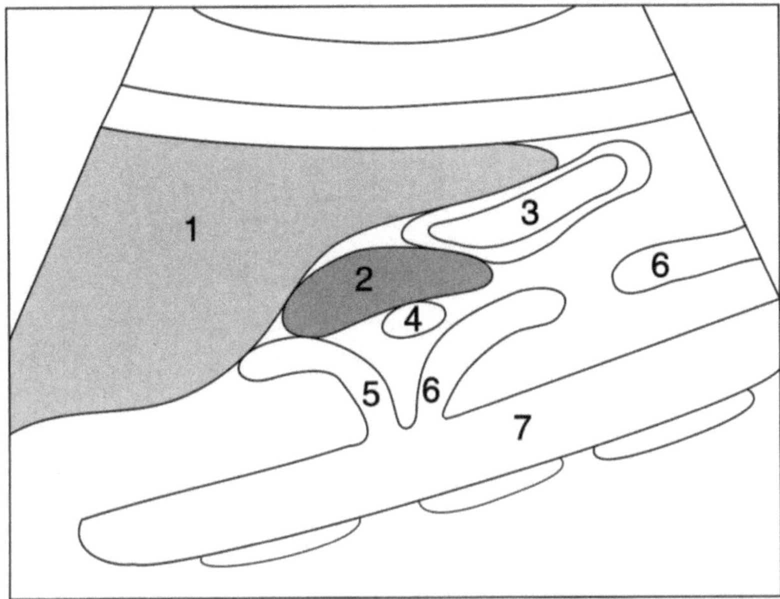

Fig. 1.15. Paramedian section on the left side. *1*, Liver; *2*, body of pancreas; *3*, antrum of stomach; *4*, splenic vein; *5*, coeliac trunk; *6*, superior mesenteric artery; *7*, aorta

Lateral Longitudinal Section on the Left Side

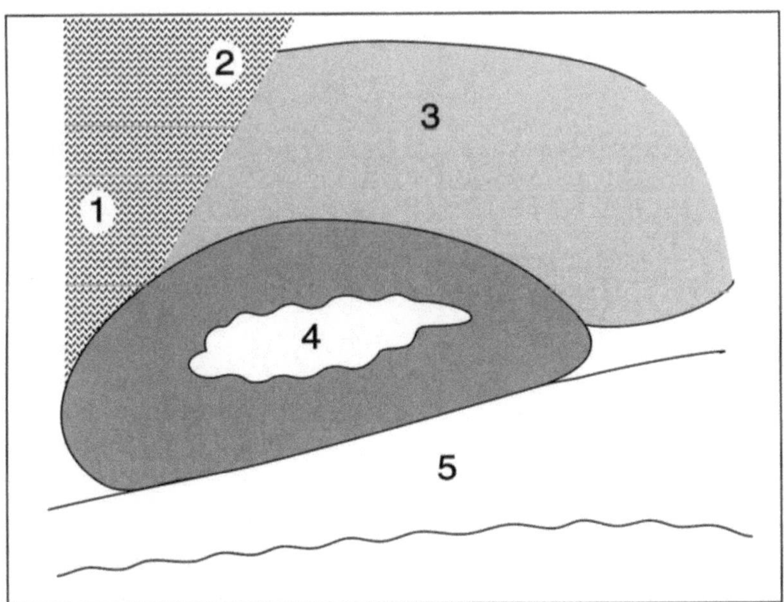

Fig. 1.16. Lateral longitudinal section on the left side. *1*, Lung; *2*, costodiaphragmatic recess; *3*, spleen; *4*, kidney; *5*, psoas muscle

Upper Transverse Section

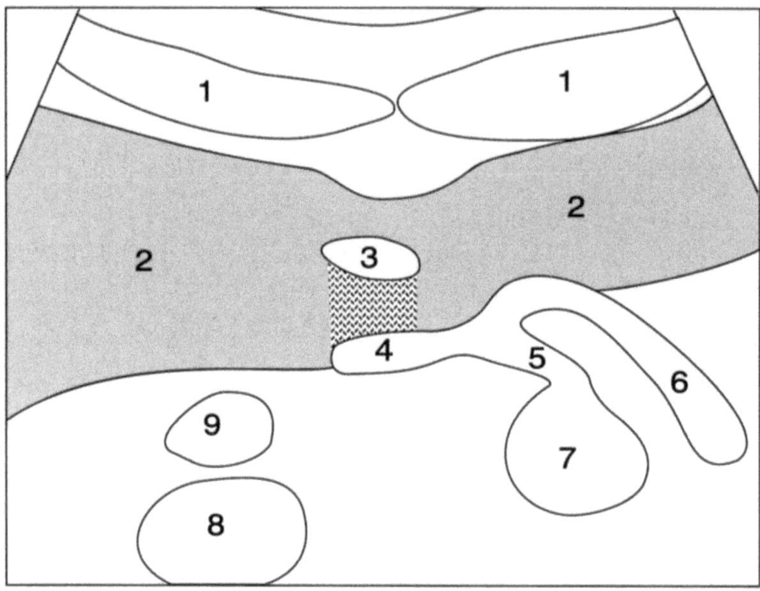

Fig. 1.17. Upper transverse section. *1*, Rectus abdominis muscle; *2*, liver; *3*, falciform ligament; *4*, hepatic artery; *5*, coeliac trunk; *6*, splenic artery; *7*, aorta; *8*, inferior vena cava; *9*, portal vein

Middle Transverse Section

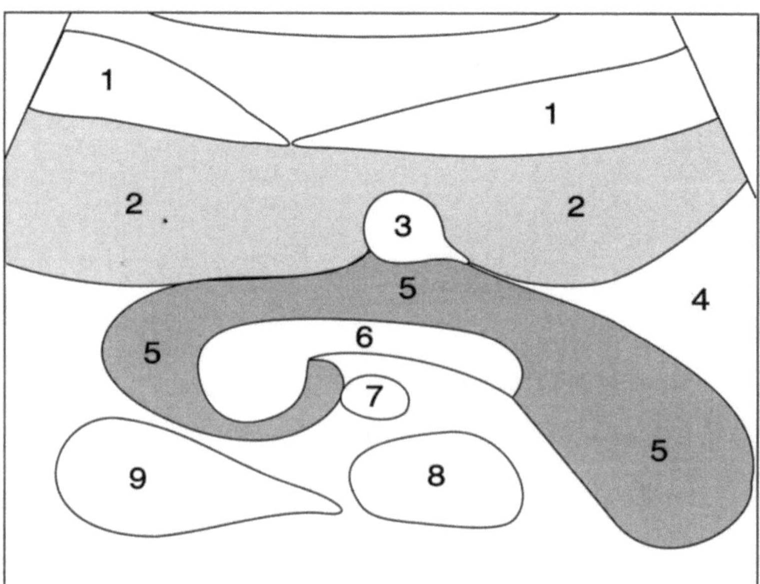

Fig. 1.18. Middle transverse section. *1*, Rectus abdominis muscle; *2*, liver; *3*, falciform ligament; *4*, antrum of stomach; *5*, pancreas; *6*, splenic vein; *7*, superior mesenteric artery; *8*, aorta; *9*, inferior vena cava

Lower Transverse Section

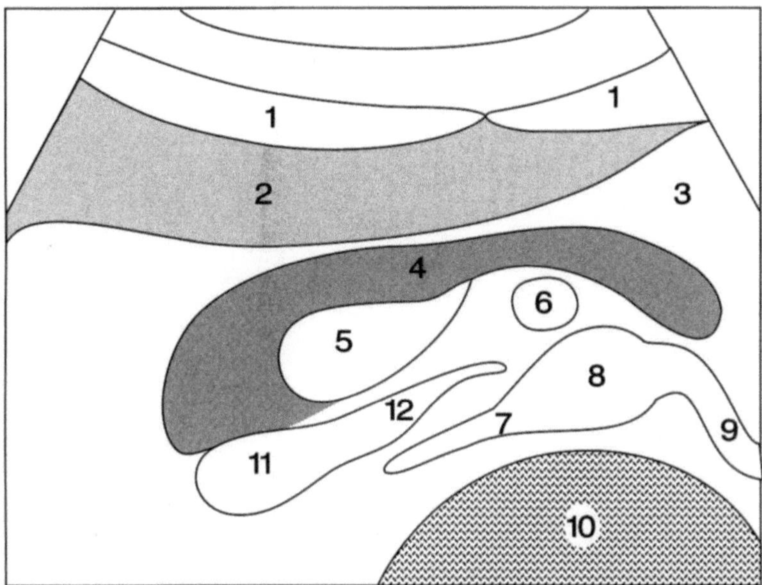

Fig. 1.19. Lower transverse section. *1*, Rectus abdominis muscle; *2*, liver; *3*, antrum of stomach; *4*, pancreas; *5*, superior mesenteric vein; *6*, superior mesenteric artery; *7*, right renal artery; *8*, aorta; *9*, left renal artery; *10*, vertebral body; *11*, inferior vena cava; *12*, left renal vein

Subcostal Section on the Right Side

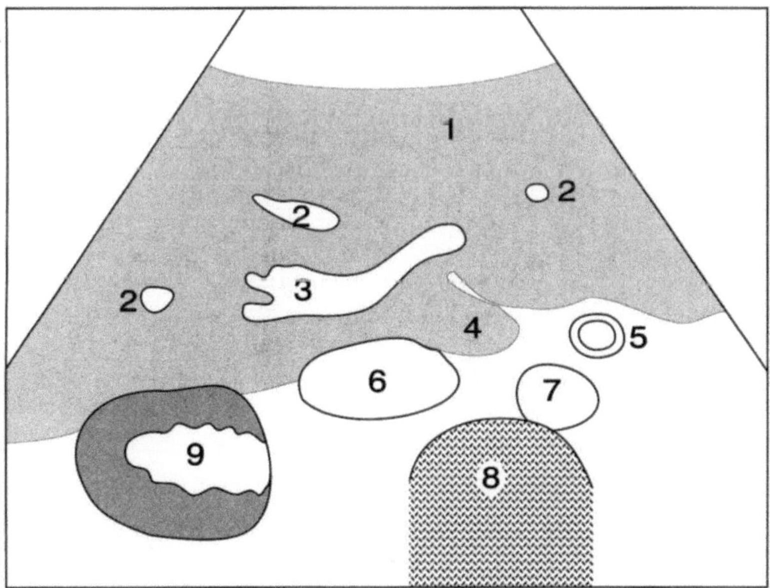

Fig. 1.20. Subcostal section on the right side. *1*, Liver; *2*, hepatic veins; *3*, portal vein; *4*, caudate lobe; *5*, cardia of stomach; *6*, inferior vena cava; *7*, aorta; *8*, vertebral body; *9*, kidney

Oblique Section on the Right Side

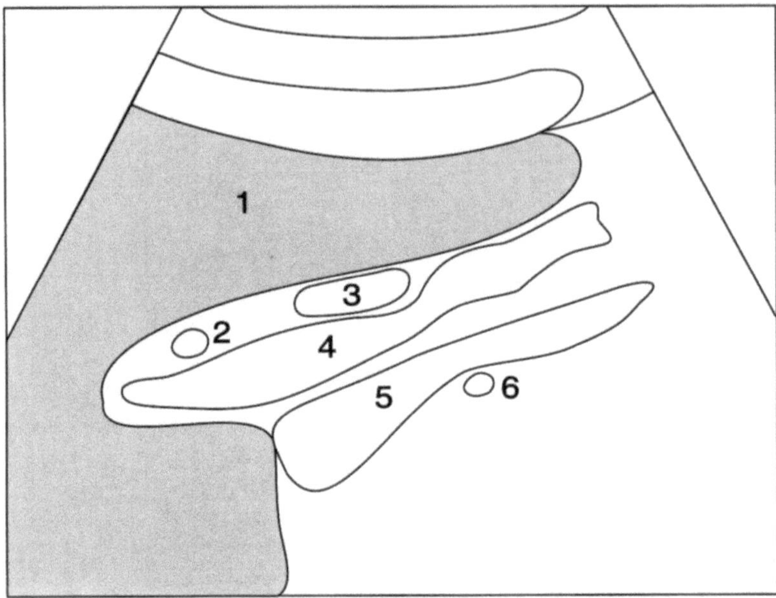

Fig. 1.21. Oblique section on the right side. *1*, Liver; *2*, hepatic artery; *3*, common bile duct; *4*, portal vein; *5*, inferior vena cava; *6*, right renal artery

Intercostal Section on the Right Side

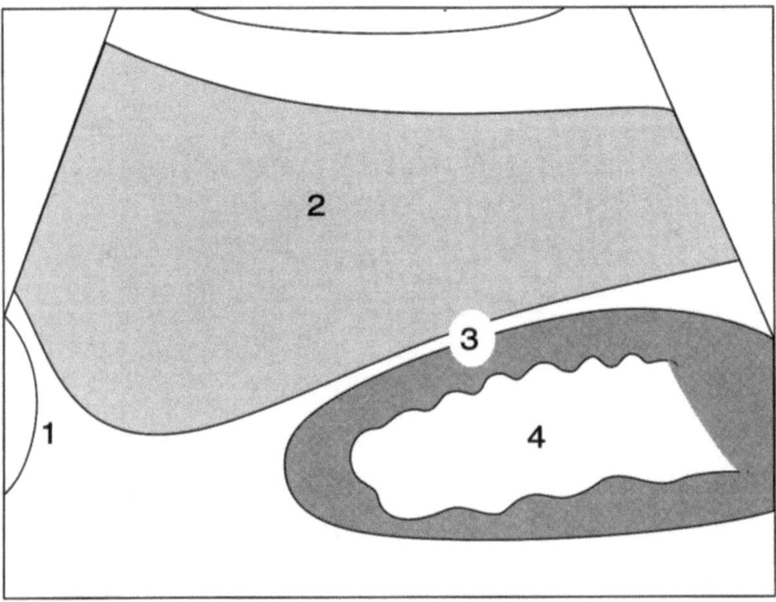

Fig. 1.22. Intercostal section on the right side. *1*, Diaphragm; *2*, liver; *3*, Morrison's pouch; *4*, kidney

Suprapubic Longitudinal Section

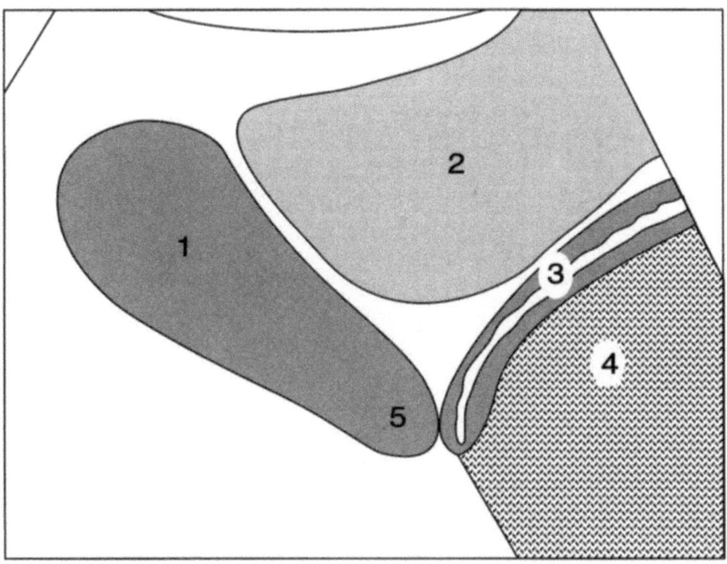

Fig. 1.23. Suprapubic longitudinal section, female. *1*, Uterus; *2*, bladder; *3*, vagina; *4*, rectosigmoid; *5*, cervix

Suprapubic Transverse Section

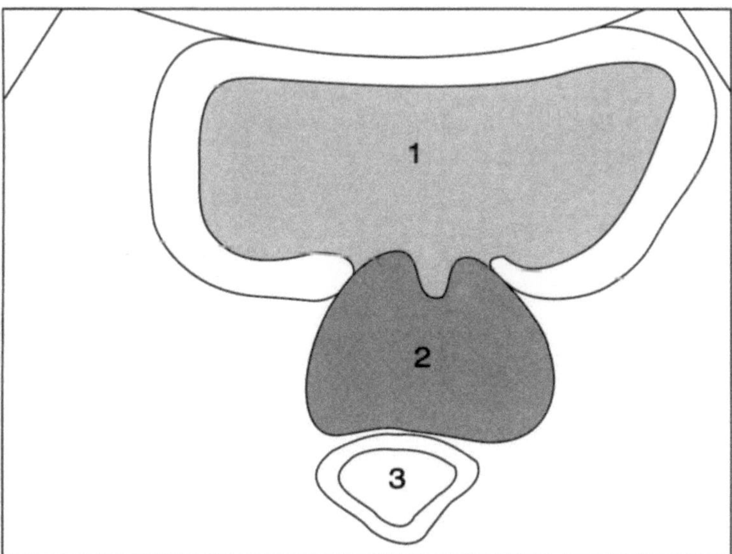

Fig. 1.24. Suprapubic transverse section, male. *1*, Bladder; *2*, prostate; *3*, rectosigmoid

Chapter ② Artefacts

Artefacts are echoes without an anatomical correlate. The sonographer should know:
- How artefacts develop.
- How artefacts look.
- How artefacts can be recognized.
- How artefacts can be avoided.

To ensure the greatest possible accuracy the sonographer must be fully aware of the physical artefacts and diagnostic pitfalls which may be encountered during scanning. In order to reduce the risk of misdiagnosis it is essential that all organs are examined in at least two planes preferably at right angles. In addition, changing the patient's position changes the position of the organs in relation to each other. This can be a valuable method of diagnosis when the sonographic appearances raise the possibility of an artefact.

Artefacts seen in everyday scanning include:
- Acoustic shadowing
- Acoustic enhancement
- Refraction artefact
- Mirror artefact
- Reverberation
- Partial volume/beam width artefact
- Comet tail artefact

Acoustic Shadowing

Tissue interfaces which are good ultrasound reflectors may completely obstruct the passage of the ultrasound beam. As the beam does not penetrate the tissues distal to this interface a shadow results. The reflecting interface is seen as a strongly echogenic band with an anechoic area running distally behind it.

Examples: gas, bone, stone

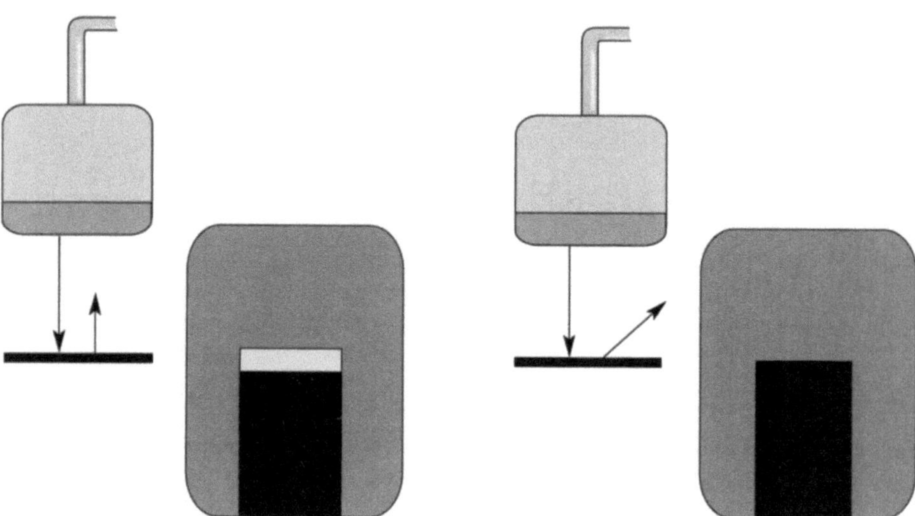

Fig. 2.1. Acoustic shadowing

Acoustic Enhancement

The ultrasound beam is attenuated as it passes through the body. When passing through semiliquid or liquid structures the ultrasound beam is subject to little if any attenuation. The beam is therefore stronger distal to a fluid-filled structure than distal to an equal thickness of soft tissue.

Examples: gallbladder, urinary bladder, cyst

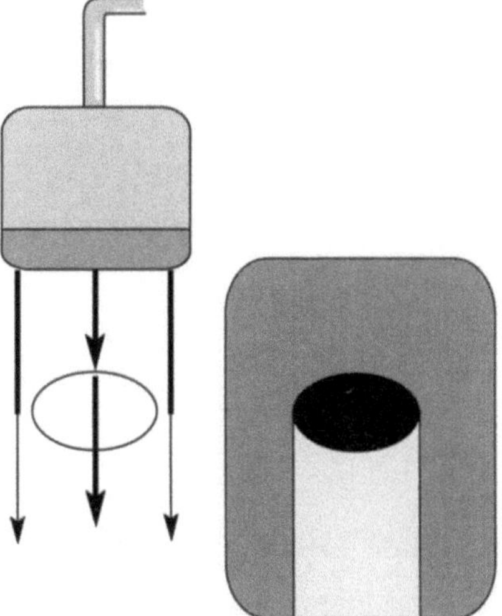

Fig. 2.2. Acoustic enhancement

Refraction Artefact

A combination of reflection and refraction causes ultrasound beam splitting, giving rise to a refraction shadow due to an area devoid of ultrasound signal. The refraction artefact must not be confused with acoustic shadowing. The presence of the refraction artefact is highly dependent upon the angle of incidence of the ultrasound beam and thus is not constant if multiple sections are taken.

Examples: gallbladder wall, urinary bladder wall, cyst wall

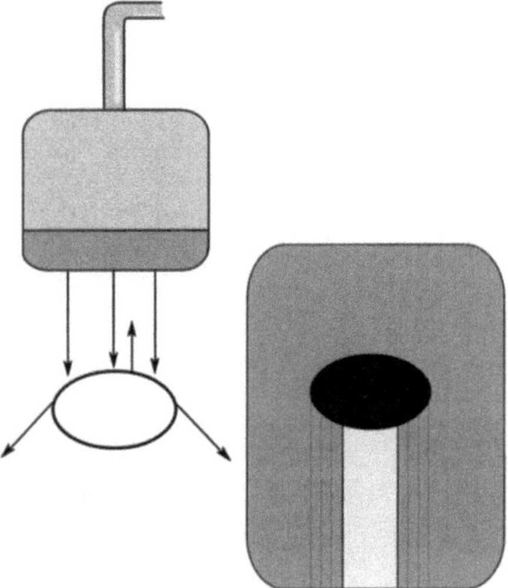

Fig. 2.3. Refraction artefact

Mirror Artefact

Mirror artefacts occur when an image arises close to a curved and strongly reflecting tissue interface. The false image is seen beyond the reflector due to the second pathway taken by the ultrasound beam.

Example: diaphragm

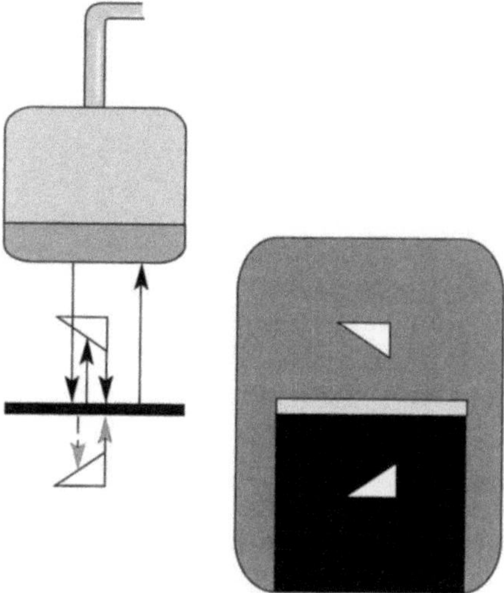

Fig. 2.4. Mirror artefact

Reverberation

The transducer face, skin, and coupling medium form acoustic interfaces. Sound passing from the probe into the body and echoes returning to the transducer from within the body may be reflected by these interfaces allowing the sound waves to be reflected back and forth.

Example: air

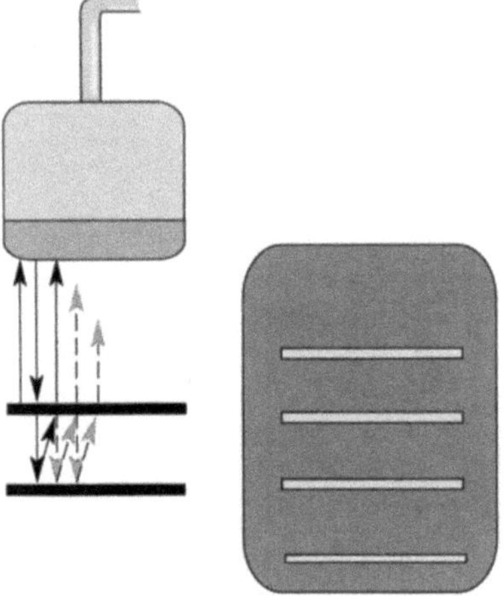

Fig. 2.5. Reverberation

Partial Volume/Beam Width Artefact

Scanning both solid tissue and the edge of a liquid structure simultaneously may give an artefactual appearance of debris within the liquid structure or a solid appearance.

Examples: gallbladder, urinary bladder

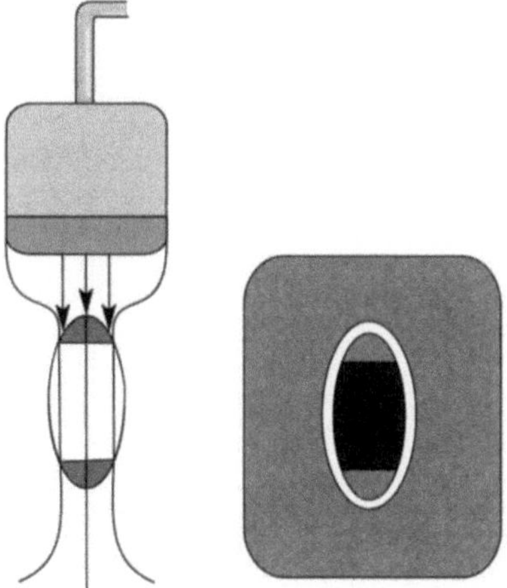

Fig. 2.6. Partial volume/beam width artefact

Comet Tail Artefact

The comet tail artefact is a form of intense reverberation which occurs between two adjacent surfaces. The resultant reverberation echoes are so close to each other that they tend to merge and give rise to a bright comet tail echo extending distally into the ultrasound field behind the structure causing the reverberation.

Example: surgical clip

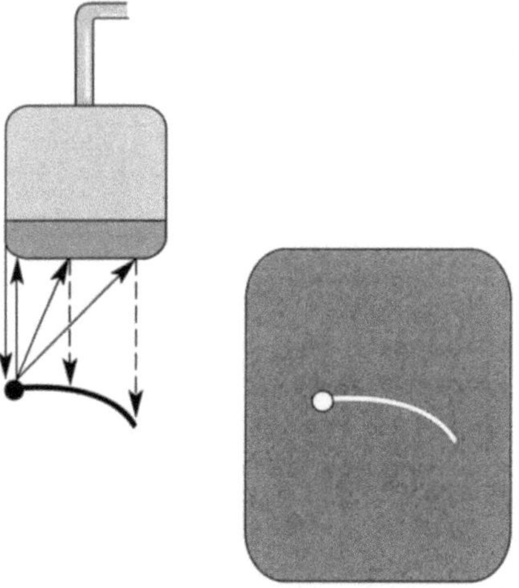

Fig. 2.7. Comet tail artefact

Chapter 3 Reporting

3.1 Image Documentation

During the course of an ultrasound examination, images should be made of every organ. The image documentation is necessary for:

- Reporting
- Follow-up
- Medical records

This calls for the following:

- Selecting of typical section levels
- Imaging of anatomical landmarks
- Showing the topographical relationship between disease process and originating organ

Only in this way can sonographic images later supply reliable diagnostic records.

3.2 Text Documentation

Completeness and thoroughness of a sonographic examination cannot be objectified through an image documentation only. The text documentation therefore plays a much bigger role in an ultrasound examination than in an X ray examination. For reporting the findings one can choose between a documentation sheet and free dictation. Normal and pathological findings must be described, while clear terminology is essential to ensure that colleagues can comprehend the results without problems:

- Anechoic, hypoechoic, isoechoic, hyperechoic
- Echofree, echopoor, echorich
- Hyporeflective, hyperreflective
- Homogeneous, heterogeneous
- Sharp, blurred, regular, irregular
- Area, structure, region, zone
- Acoustic shadowing, acoustic enhancement
- Normal appearance, no abnormality found

The findings must be documented, described, and interpreted in the light of any clinical information given (clinical history, physical examination) and the results of other investigations (laboratory tests, X-ray).

An organ must never be described as normal if it was not seen adequately. In the report it can then be described as:

- Inadequately imaged
- Not visible
- Not assessable

Pathological processes must be described precisely, especially with regard to:
- Localization
- Size
- Shape
- Contour
- Echogenicity
- Echopattern
- Tenderness
- Consistency

This limited number of parameters may be affected by a wide range of diseases and thus it is not surprising that many sonographic features are non-specific. In this book, a checklist follows each chapter for reference during reporting.

The ultrasound report consists of:

Patient
- **Surname**
- **Christian name**
- **Date of birth**
- **Hospital number**

Examination number

Examination type

Examination date

Clinical data
- **Clinical history**
- **Physical examination**
- **Laboratory tests**
- **X-ray**

Examination technique

Findings

Conclusion
- **Diagnosis**
- **Differential diagnosis**
- **Recommendation of further relevant investigations**

Part II

Chapter 4 Liver

4.1 Imaging Modalities

Sonography is the method of choice to image the liver. Imaging modalities are:

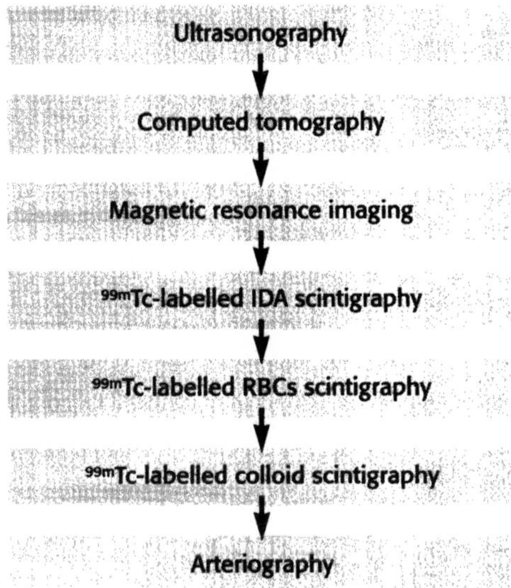

4.2 Ultrasonography

4.2.1 Examination Technique

Special preparation of the patient is unnecessary. The examination takes place with a 3.5-MHz probe; a 5-MHz transducer is better for thin patients. The convex transducer, as a compromise between the linear and the sector techniques, has the benefit of mostly good images of the near field as well as of the far field. If a convex transducer is not available, the following examination technique is recommended:

◆ Examination of the superficial liver structures with a 5-MHz linear probe
◆ Examination of the deep liver structures with a 3.5-MHz sector probe

More important than the kind of transducer is the comprehensive examination of the organ in several sections:

- Longitudinal section
- Transverse section
- Subcostal section
- Oblique section
- Intercostal section

The right lobe of the liver can be examined particularly well in the subcostal section; the probe is then tilted from far cranial to caudal. Sound obstacles such as ribs, the falciform ligament, and intestines should be bypassed to avoid missing any pathology of underlying structures. For this reason, organ boundaries also should be examined carefully. For the examination of the liver the patient should be lying:

- In the supine position or with the right side slightly raised
- With the right arm behind the head to enlarge the intercostal space
- In deep inspiration, with abdominal pressure

The examination technique must be modified from patient to patient and from section level to section level, according to individual requirements. Limiting factors are:

- Obesity
- Fatty change
- Elevation of the diaphragm
- Intestinal superimposition

Depression of the diaphragm can simulate hepatomegaly. A small, elevated liver can be best examined in the intercostal section.

4.2.2 Sonoanatomy

The normal liver displays considerable variation in size and shape. It consists of a larger right lobe and a smaller left lobe separated by the interlobar fissure. There are two smaller lobes, the caudate lobe posteriorly and the quadrate lobe inferiorly.

Anatomical relationships:
- Caudate lobe
    - Portal vein
    - Inferior vena cava
    - Ligamentum teres
- Quadrate lobe
    - Portal vein
    - Falciform ligament
    - Gallbladder

The falciform ligament frequently contains fat and may appear strikingly hyperechoic. Inferiorly it is continuous with the ligamentum teres. About 25% of the blood supply is via the hepatic artery and 75% via the portal vein which drains the stomach, intestines, and spleen. Hepatic artery and portal vein enter the liver at the porta hepatis and divide into major right and left branches. The division between the territories supplied by the two branches does not correspond to the anatomical right and left lobes.

Porta hepatis:
- Hepatic artery
- Portal vein
- Bile duct

Surrounding these portal triads is an hyperechoic sheath of fibrous and fatty tissue. The venous drainage forms three major veins which follow different paths from the arteries and terminate in the inferior vena cava within the upper part of the liver posteriorly. In contrast to the portal vein and its branches, the hepatic veins may be identified within the liver as anechoic tubes without identifiable walls. The normal hepatic parenchyma has a homogeneous echopattern of relatively fine echoes, interspersed with the bright echoes of the portal triads and anechoic areas corresponding to hepatic veins.

4.2.2.1 Normal Dimensions

Liver:
- Left lobe < 5 cm
- Right lobe < 15 cm
- Portal vein < 1.5 cm
- Hepatic veins < 0.5 cm

For the left lobe, the antero-posterior diameter is measured in the paravertebral line and for the right lobe, the cranio-caudal diameter is measured in the mid-clavicular line.

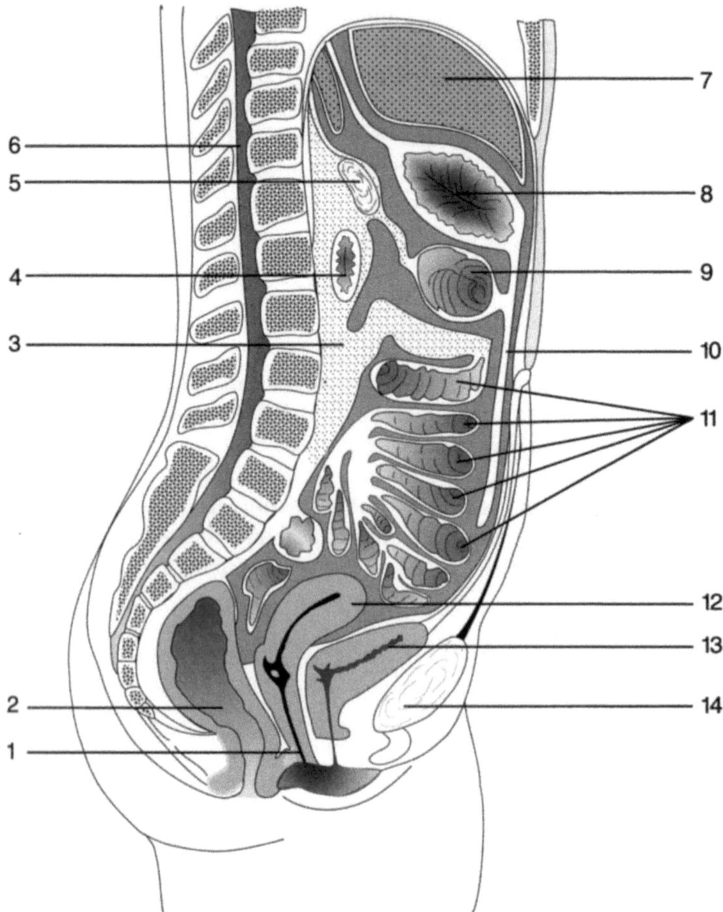

Fig. 4.1. Sagittal section of the abdomen. *1*, Vagina; *2*, rectum; *3*, root of the mesentery; *4*, duodenum; *5*, head of pancreas; *6*, spinal canal; *7*, liver; *8*, stomach; *9*, transverse colon; *10*, greater omentum; *11*, bowel loops; *12*, uterus; *13*, bladder; *14*, symphysis

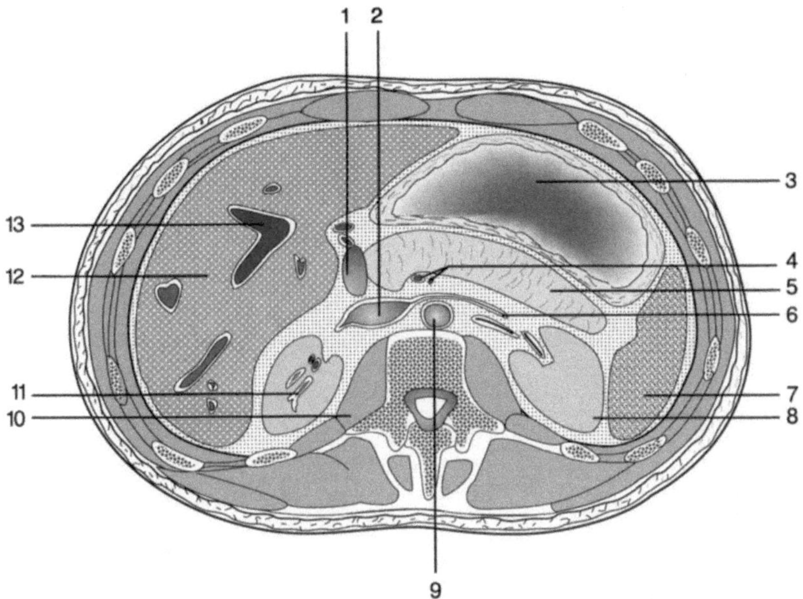

Fig. 4.2. Transverse section of the abdomen. *1*, duodenum; *2*, inferior vena cava; *3*, stomach; *4*, superior mesenteric vein and superior mesenteric artery; *5*, pancreas; *6*, left renal vein; *7*, spleen; *8*, left kidney; *9*, aorta; *10*, psoas muscle; *11*, right kidney; *12*, liver; *13*, portal vein branches

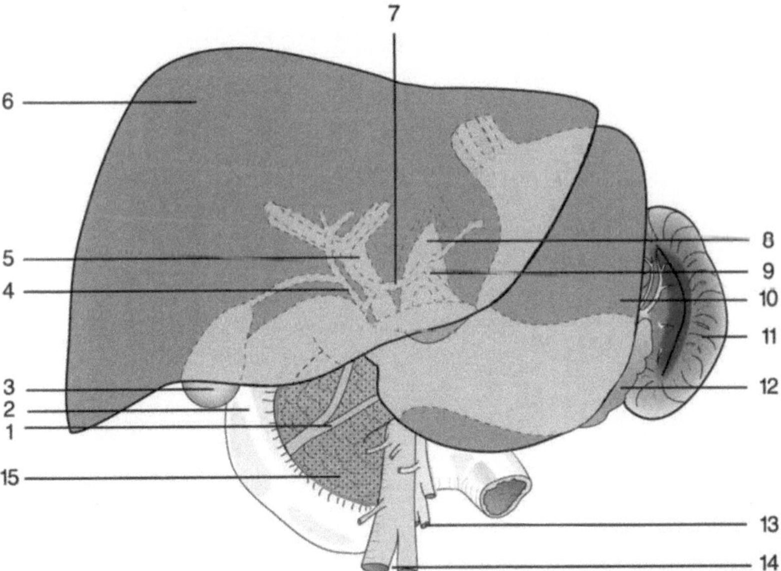

Fig. 4.3. Upper abdominal region. *1*, Common bile duct and pancreatic duct; *2*, duodenum; *3*, gallbladder; *4*, common bile duct; *5*, portal vein; *6*, liver; *7*, hepatic artery; *8*, aorta; *9*, coeliac trunk; *10*, stomach; *11*, spleen; *12*, tail of pancreas; *13*, superior mesenteric artery; *14*, superior mesenteric vein; *15*, head of pancreas

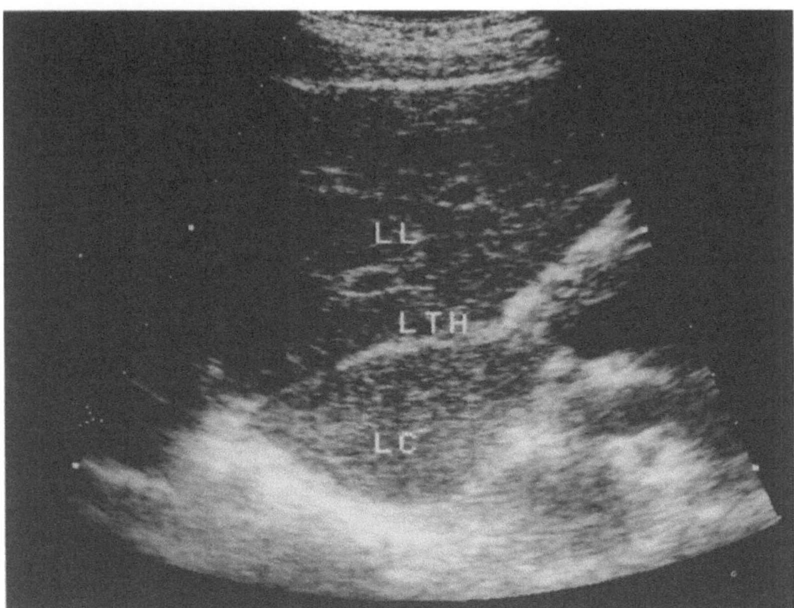

Fig. 4.4. Liver. Longitudinal scan of the left lobe. *LL*, Left lobe; *LTH*, ligamentum teres; *LC*, caudate lobe

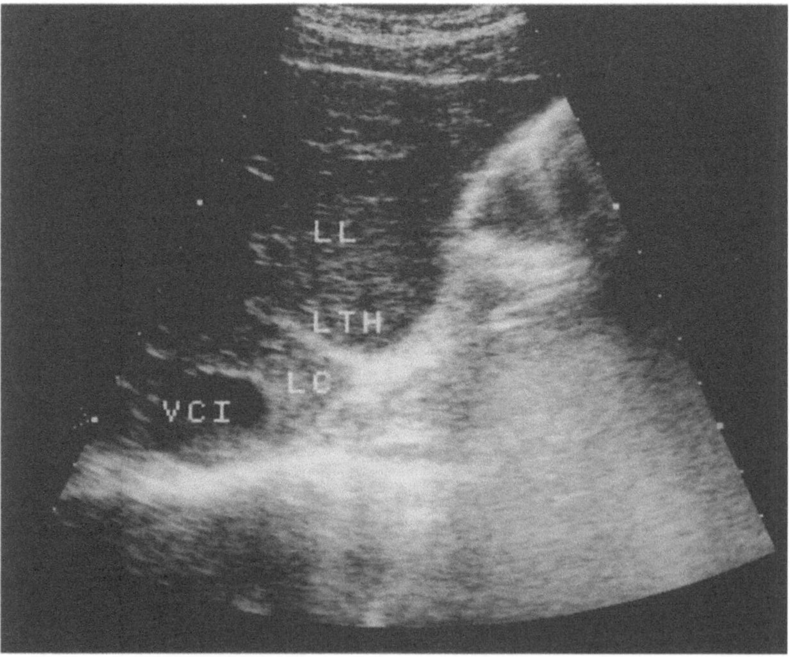

Fig. 4.5. Liver. Transverse scan of the left lobe. *LL*, Left lobe; *LTH*, ligamentum teres; *LC*, caudate lobe; *VCI*, inferior vena cava

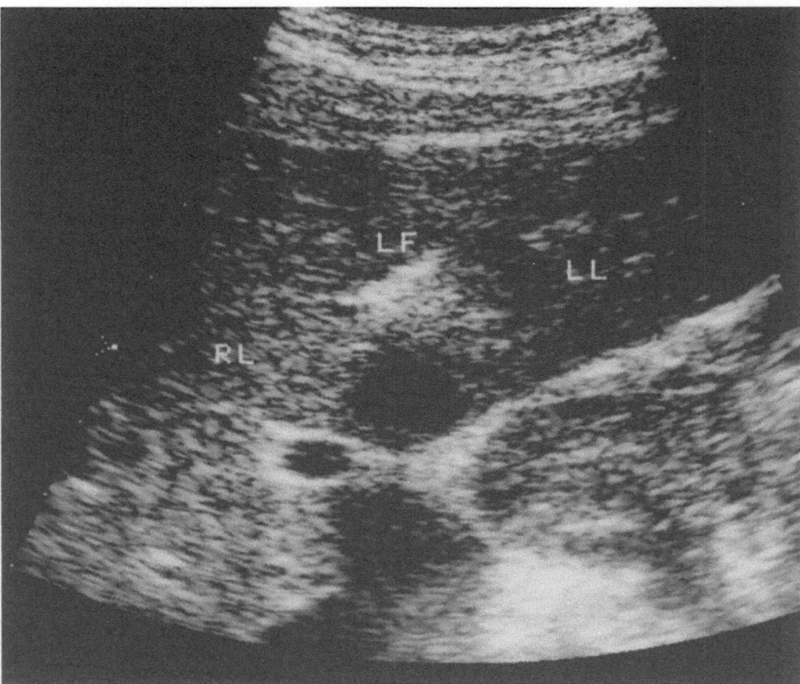

Fig. 4.6. Liver. Transverse scan showing the falciform ligament as an echogenic structure with distal acoustic shadowing. The ligament must not be confused with a mass. *LF,* Falciform ligament; *LL,* left lobe; *RL,* right lobe

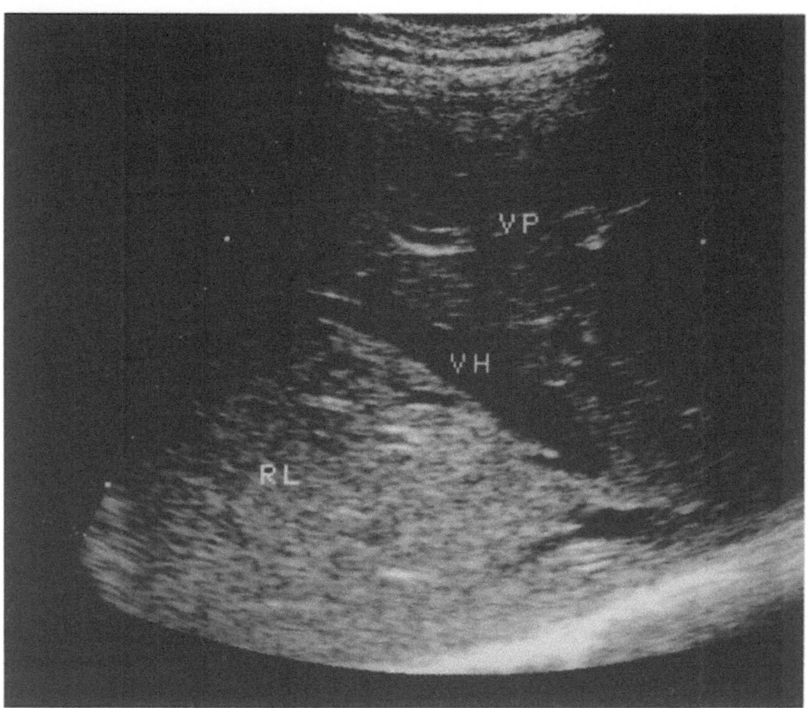

Fig. 4.7. Liver. Subcostal scan. Uniform echopattern interspersed with bright echoes of portal triads and anechoic areas of hepatic veins. The hyperechoic band-shaped structure at the bottom of the image is the diaphragm. *RL*, Right lobe; *VP*, portal vein; *VH*, hepatic vein

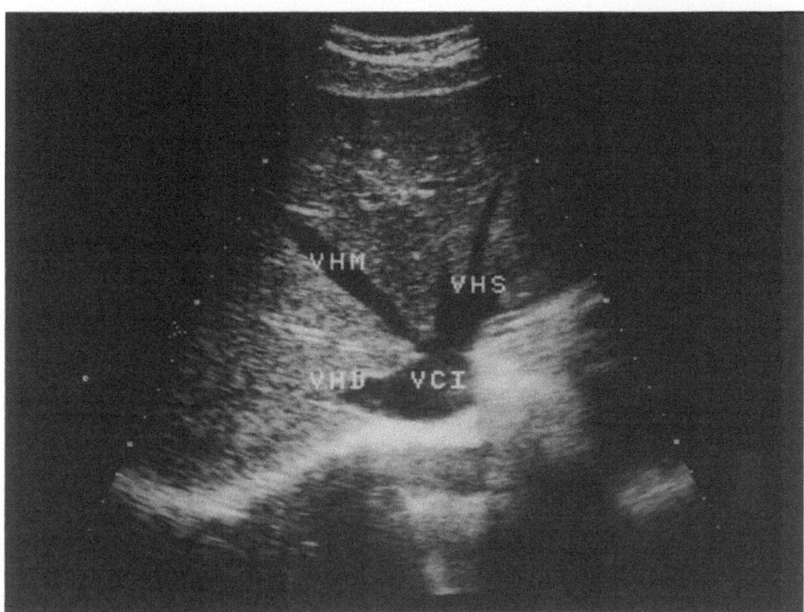

Fig. 4.8. Liver. Subcostal scan through the superior portion of the liver showing the right, middle, and left hepatic veins draining into the inferior vena cava as it penetrates the diaphragm to enter the chest. *VHD*, Right hepatic vein; *VHM*, middle hepatic vein; *VHS*, left hepatic vein; *VCI*, inferior vena cava

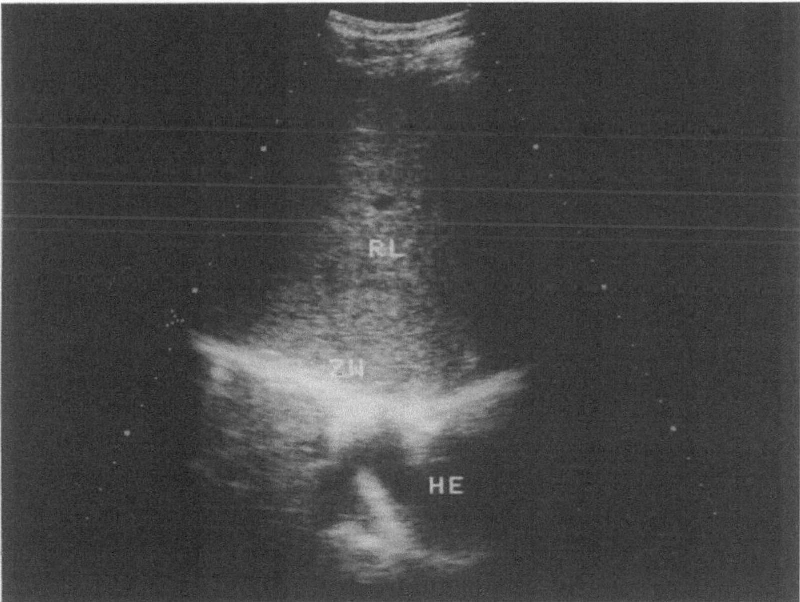

Fig. 4.9. Liver. Intercostal scan. Acoustic shadowing due to ribs. *RL*, Right lobe; *ZW*, diaphragm; *HE*, heart

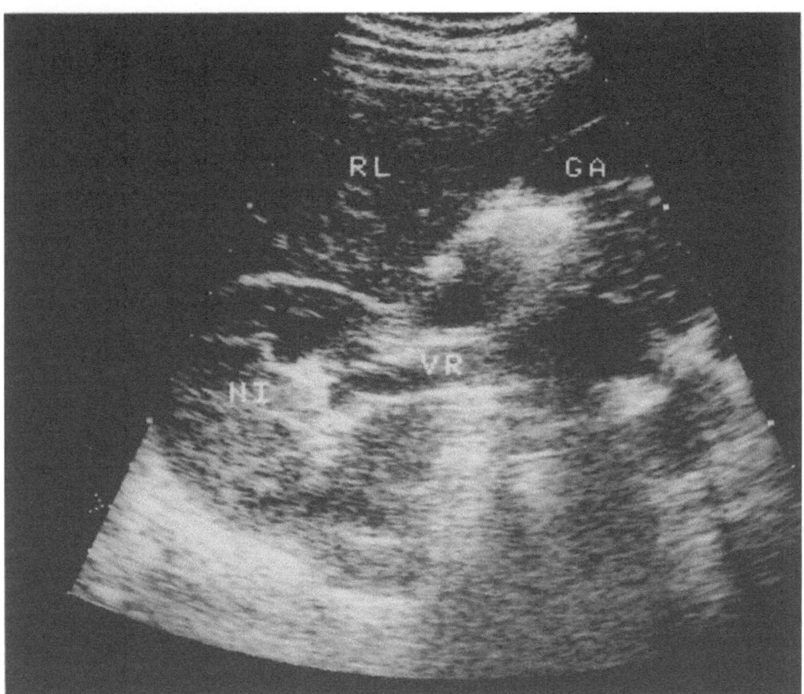

Fig. 4.10. Liver. Transverse scan of the liver, gallbladder, and kidney. *RL*, Right lobe; *GA*, gallbladder; *NI*, kidney; *VR*, renal vein

4.2.3 Sonopathology

4.2.3.1 Fatty Infiltration

Clinical Data

Aetiology:
◆ Alcohol
◆ Viral hepatitis
◆ Diabetes mellitus
◆ Hyperlipidaemia
◆ Obesity
◆ Starvation
◆ Drugs
◆ Pregnancy

The accumulation of fat in the liver is a non-specific response to a wide variety of aetiologies. Simple steatosis is often asymptomatic and may present with hepatomegaly or abnormal liver function tests as chance findings.

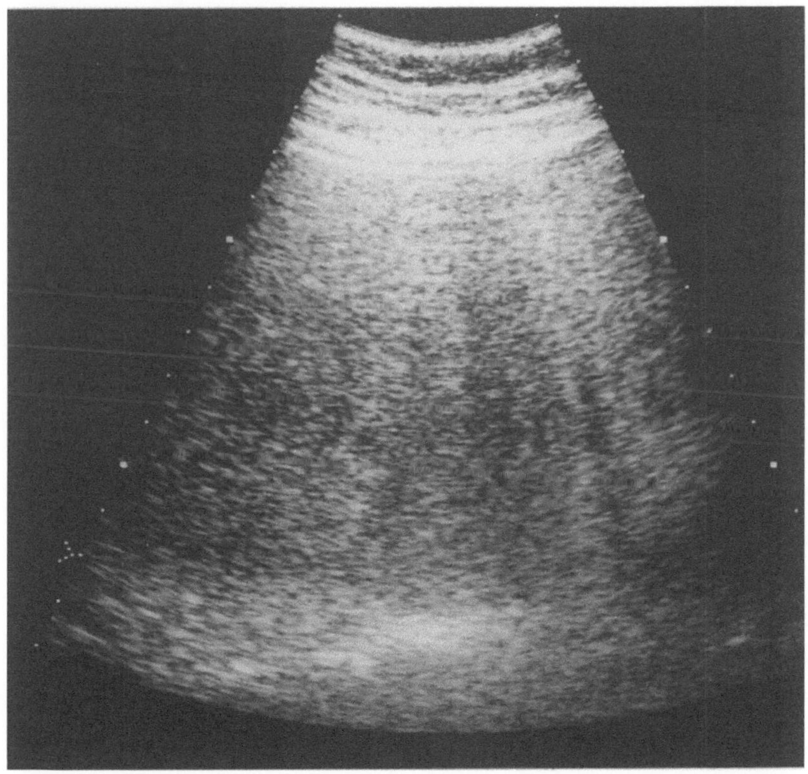

Fig. 4.11. Fatty infiltration. The diaphragm is barely visible

Sonographic Diagnosis

Criteria

→ Enlarged liver
→ Hyperechoic echopattern
→ Reduced ultrasound beam penetration
→ Less prominent hepatic veins

Sonographic Differential Diagnosis

Diffusely hyperechoic liver:
◆ Fatty infiltration
◆ Cirrhosis
◆ Hepatitis
◆ Deposition
◆ Malignant infiltration

4.2.3.2 Focal Fatty Infiltration

Clinical Data

This finding has differential diagnostic importance.

Sonographic Diagnosis

Criteria

→ Hyperechoic area
→ Interdigitation with normal liver tissue
→ Angulated margins

Sites of focal fatty infiltration are usually around the gallbladder, the portal vein branching, and the inferior vena cava.

Sonographic Differential Diagnosis

Focally hyperechoic liver:
◆ Focal fatty infiltration
◆ Adenoma
◆ Haemangioma
◆ Tumour
◆ Metastasis

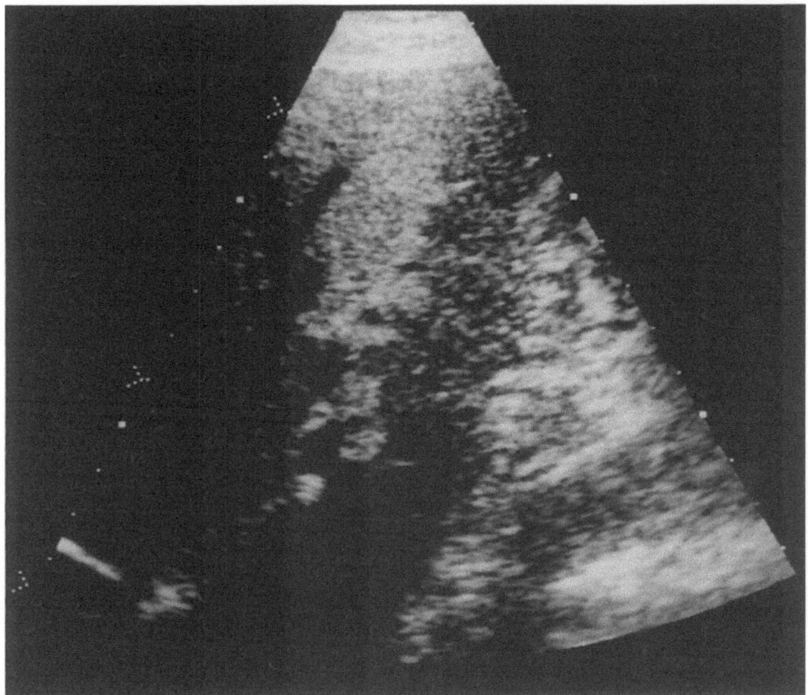

Fig. 4.12. Focal fatty infiltration. Uneven distribution of the liver fat giving rise to an area of increased reflectivity against a background of normal parenchymal echopattern

4.2.3.3 Focal Sparing in Fatty Infiltration

Clinical Data

Focal sparing in fatty infiltration is an important finding in the sonographic differential diagnosis of focal liver lesions.

Sonographic Diagnosis

Criterion

→ Irregular, hypoechoic area

Focal sparing in fatty infiltration frequently occurs at the porta hepatis.

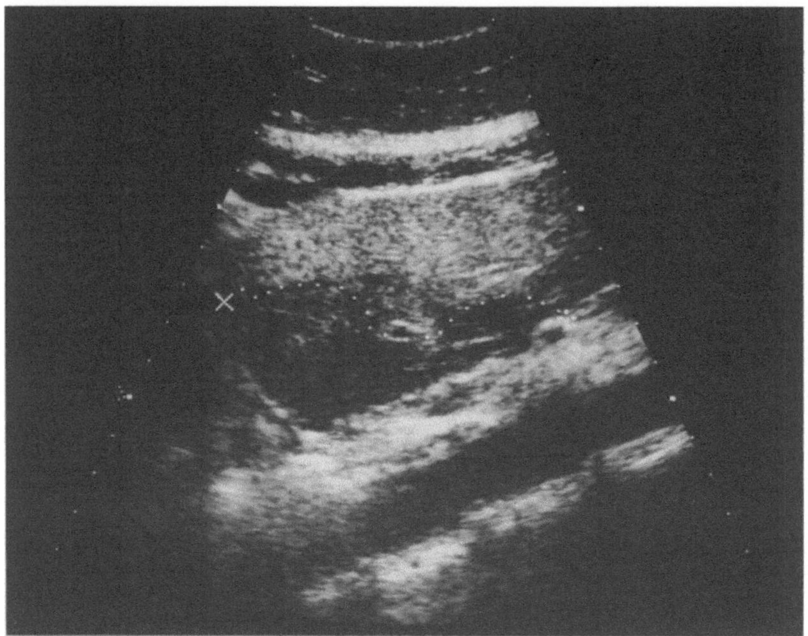

Fig. 4.13. Focal sparing in fatty infiltration

Sonographic Differential Diagnosis

Focally hypoechoic liver:
◆ Focal sparing in fatty infiltration
◆ Focal nodular hyperplasia
◆ Abscess
◆ Haematoma
◆ Complex cyst
◆ Tumour
◆ Lymphoma
◆ Metastasis

4.2.3.4 Cirrhosis

Clinical Data

Aetiology:
◆ Alcohol
◆ Viral hepatitis

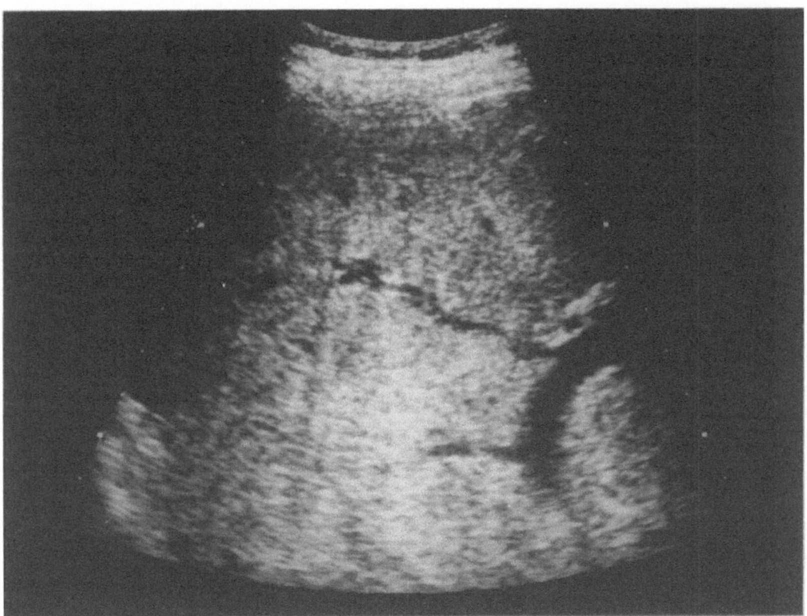

Fig. 4.14. Cirrhosis. Early stage. Note the irregular course of the portal vein branches. Increased hepatic echogenicity reduced the apparent echogenicity of the portal vein walls

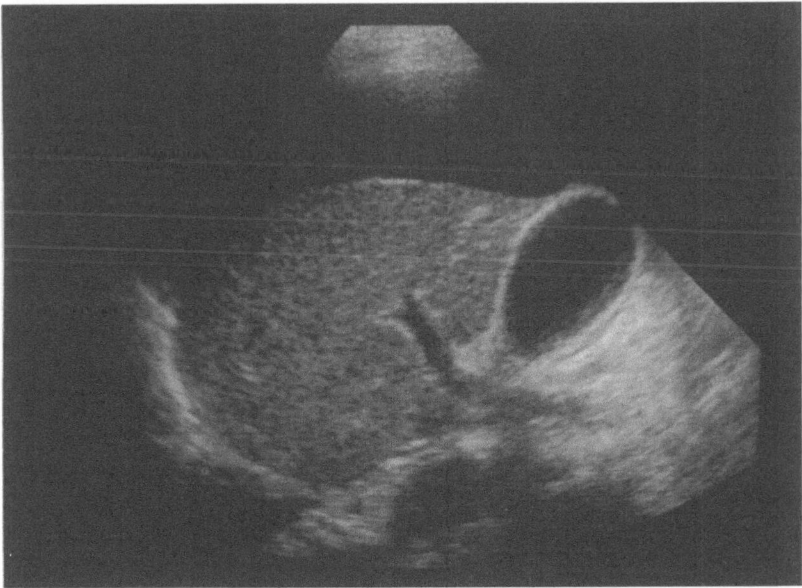

Fig. 4.15. Cirrhosis. Late stage. The scan shows a shrunken liver surrounded by ascites. Increased gallbladder wall thickness

Cirrhosis presents insidiously with non-specific symptoms and the gradual development of the characteristic signs of chronic liver disease: spider naevi, pink palms, Dupuytren's contracture, white nails, prominent veins. Hepatosplenomegaly. Feminization with gynaecomastia and impotence are common in men. The major complications of cirrhosis are ascites, bleeding from oesophageal varices, and encephalopathy.

Sonographic Diagnosis

Criteria

→ Enlarged, normal or shrunken liver
→ Enlarged, hypoechoic caudate lobe
→ Uneven liver surface
→ Heterogeneous, hyperechoic echopattern

Sonographic features of portal hypertension may include:
◆ Dilated portal vein
◆ Dilated splenic vein
◆ Dilated superior mesenteric vein
◆ Dilated veins along the course of the umbilical vein
◆ Increased gallbladder wall thickness
◆ Ascites
◆ Splenomegaly
◆ Lienorenal anastomoses

Sonographic Differential Diagnosis

Cirrhosis in an early stage and fatty infiltration cannot be reliably differentiated sonographically.

Enlargement of the liver:
◆ Fatty infiltration
◆ Cirrhosis
◆ Liver congestion
◆ Tumour
◆ Metastatic infiltration

4.2.3.5 Ascites

Clinical Data

Aetiology:
◆ Portal hypertension
◆ Renal disease
◆ Right-sided heart failure

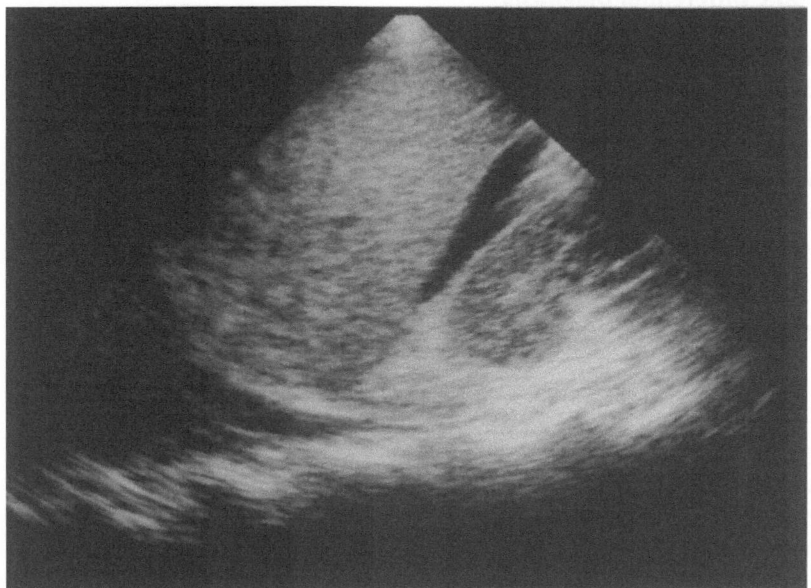

Fig. 4.16. Ascites between the liver and right kidney (Morrison's pouch)

◆ Malignancy
◆ Hypoproteinaemia

A collection of fluid in the peritoneal cavity is a common clinical finding, and a thorough investigation of the patient should be made in order to discover the cause.

Sonographic Diagnosis

Criterion

→ Anechoic fluid
   – Around the liver
   – Around the spleen
   – Between the bowel loops
   – In the flanks
   – In the pelvis

The location of the fluid depends upon the patient's position.

Sonographic Differential Diagnosis

Differential diagnosis:
◆ Blood
◆ Urine
◆ Gallbladder hydrops
◆ Ovarian cyst
◆ Abscess
◆ Aneurysm

4.2.3.6 Pleural Effusion

Clinical Data

Aetiology:
◆ Heart failure
◆ Trauma
◆ Infection
◆ Carcinoma

Pain and dyspnoea are the major symptoms.

Sonographic Diagnosis

Criteria

→ Anechoic fluid
→ Impaired diaphragmatic movement

Sonographic Differential Diagnosis

Findings are typical.

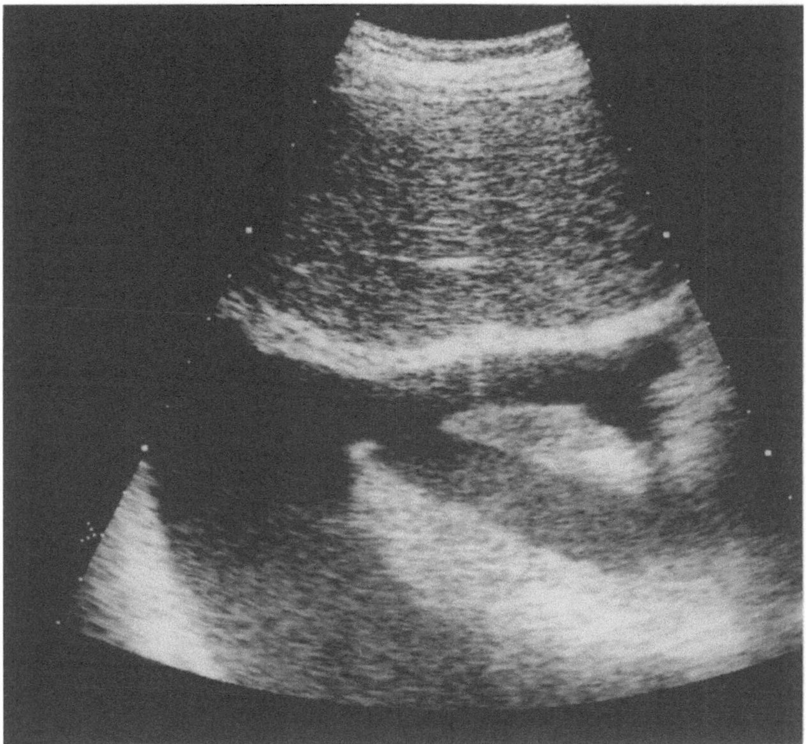

Fig. 4.17. Pleural effusion. The atelectatic lung is surrounded by fluid

4.2.3.7 Abscess

Clinical Data

Infection may reach the liver by three different routes:
◆ Ascending the bile ducts
◆ Blood-borne infection via the hepatic artery
◆ Blood-borne infection via the portal vein

There is tender enlargement of the liver, with pain referred to the back and shoulder; fever, general malaise, anorexia.

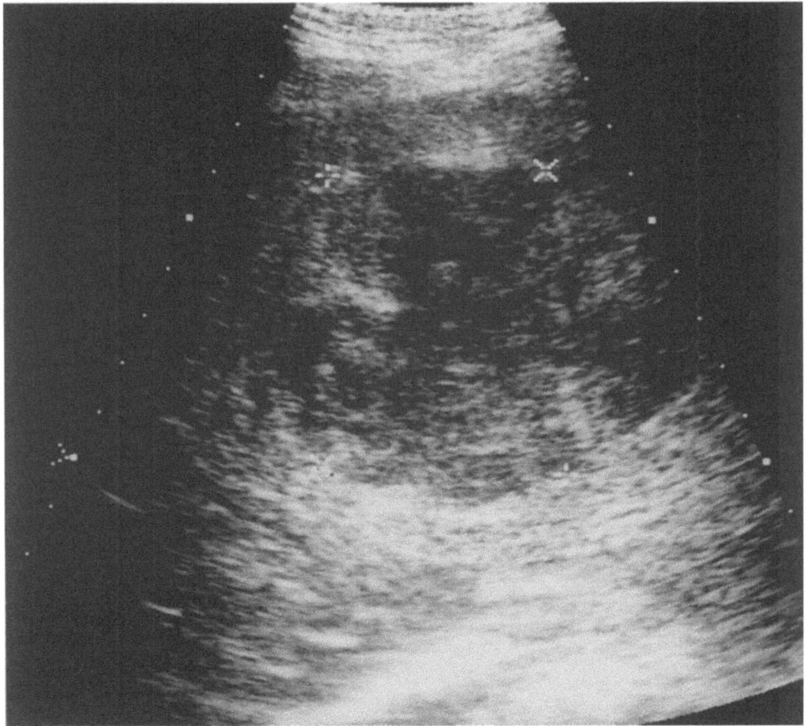

Fig. 4.18. Liver abscess. Liquefaction has just started to form centrally within the abscess

Sonographic Diagnosis

Criteria

→ Irregular wall
→ Heterogeneous, hypoechoic echopattern
→ Anechoic areas with acoustic enhancement due to necrosis or pus
→ Echogenic areas with acoustic shadowing due to calcification or gas

A hypoechoic rim may surround the outer margin of the abscess. As a fibrous reaction occurs around the abscess an increasingly hyperechoic wall forms which may calcify in long-standing cases.

Ultrasound is helpful not only in confirming the diagnosis but also in guiding the aspirating needle to identify the organism and in monitoring the response to therapy.

Sonographic Differential Diagnosis

Fungal abscesses may be seen as multiple target lesions and thus may be indistinguishable from multiple liver metastases.

4.2.3.8 Haematoma

Clinical Data

Trauma may cause acute or delayed haemorrhage with parenchymal laceration. The signs are those of shock and intraperitoneal bleeding. Pain. Rigidity of the abdominal wall.

Sonographic Diagnosis

Criteria
→ Initially anechoic collections
→ Hyperechoic lesion as the blood clots
→ Later complex appearance

Resolving haematomas may give rise to hepatic cysts.

Sonographic Differential Diagnosis

Haematomas are anechoic during acute haemorrhage and during clot liquefaction.

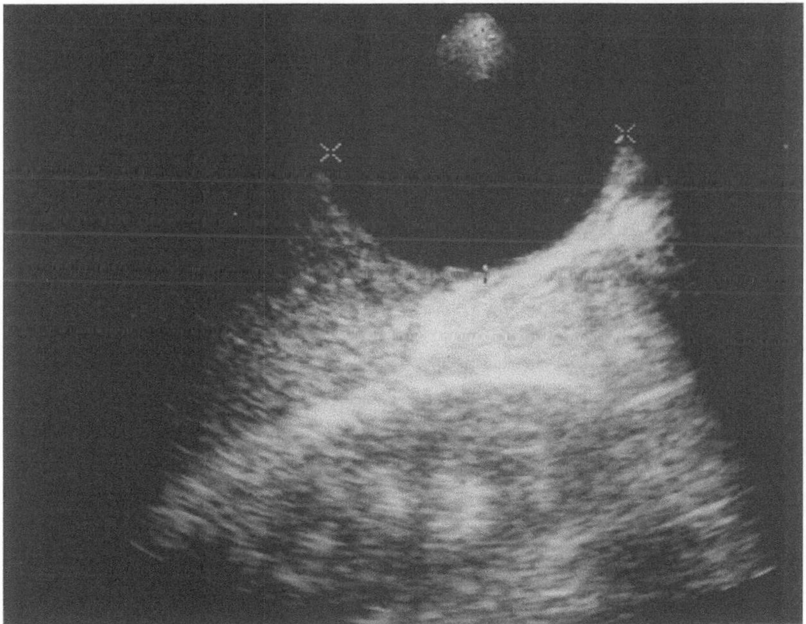

Fig. 4.19. Liver haematoma. Early stage

4.2.3.9 Cysts

Clinical Data

Although liver cysts are found less frequently than renal cysts they are not uncommon. When multiple they are often associated with cystic disease in other organs (kidney, pancreas, spleen, lung). The incidence of liver cysts rises with age. When large they may compress liver parenchyma and bile ducts but they are usually asymptomatic.

Sonographic Diagnosis

Criteria

→ Spherical or oval anechoic lesion
→ Sharp and well-defined border
→ Distal acoustic enhancement
→ Prominent posterior border

Sonographic features of hydatid disease may include cysts within a cyst, a multilocular cyst with hyperechoic material, a complex mass with solid areas, and cysts with undulating membranes. Some masses are densely calcified and show distal acoustic shadowing. Hydatid cysts are usually spherical or oval, well defined and have a demonstrable wall.

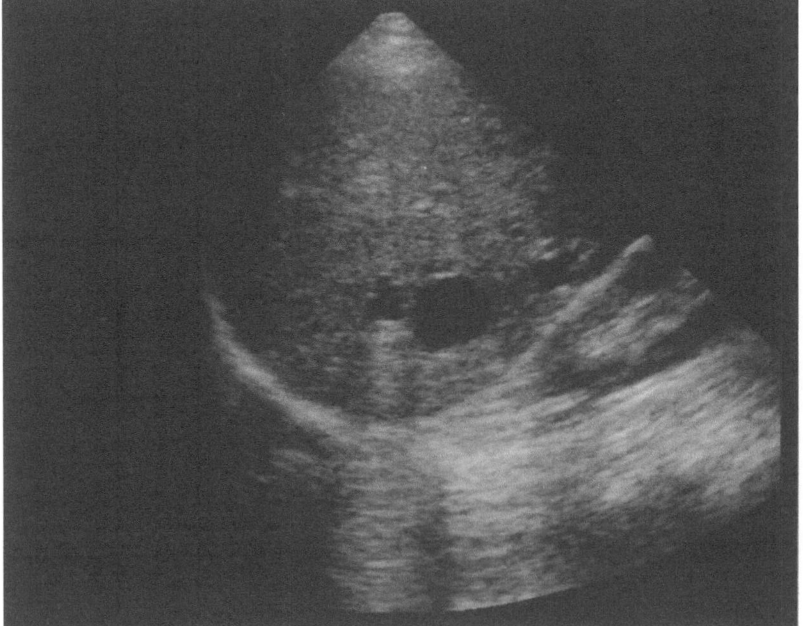

Fig. 4.20. Liver cysts

Sonographic Differential Diagnosis

Irregular Cyst Wall:
- Haemorrhagic cyst
- Hydatid disease
- Tumour necrosis
- Metastasis
- Abscess
- Lymphoma

4.2.3.10 Focal Nodular Hyperplasia

Clinical Data

Focal nodular hyperplasia is a tumour-like disorder which histologically may resemble macronodular cirrhosis and is a hamartoma rather than a true neoplasm. Oral contraceptives have been implicated in enhancing the size of the lesion, but are probably not causative. Related variants exist, and histopathological overlap with adenoma may occur.

Sonographic Diagnosis

Criteria
- → Well-defined mass
- → Hypoechoic or isoechoic echopattern
- → May be multiple
- → May be pedunculate

An adenoma is usually seen as a hyperechoic mass which is well defined and of relatively uniform appearance. If the echopattern is similar to that of adjacent liver tissue, the adenoma may be difficult to identify.

Sonographic Differential Diagnosis

Liver metastasis.

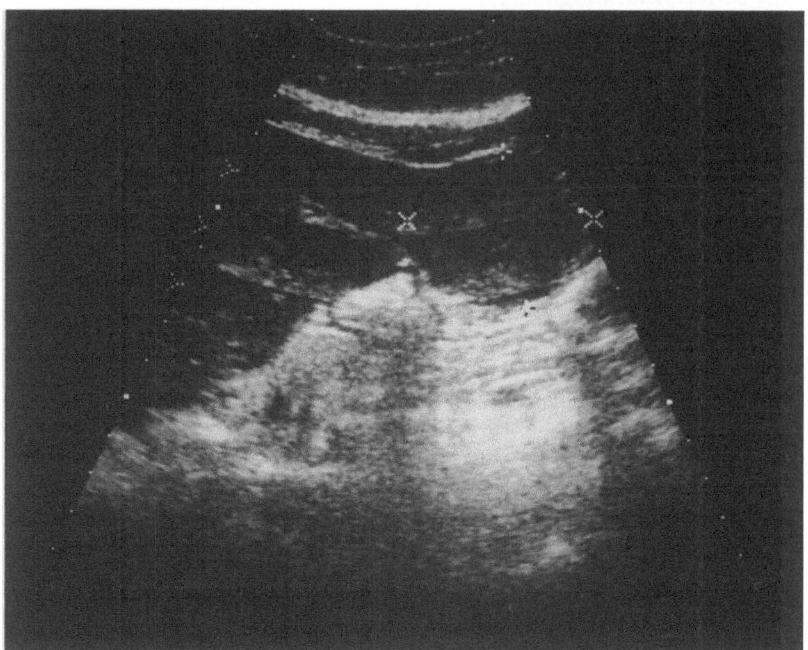

Fig. 4.21. Focal nodular hyperplasia

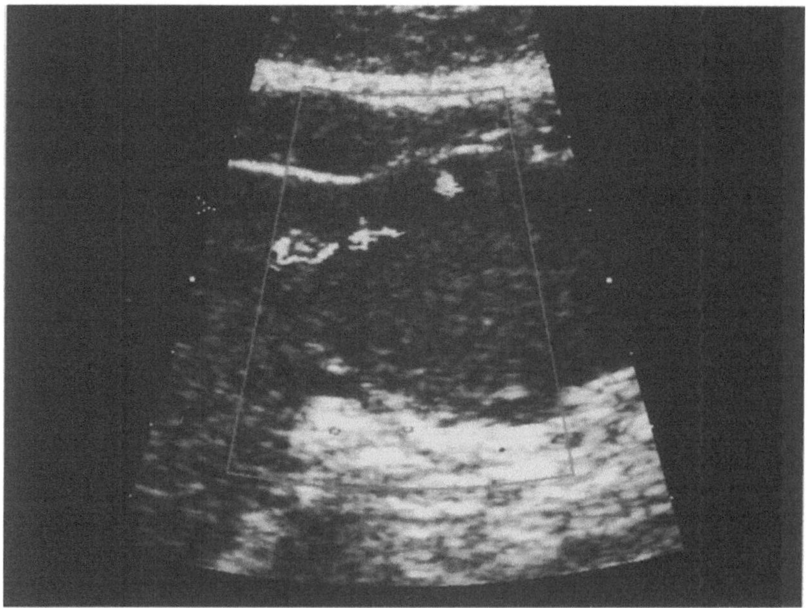

Fig. 4.22. Focal nodular hyperplasia. The majority are vascular on colour Doppler

4.2.3.11 Haemangioma

Clinical Data

Haemangiomas are commonly seen in the liver. Rarely they are large enough to cause symptoms.

Sonographic Diagnosis

Criteria

→ Well-defined, highly echogenic mass
→ Frequently superficial within the liver
→ Variable form and size
→ No halo sign
→ No acoustic shadowing
→ May be multiple
→ May cause mirror artefacts

Haemangiomas usually show little change in appearance over prolonged periods. Haemorrhage, however, may give rise to a complex appearance.

There is only very limited blood flow through haemangiomas and colour Doppler studies are usually of no value in confirming the diagnosis.

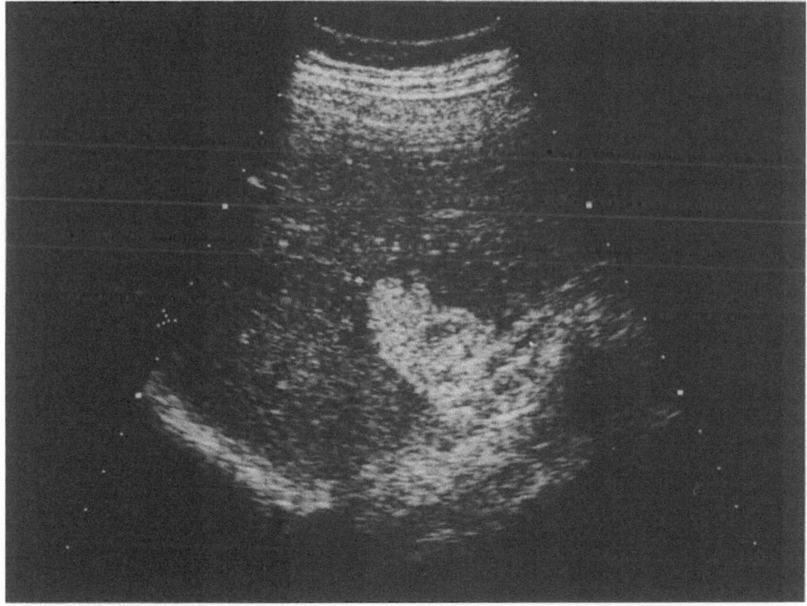

Fig. 4.23. Haemangioma lying on the liver capsule

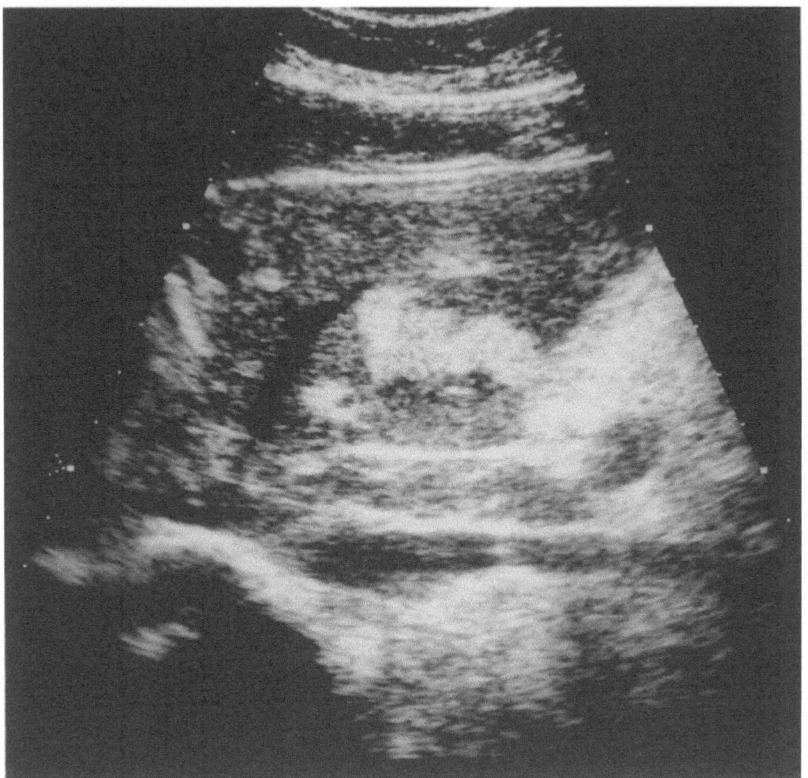

Fig. 4.24. Multiple haemangiomas in the left lobe

Sonographic Differential Diagnosis

Hyperechoic liver metastasis.

4.2.3.12 Metastases

Clinical Data

The liver is one of the commonest sites of metastatic cancer, particularly stomach, pancreas, colon, rectum, lung, breast, oesophagus, and thyroid. Secondary liver tumours are far more common than primary growths (hepatocellular carcinoma, cholangiocarcinoma). Enlargement of the liver, accompanied by continuous pain, suggests the presense of a liver tumour.

Sonographic Diagnosis

Criteria

→   I   Cystic lesion
→   II   Hypoechoic lesion
→ III   Hyperechoic lesion
→ IV   Bull's eye lesion (hyperechoic margin)
→   V   Target lesion (hypoechoic margin)
→ VI   Calcified lesion
→ VII   Complex lesion
→ VIII Miliary metastatic deposits

General signs include:
- Altered hepatic shape
- Nodular liver surface
- Compressed adjacent parenchyma

There is poor correlation between the sonographic appearance and tumour histology. Chemotherapy may give rise to increased or decreased echogenicity of metastases. Cystic change may occur in any metastasis undergoing central necrosis.

Lymphoma and leukaemia are particularly prone to diffuse hepatic malignancy which usually appears hypoechoic.

In hepatocellular carcinoma, most patients present with a history of underlying cirrhosis or other liver disorder. Sonographic appearances are variable and there are no pathognomonic findings.

Sonographic Differential Diagnosis

Sonographic signs indicating malignancy:
- Growth
- Infiltration
- Halo sign
- Central necrosis

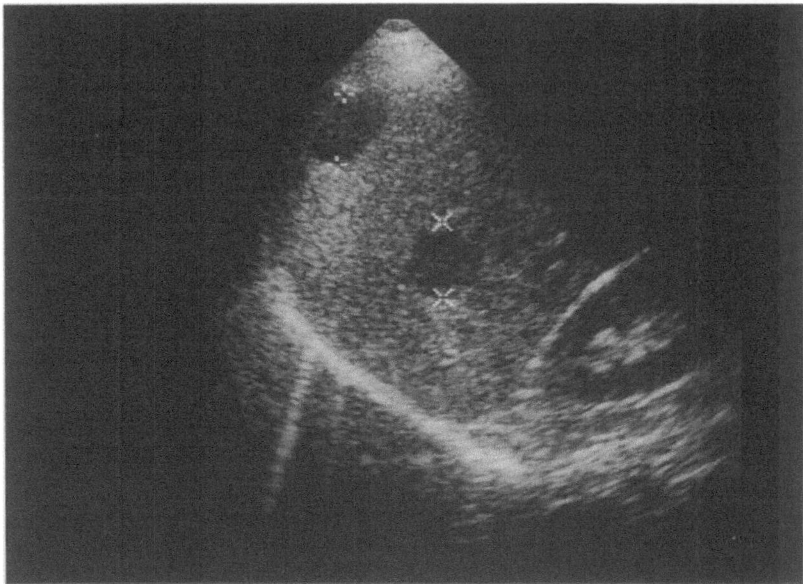

Fig. 4.25. Hypoechoic liver metastases

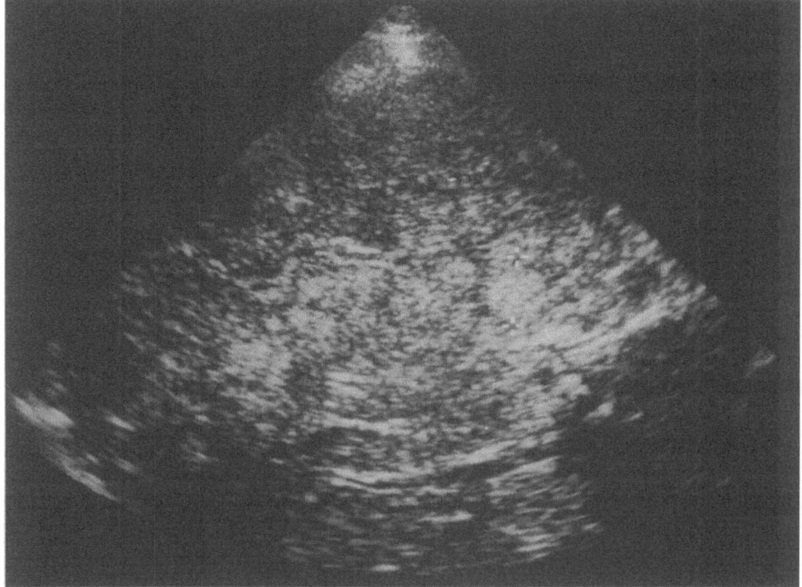

Fig. 4.26. Hyperechoic liver metastases

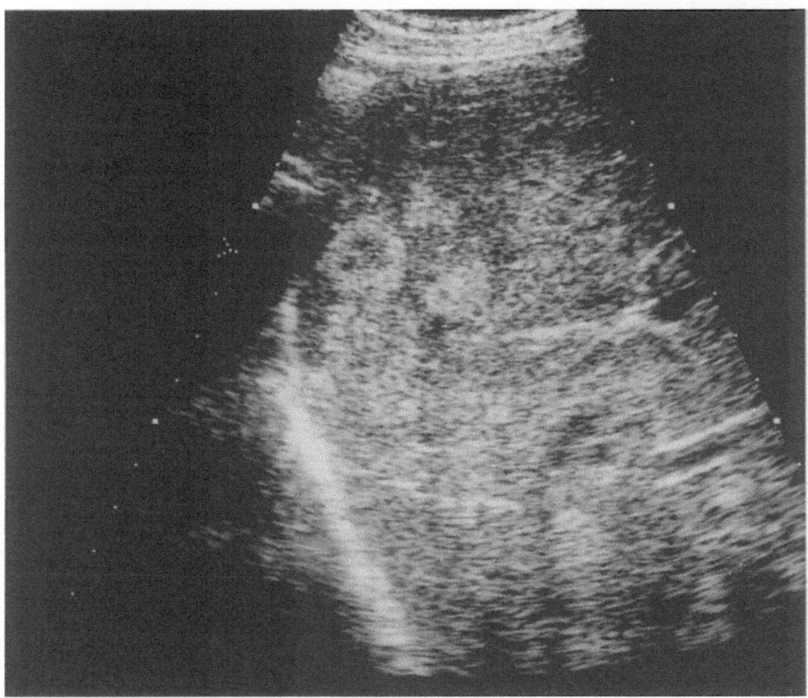

Fig. 4.27. Bull's eye lesions. The margin of the lesion is hyperechoic

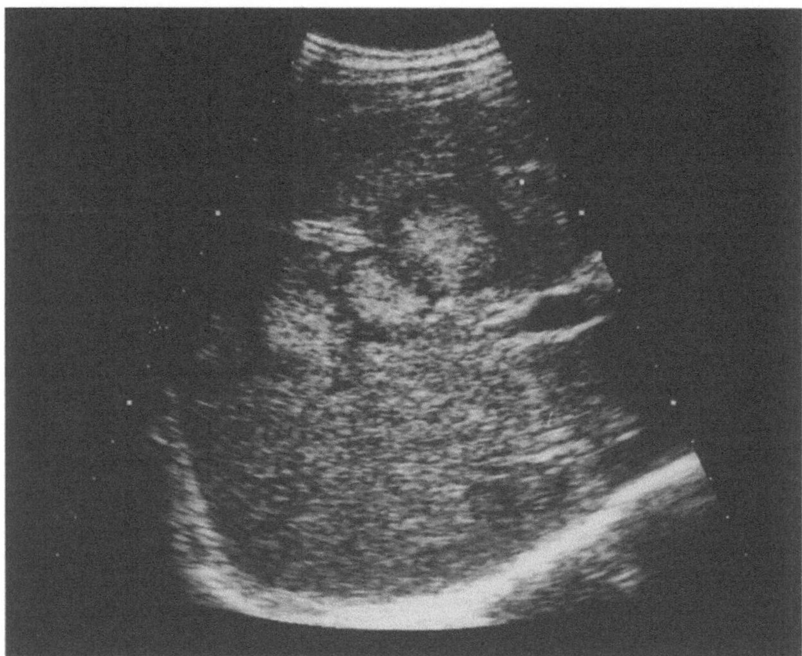

Fig. 4.28. Target lesions. The margin of the lesion is hypoechoic (halo sign)

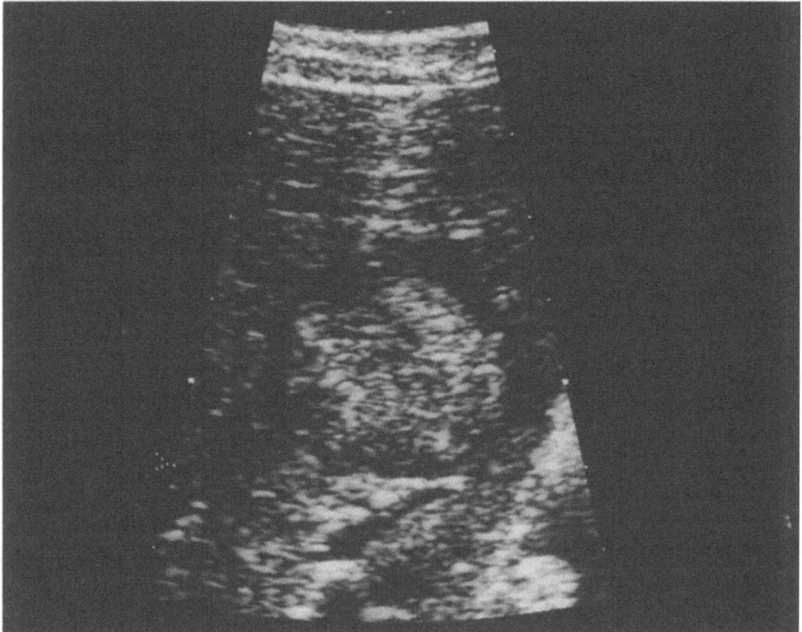

Fig. 4.29. Target lesion (magnification)

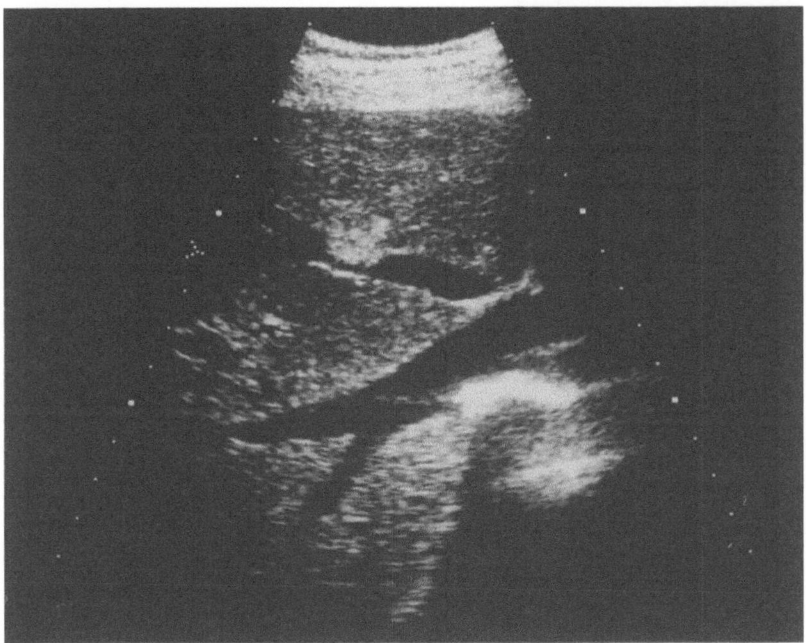

Fig. 4.30. Hyperechoic metastasis infiltrating a hepatic vein

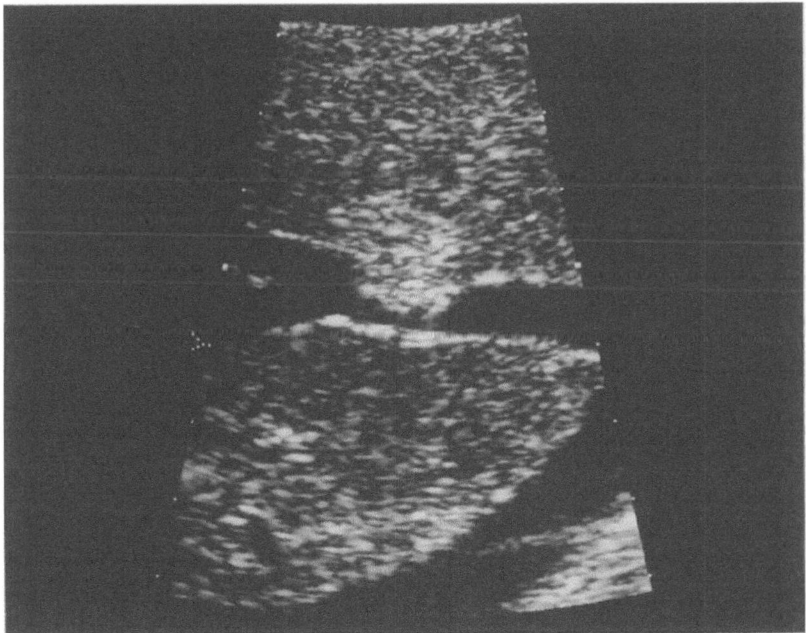

Fig. 4.31. Hyperechoic metastasis infiltrating a hepatic vein (magnification)

4.2.4 Checklist for Reporting

Liver
- Size
- Contour
- Echopattern

Vessels
- Portal vein
- Hepatic veins
- Splenic vein
- Inferior vena cava

Bile ducts

Spleen
- Size

Ascites

Pleural effusion

Chapter 5 Biliary System

5.1 Imaging Modalities

Sonography is the method of choice to image the biliary system. Imaging modalities are:

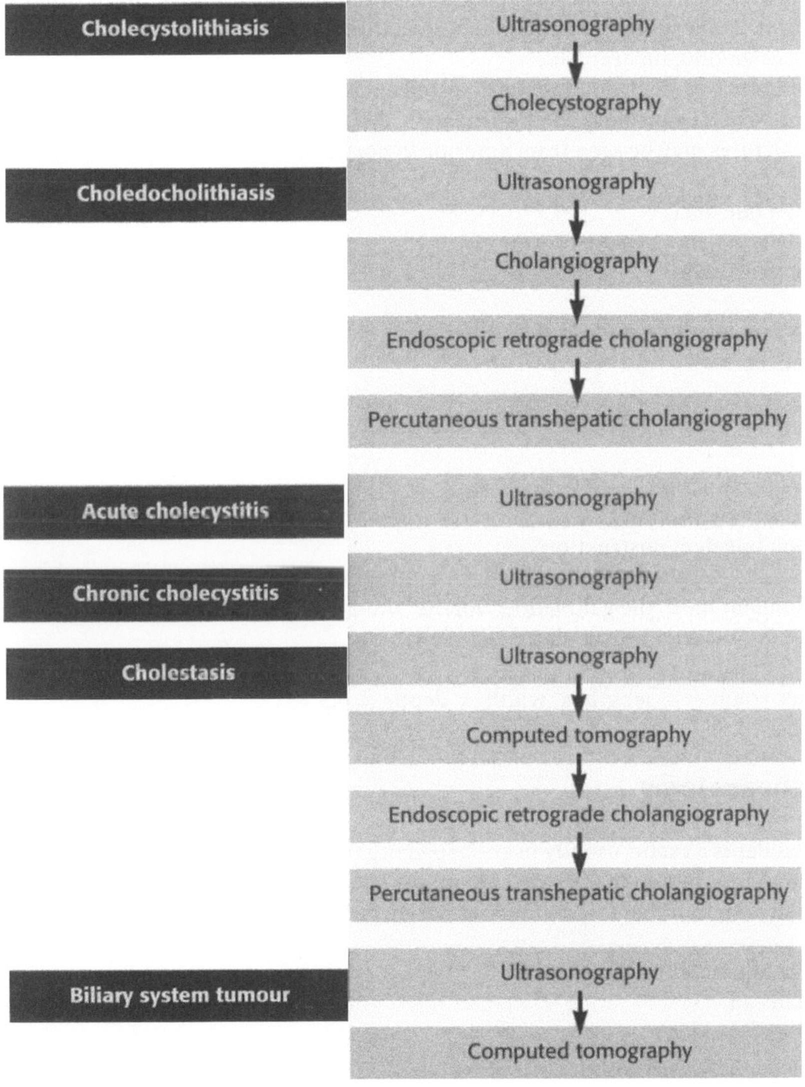

5.2 Ultrasonography

5.2.1 Examination Technique

The information from abdominal examinations may be significantly impaired by gas in the bowel which interferes with the transmission of sound. Intestinal gases are expelled from the examination area if the patient drinks 500–1000 ml water immediately before the examination. For the display of the gallbladder a 3.5-MHz sector or convex probe is recommended and for the display of the bile ducts a 5-MHz sector probe. A 3.5- or 5-MHz convex transducer can also be used. It is important that the gallbladder be full, so the patient fasts to prevent contraction.

The landmark to find the gallbladder in the subcostal section is the right main branch of the portal vein. Longitudinal, transverse, and intercostal sections should also be performed. The image obtained from ultrasound is that of a slice, so in order to obtain a three dimensional assessment of a structure, a number of slices must be made by moving or angling the transducer.

The common bile duct can only be assessed sonographically from a diameter of at least 2 mm. When examining the patient with the right side elevated three adjacent tubular structures may be seen from anterior to posterior:

◆ Common bile duct
◆ Portal vein
◆ Inferior vena cava

The distal common bile duct may be obscured by bowel gas as it passes behind the duodenum.

The examination of the gallbladder after a stimulant meal allows the demonstration of:

◆ Gallbladder function
◆ Cystic duct obstruction
◆ Common bile duct obstruction

After a stimulant meal, the gallbladder volume should be reduced by at least 30%. The gallbladder volume can be calculated as follows:

Gallbladder volume = length x width x depth x 0.5

5.2.2 Sonoanatomy

The gallbladder is a cystic, usually pear-shaped organ lying in the gallbladder bed posteromedial to the right lobe of liver. The fundus is often folded over. The normal gallbladder wall is so thin that it is sometimes barely perceptible.

Gallbladder anomalies:
◆ Phrygian cap
◆ Septate gallbladder

Structures mimicking the gallbladder:
◆ Bowel loop
◆ Vessel
◆ Cyst
◆ Haematoma
◆ Abscess
◆ Ascites

Non-visualization of the gallbladder:
◆ Agenesis
◆ Postprandial contraction
◆ Gas
◆ Obesity
◆ Cholecystectomy
◆ Sludge
◆ Porcelain gallbladder
◆ Carcinoma

The bile ducts drain into the right and left hepatic ducts which unite at the porta hepatis to form the common hepatic duct. The cystic duct connects the gallbladder to the common hepatic duct to form the common bile duct which drains into the duodenum.

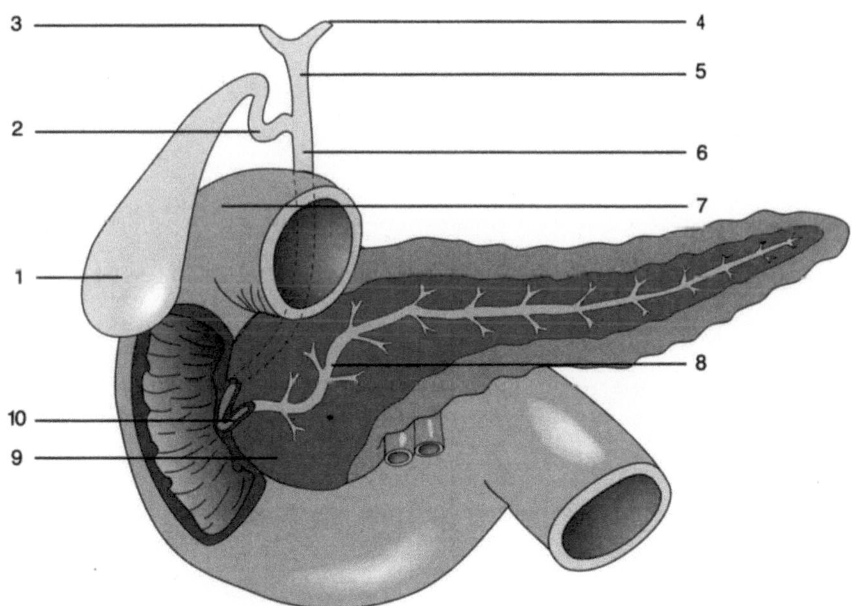

Fig. 5.1. Bile duct region. *1*, Gallbladder; *2*, cystic duct; *3*, right hepatic duct; *4*, left hepatic duct; *5*, common hepatic duct; *6*, common bile duct; *7*, duodenum; *8*, pancreatic duct; *9*, head of pancreas; *10*, greater duodenal papilla

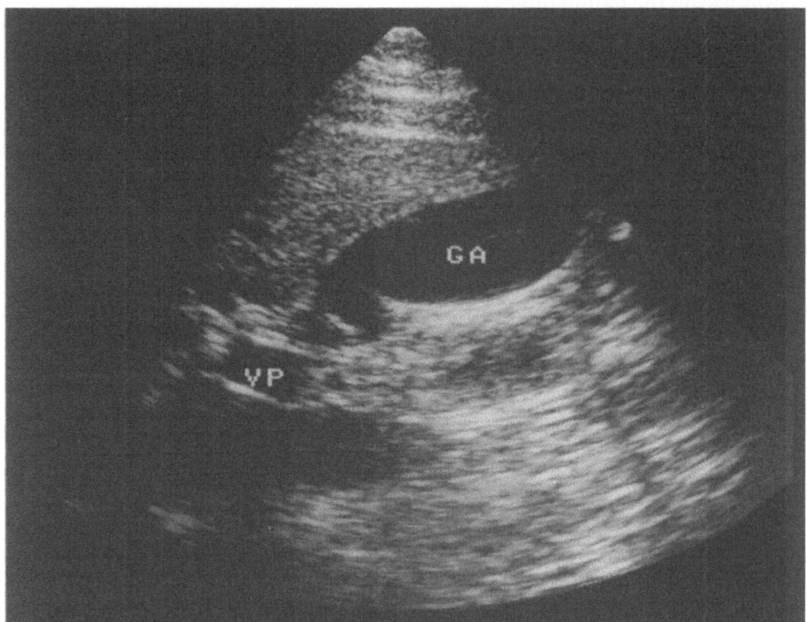

Fig. 5.2. Gallbladder. Note the thin wall, absence of internal echoes, and acoustic enhancement behind the gallbladder. *GA*, Gallbladder; *VP*, portal vein

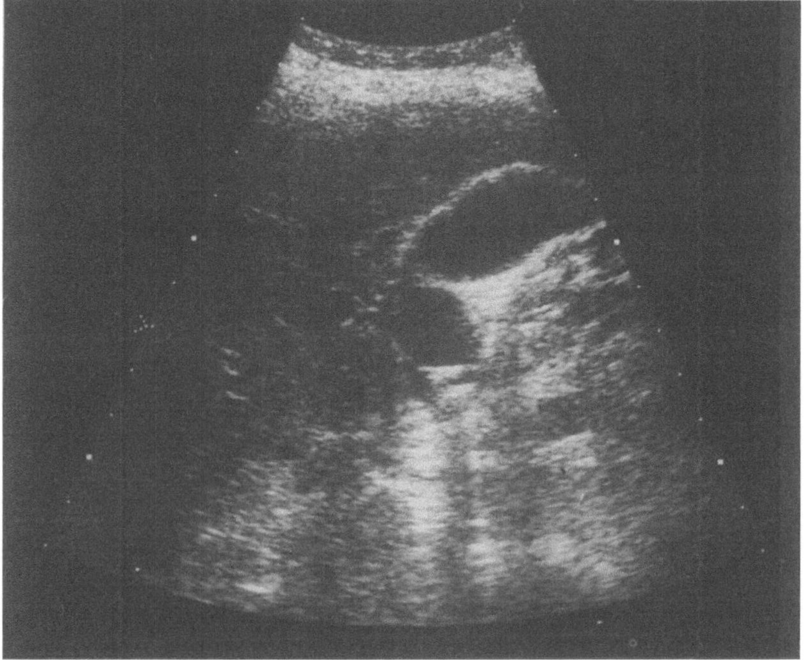

Fig. 5.3. Septate gallbladder. This appearance is usually due to gallbladder folding

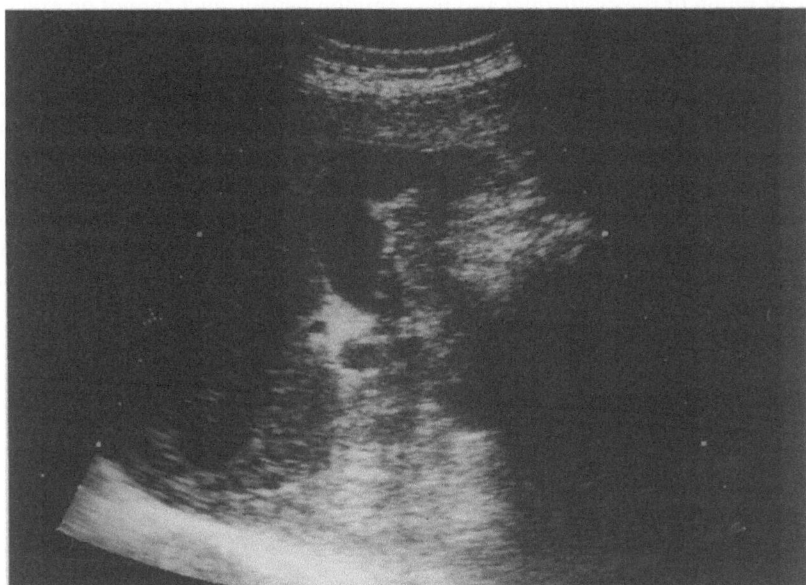

Fig. 5.4. Phrygian cap. Gallbladder cap folded back on itself

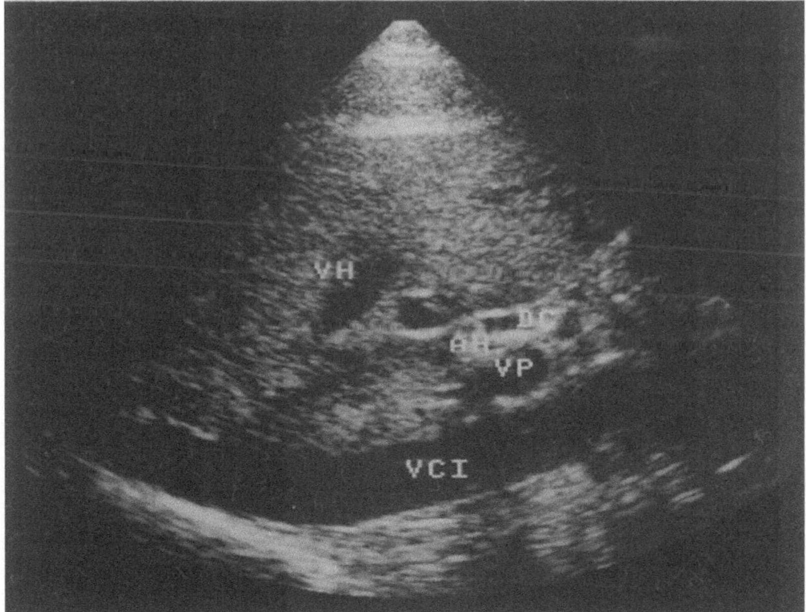

Fig. 5.5. Porta hepatis. The common bile duct can be visualized anterior to the portal vein and the inferior vena cava. *DC*, Common bile duct; *VP*, portal vein; *VCI*, inferior vena cava; *AH*, hepatic artery; *VH*, hepatic vein

The point of union of the cystic duct and the common hepatic duct cannot be exactly defined on sonography and thus the point of transition from common hepatic duct to common bile duct cannot be accurately demarcated.

The common hepatic and the common bile duct can be seen as small tubular structures lying anterior to the portal vein in the porta hepatis. The lower end of the common bile duct is often obscured by gas in the duodenum which lies just in front of it. The intrahepatic biliary tree is normally of such small calibre as to be almost invisible though small portions of it may be seen occasionally over lengths of a few millimetres.

The hepatic artery is very variable in its extrahepatic course. The right branch of the hepatic artery crosses anterior to the portal vein and lies between the portal vein and common bile duct.

5.2.2.1 Normal Dimensions

Biliary system:
- Gallbladder
  - Length < 10 cm
  - Diameter < 4 cm
  - Wall thickness < 3 mm
- Common bile duct
  - Diameter < 6 mm
  - Diameter after cholecystectomy < 8 mm

Simple measurement of the gallbladder area in a single plane is usually adequate for the comparison of pre- and post-prandial gallbladder sizes. The gallbladder and the common bile duct are physiologically wider in older people.

5.2.3 Sonopathology

5.2.3.1 Sludge

Clinical Data

Aetiology:
- Prolonged fasting
- Parenteral nutrition
- Bile duct obstruction

Normally, sludge is a transient phenomenon which passes as the patient's health improves.

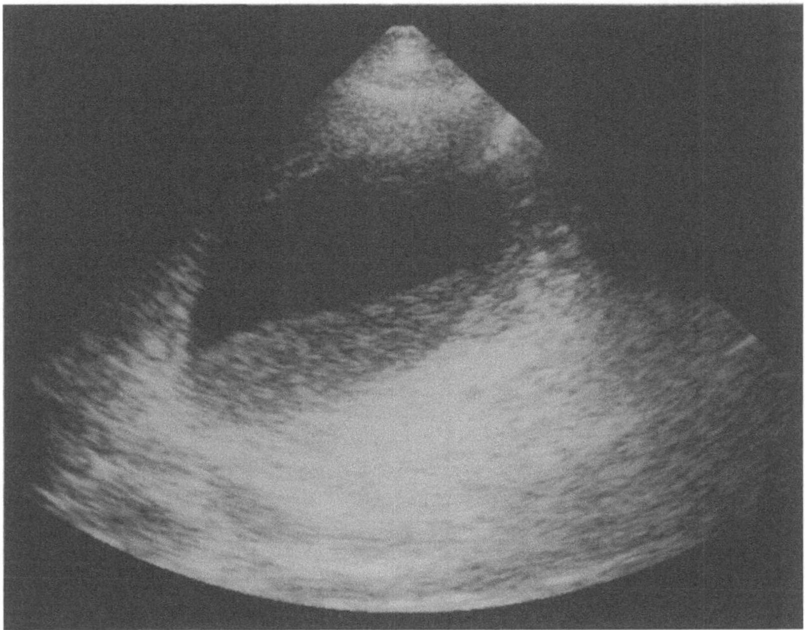

Fig. 5.6. Sludge

Sonographic Diagnosis

Criteria

→ Slightly hyperechoic sediment
→ Fluid/sludge level

Inspissated bile sludge may mimic polyps and tumours.

Sonographic Differential Diagnosis

Hyperechoic gallbladder:
◆ Partial volume/beam width artefact
◆ Sludge
◆ Gravel
◆ Cholecystitis
◆ Empyema
◆ Tumour

5.2.3.2 Cholelithiasis

Clinical Data

Many gallstones produce no symptoms – so-called silent stones – and are usually discovered sonographically. The typical symptom of uncomplicated stones is the pain of biliary colic. Other symptoms are those of complications and include obstructive jaundice, cholangitis, and acute pancreatitis. Flatulent dyspepsia, fat intolerance.

Sonographic Diagnosis

Criteria
- → Mobile echogenic focus
- → Distal acoustic shadowing

Scans should be made in two planes at right angles. The patient should be turned from side to side during the examination.

Gallstones of a diameter of 2–3 mm or more usually cause shadowing. They are usually found in the most dependent part of the gallbladder but can also float in the bile. The sensitivity of sonography in the diagnosis of gallstones is limited with:

- ◆ Very small stones
- ◆ Empyema
- ◆ Impacted stones

It is not possible to determine the age of a stone. The number and size of gallstones may be difficult to assess, but an estimation should always be attempted. Stones in the cystic duct are difficult to visualize.

Sonographic Differential Diagnosis

Differential diagnosis:
- ◆ Refraction
- ◆ Inspissated bile sludge
- ◆ Bowel gas
- ◆ Mucosal fold
- ◆ Rib
- ◆ Pus
- ◆ Clot
- ◆ Polyp
- ◆ Tumour

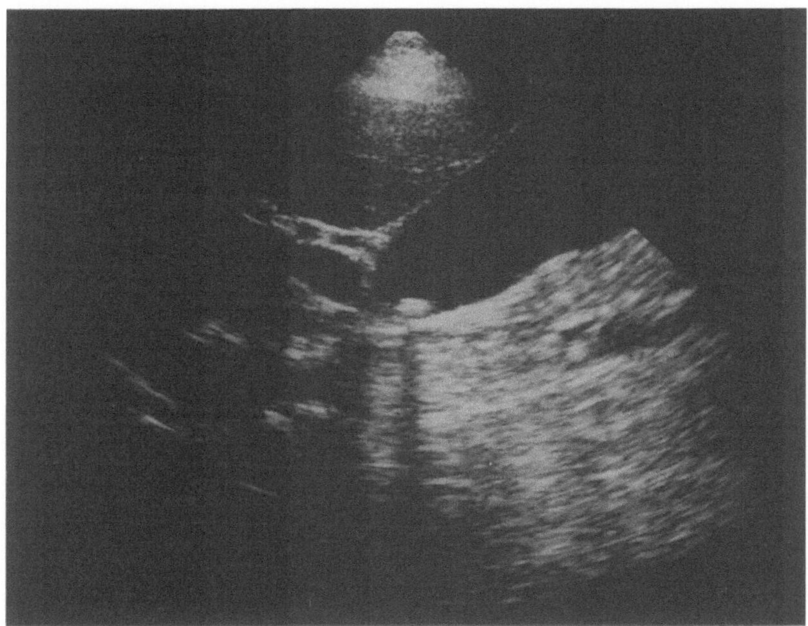

Fig. 5.7. Cholecystolithiasis. A single gallstone seen as an echogenic structure with acoustic shadowing

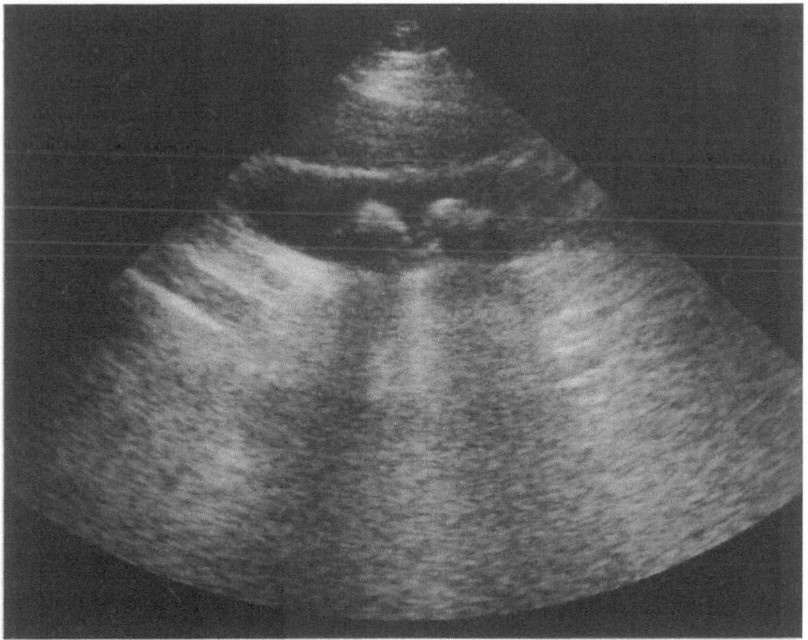

Fig. 5.8. Cholecystolithiasis. Two gallstones floating in the bile

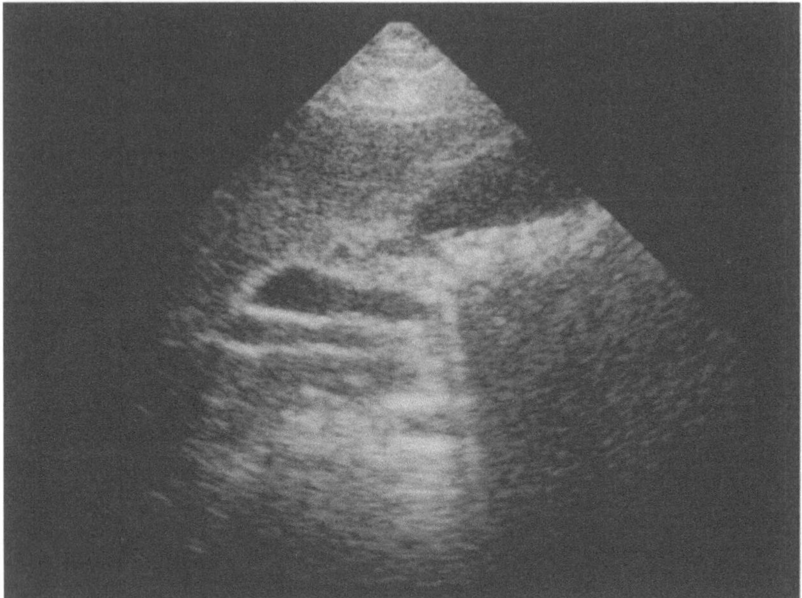

Fig. 5.9. Cholecystolithiasis. Multiple small gallstones

5.2.3.3 Pneumobilia

Clinical Data

Aetiology:
- ◆ Air ascending from the duodenum
    - After ERCP
    - After sphincterotomy
    - After gallstone passage
- ◆ Cholangitis

Pneumobilia is the presence of air within the biliary tree.

Sonographic Diagnosis

Criteria

- → Densely echogenic line
- → Acoustic shadowing along the course of the biliary system

Sonographic Differential Diagnosis

Stones.

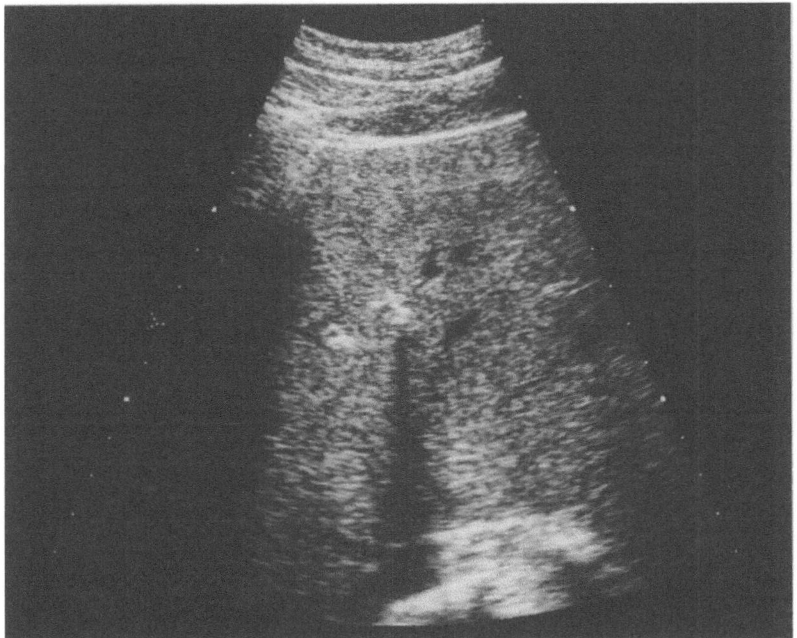

Fig. 5.10. Pneumobilia

5.2.3.4 Gallbladder Hydrops

Clinical Data

Tense gallbladder distension occurs in gallstone disease, inflammation, lymphadenopathy, and congenital malformation.

Sonographic Diagnosis

Criterion

→ Tense gallbladder distension

A diseased gallbladder may be incapable of contraction or distension. Some patients with obstruction of the cystic duct or the common bile duct show only slight gallbladder distension.

Sonographic Differential Diagnosis

The normal gallbladder may show marked enlargement in a fasting patient. Therefore, pre- and postprandial examinations should be performed to confirm a gallbladder

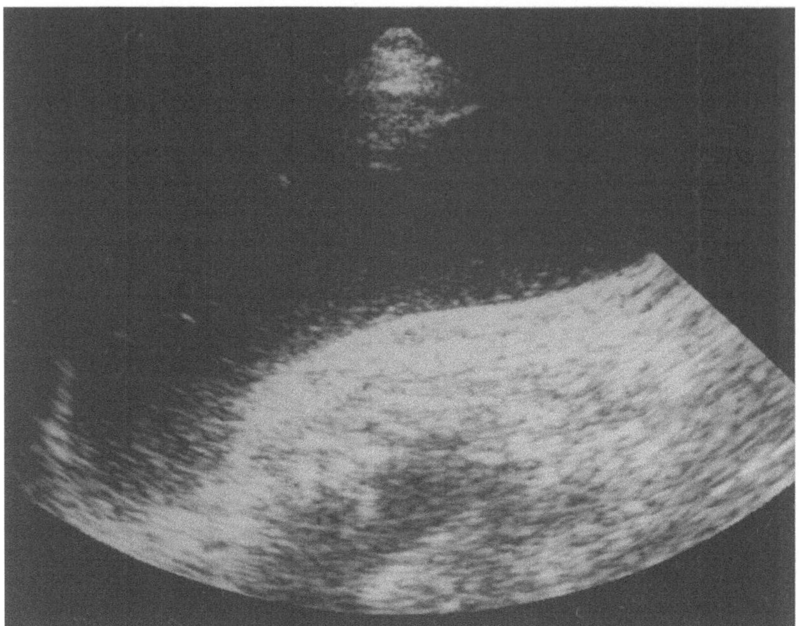

Fig. 5.11. Gallbladder hydrops

hydrops. Biliary stasis also occurs after surgery and in diabetes mellitus and may give rise to cholecystomegaly.

5.2.3.5 Choledocholithiasis

Clinical Data

Stones in bile ducts, although present less often than in the gallbladder, are the most common cause of extrahepatic obstructive jaundice. Ductal calculi may pass quietly into the duodenum, may remain silent for long periods in the duct, or may at some time partially obstruct the terminal duct, producing either transient or persistent pain, jaundice, and infection.

Sonographic Diagnosis

Criteria

→ Echogenic focus
→ Distal acoustic shadowing
→ Usually dilated common bile duct

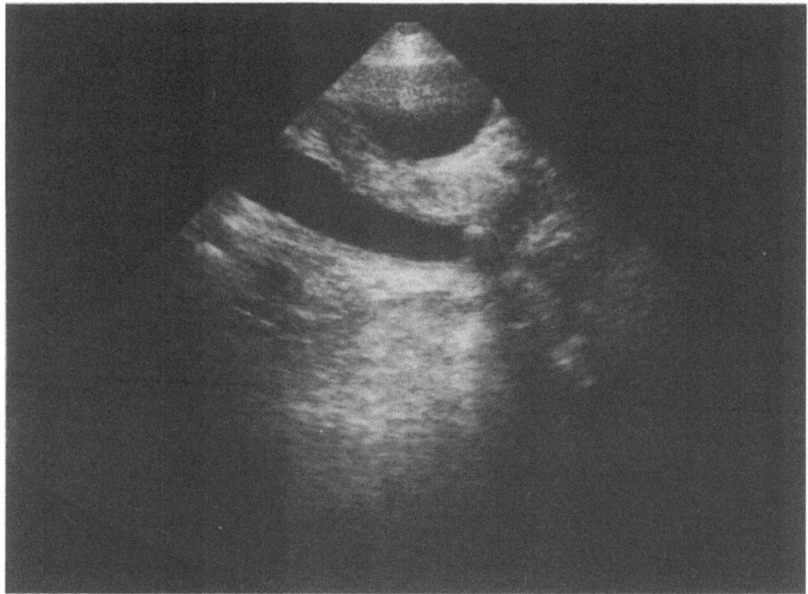

Fig. 5.12. Choledocholithiasis. The scan shows a single gallstone in the dilated common bile duct

Sonographic Differential Diagnosis

In a non-dilated common bile duct, especially small gallstones may be missed.

5.2.3.6 Biliary Dilatation

Clinical Data

Biliary dilatation usually precedes biochemical evidence of biliary obstruction. The degree of dilatation depends upon:

- Speed of onset
- Duration
- Degree of obstruction

Aetiology:
- Normal variant
- Age
- Gallstones
- After cholecystectomy
- Neoplasm

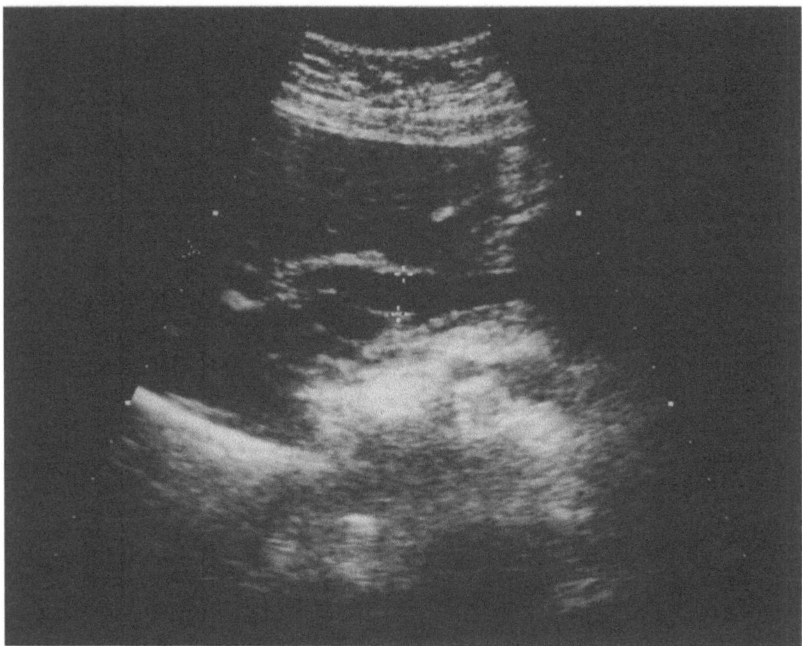

Fig. 5.13. Extrahepatic biliary dilatation. Dilatation of the common hepatic and bile ducts lying anterolateral to the portal vein in the porta hepatis

◆ Lymphadenopathy
◆ Fibrosis
◆ Parasites

The dilated common bile duct lies anterolateral to the portal vein.

Sonographic Diagnosis

Criteria

→ Extrahepatic
  - Dilated common hepatic duct
  - Dilated common bile duct
→ Intrahepatic
  - Parallel channel sign in the longitudinal scan
    • Portal vein and bile duct as anechoic tubes side by side
  - Double-barrel shotgun sign in the transverse scan
    • Portal vein and bile duct as adjacent anechoic circles
  - Tortuous course of bile ducts
  - Focal areas of acoustic enhancement

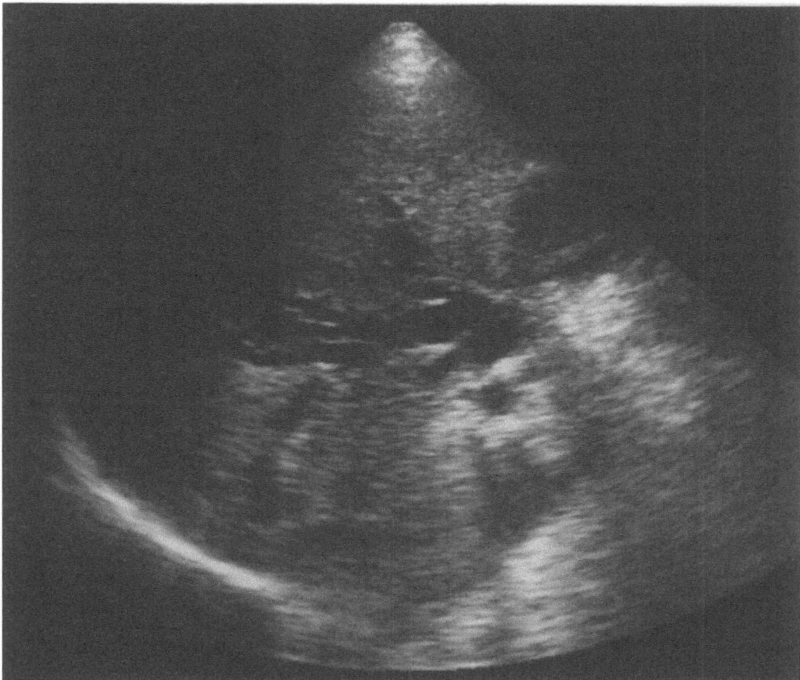

Fig. 5.14. Intrahepatic biliary dilatation. When intrahepatic bile ducts are dilated they become visible and are seen as tubes which lie directly adjacent to the portal vein branches. The tube with the echogenic walls is the portal vein branch

A common bile duct obstruction due to a stone impacted in the cystic duct is called Mirizzi's syndrome.

Sonographic Differential Diagnosis

The findings are typical.

5.2.3.7 After Cholecystectomy Haematoma

Clinical Data

Early complications after cholecystectomy include bleeding from the cystic artery and the liver bed.

Sonographic Diagnosis

Criteria

→ Initially anechoic collections
→ Hyperechoic lesion as the blood clots
→ Later complex appearance

Sonographic Differential Diagnosis

Because the haematoma occurs after surgery, the diagnosis is normally not difficult.

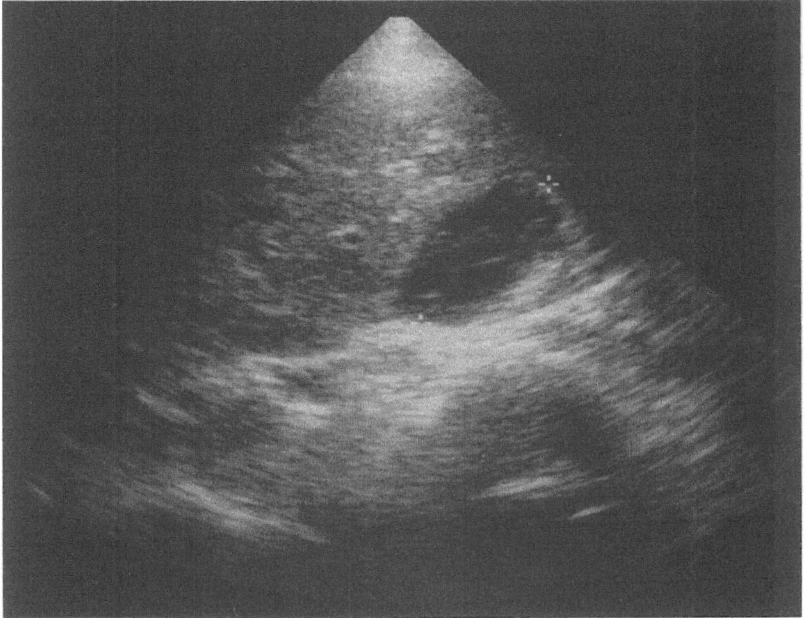

Fig. 5.15. After cholecystectomy haematoma

5.2.3.8 Acute Cholecystitis

Clinical Data

Acute cholecystitis is associated with marked local tenderness, guarding, and fever.

Sonographic Diagnosis

Criteria

→ Enlarged gallbladder
→ Increased gallbladder wall thickness
→ Hypoechoic halo around the gallbladder wall
→ Occasionally pericholecystic fluid collections
→ Usually gallstones

Sonographic Differential Diagnosis

Pericholecystic fluid collections:
◆ Acute cholecystitis
◆ Pericholecystic abscess
◆ Ascites
◆ Pancreatitis

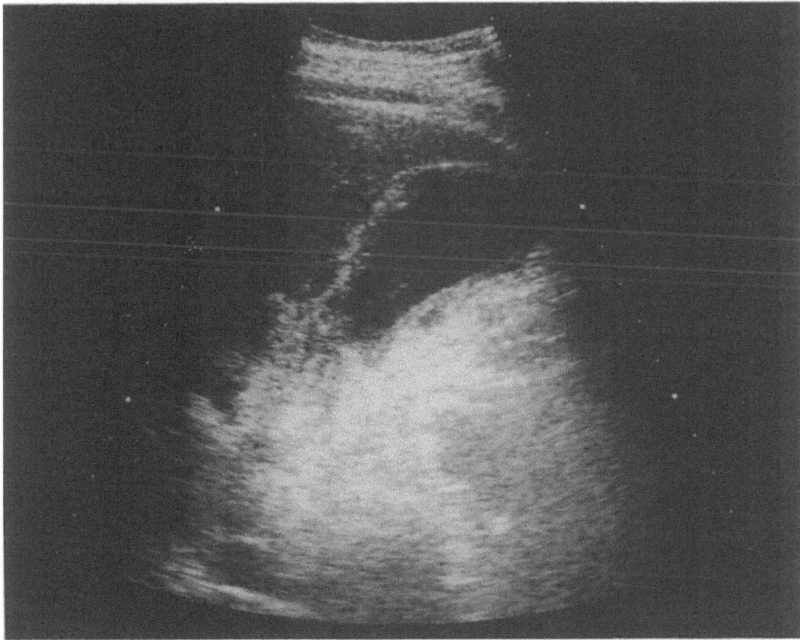

Fig. 5.16. Acute cholecystitis. The gallbladder is tender on examination (sonographic Murphy's sign)

5.2.3.9 Gallbladder Empyema

Clinical Data

Acute cholecystitis can be complicated by secondary infection with pus formation and septicaemia. The patient is very ill with high fever and marked tenderness over the gallbladder.

Sonographic Diagnosis

Criteria

→ Appearance of acute cholecystitis
→ Inhomogeneous debris and pus in the gallbladder lumen

Sonographic Differential Diagnosis

The findings are pathognomonic.

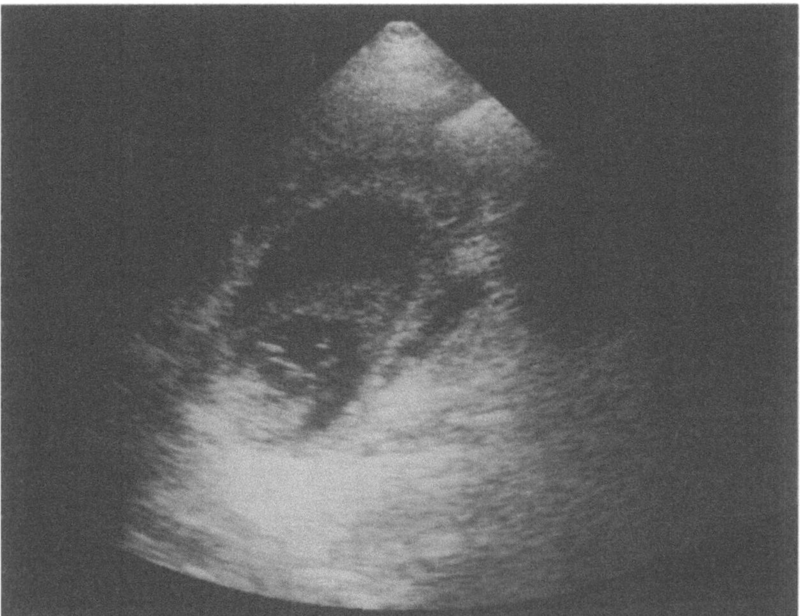

Fig. 5.17. Gallbladder empyema

5.2.3.10 Chronic Cholecystitis

Clinical Data

The gallbladder contains stones and is found to be thickened and fibrotic with loss of normal mucosal pattern. Repeated attacks of flatulent dyspepsia or biliary colic.

Sonographic Diagnosis

Criteria

→ Shrunken gallbladder
→ Usually increased gallbladder wall thickness
→ Gallstones

The porcelain gallbladder is usually associated with chronic inflammation. There is an increased risk of gallbladder carcinoma.

Sonographic Differential Diagnosis

Increased gallbladder wall thickness:
◆ Fasting
◆ Sludge
◆ Cholecystitis
◆ Right-heart failure
◆ Renal failure
◆ Cirrhosis
◆ Hepatitis
◆ Ascites
◆ Hypoproteinaemia
◆ Lymphoma
◆ Tumour

Differential diagnosis of porcelain gallbladder:
◆ Bowel loops
◆ Cholelithiasis
◆ Chronic cholecystitis

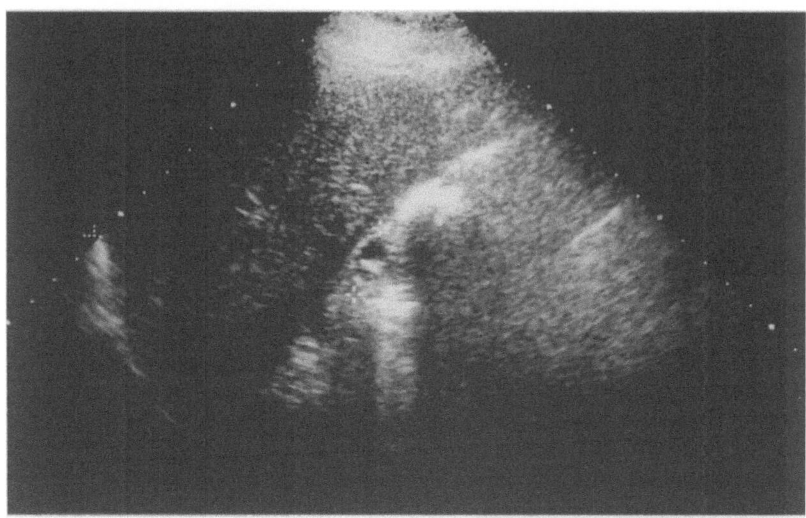

Fig. 5.18. Chronic cholecystitis on a patient with cholelithiasis

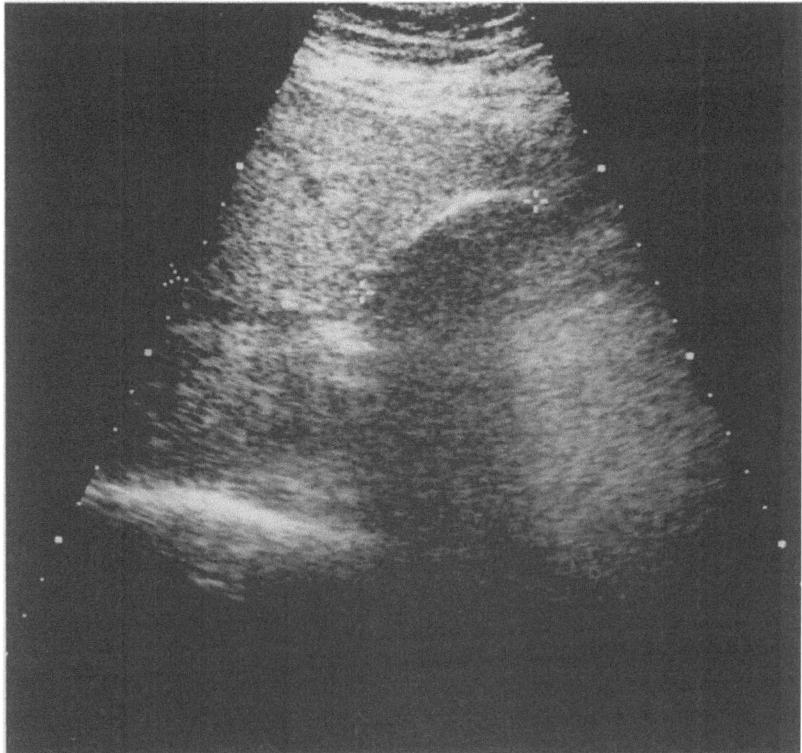

Fig. 5.19. Porcelain gallbladder. Note the curvilinear echogenic area with distal acoustic shadowing due to diffuse wall calcification

5.2.3.11 Gallbladder Polyps

Clinical Data

Polyps may be single or multiple, occur anywhere in the gallbladder, and do not change with position of the patient. Stones may coexist. Pain is irregularly associated with this condition.

Sonographic Diagnosis

Criteria

→ Well-defined, homogeneous, slightly hyperechoic mass
→ No acoustic shadowing

Sonographic Differential Diagnosis

Differential diagnosis:
- Carcinoma
- Adherent gallstone
- Inspissated sludge

Rapid growth, irregular border, and inhomogeneous echopattern may indicate malignancy.

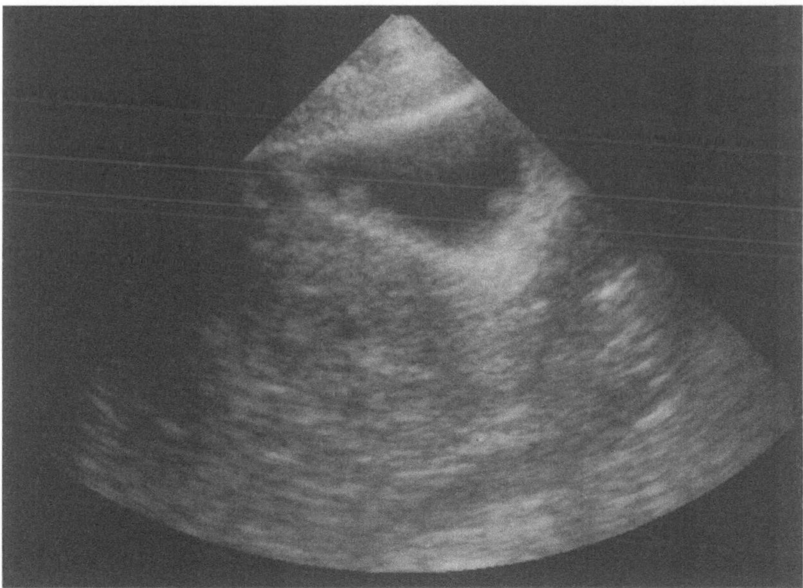

Fig. 5.20. Gallbladder polyps

5.2.3.12 Gallbladder Carcinoma

Clinical Data

Carcinoma of the gallbladder is rare, but is invariably found associated with gallstones. The patient may present with painless jaundice and weight loss.

Sonographic Diagnosis

Criteria

→ Usually hypoechoic mass
→ Gallbladder wall thickening and invasion
  - Focal
  - Generalized
→ Gallstones
→ Extensive tumour spread
  - Liver
  - Hepatic veins
  - Common bile duct
  - Portal vein
  - Lymph nodes

A carcinoma which fills the gallbladder lumen completely can be difficult to detect as it may be indistinguishable from the adjacent liver parenchyma. Gallstones within a mass is strongly suspicious of gallbladder carcinoma.

Bile duct carcinomas are rare. Klatskin's tumours arise at the porta hepatis and have a characteristic appearance:

◆ Usually hyperechoic mass
◆ Intrahepatic biliary dilatation without extrahepatic biliary dilatation
◆ No communication of right and left hepatic ducts
◆ Invasion of liver

Sonographic Differential Diagnosis

The differential diagnosis includes nearly all filling defects in the gallbladder.

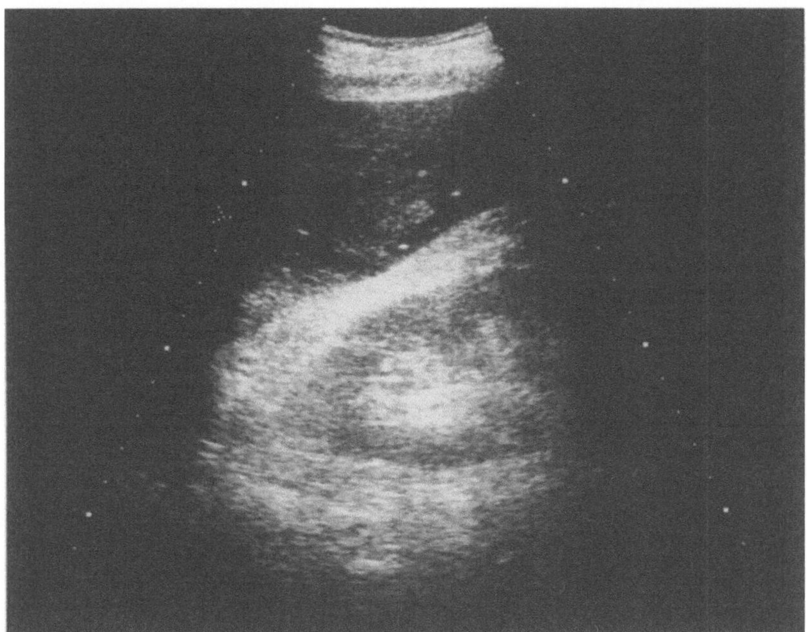

Fig. 5.21. Gallbladder carcinoma

5.2.4 Checklist for Reporting

Gallbladder
- Position
- Size
- Contour
- Wall thickness
- Echopattern

Bile ducts
- Diameter

Head of pancreas
- Size

Pancreatic duct
- Diameter

Chapter 6 Pancreas

6.1 Imaging Modalities

Sonography is the method of choice to image the pancreas. Imaging modalities are:

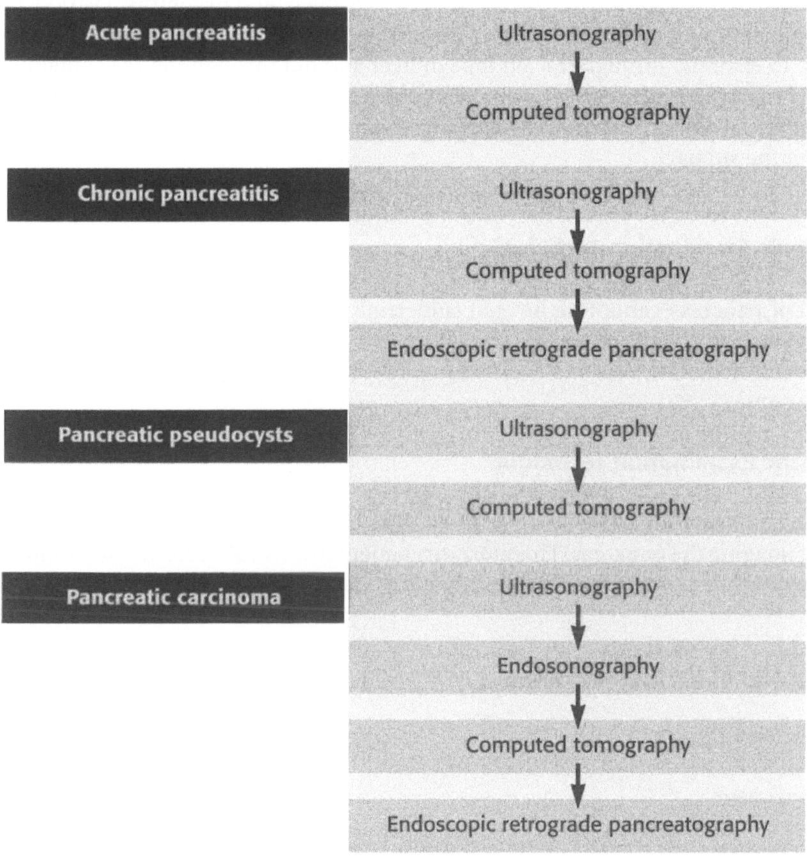

6.2 Ultrasonography

6.2.1 Examination Technique

Because of its retroperitoneal position, intestinal gas, and omental fat the pancreas is the most difficult of all the abdominal organs to image. Ultrasonography is an accurate method for the assessment of the pancreatic head and body but visualization of the pancreatic tail is less reliable. The patient must have an empty stomach for the examination.

Transhepatic Examination Technique

An alternative to the supine position of the patient is the lateral decubitus position, i.e. with the patient lying on his or her left side. In this position, the liver is ventral to the pancreas. To examine through the left lobe of liver and not through the gas containing intestinal loops, the transducer must be placed directly below the xiphoid process and slightly tilted caudally. The left lobe moves further caudally if the patient inspires and pushes out the stomach.

Transsplenic Examination Technique

If the tail of pancreas cannot be imaged sufficiently because of intestinal gas, the left intercostal section is recommended. The spleen then serves as an acoustic window. The patient should either be in prone position or lie on his or her right side.

Transgastric Examination Technique

The stomach filled with liquid as an acoustic window increases considerably the possibility of imaging the pancreas. Therefore, the patient drinks 500–1000 ml water immediately before the examination. The examination takes place with the patient sitting or standing.

The landmarks of the pancreas are:
- ◆ Head
  - Inferior vena cava
- ◆ Body
  - Splenic vein
  - Superior mesenteric artery
  - Aorta
- ◆ Tail
  - Splenic vein

If the pancreas is, despite an adequate examination technique, not sufficiently assessable, the examination must be repeated at a later date.

Endosonographically, the head of pancreas can be assessed well from the duodenum, and the body of pancreas from the stomach; the examination is performed with high frequency transducers. This means that in comparison with the transabdominal examination there is no gas superimposition and much better resolution.

6.2.2 Sonoanatomy

The normal pancreas is an elongated retroperitoneal organ surrounded by a variable amount of fat. The head nestles in the duodenal loop and the uncinate process folds behind the superior mesenteric artery and vein. The body of the pancreas lies in front of the superior mesenteric artery and vein and passes behind the stomach, with the tail situated near the hilum of the spleen. The splenic vein, which can be a surprisingly large structure, is another useful landmark; lying behind the pancreas, it joins the superior mesenteric vein posterior to the neck of the pancreas to form the portal vein.

The pancreas should have homogeneous echogenicity. In children, the gland is less echogenic than in adults. Generally, the pancreas decreases in size with age and becomes more echogenic.

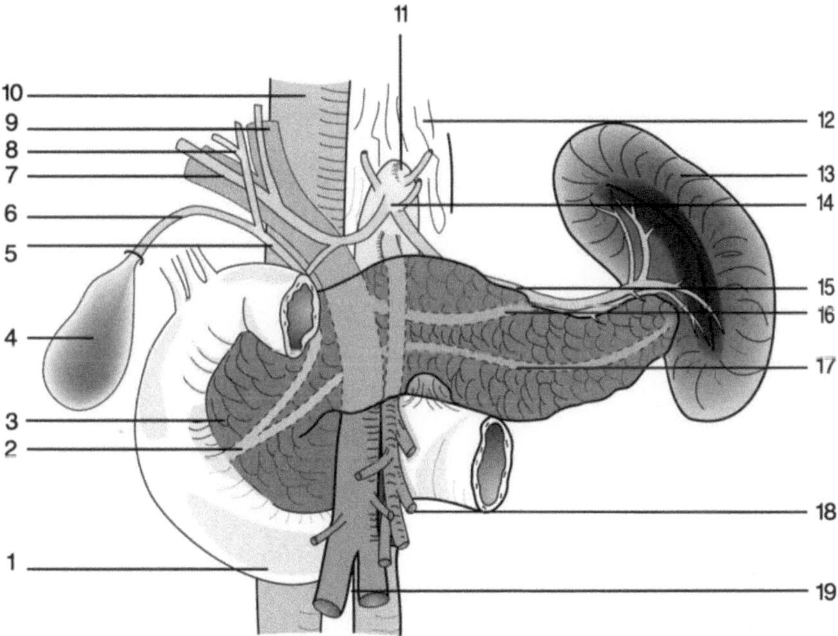

Fig. 6.1. Pancreatic region. *1*, Duodenum; *2*, common bile duct and pancreatic duct; *3*, head of pancreas; *4*, gallbladder; *5*, common bile duct; *6*, cystic duct; *7*, hepatic artery; *8*, common hepatic duct; *9*, portal vein; *10*, inferior vena cava; *11*, aorta; *12*, crus of diaphragm; *13*, spleen; *14*, coeliac trunk; *15*, splenic artery; *16*, splenic vein; *17*, pancreatic duct; *18*, superior mesenteric artery; *19*, superior mesenteric vein

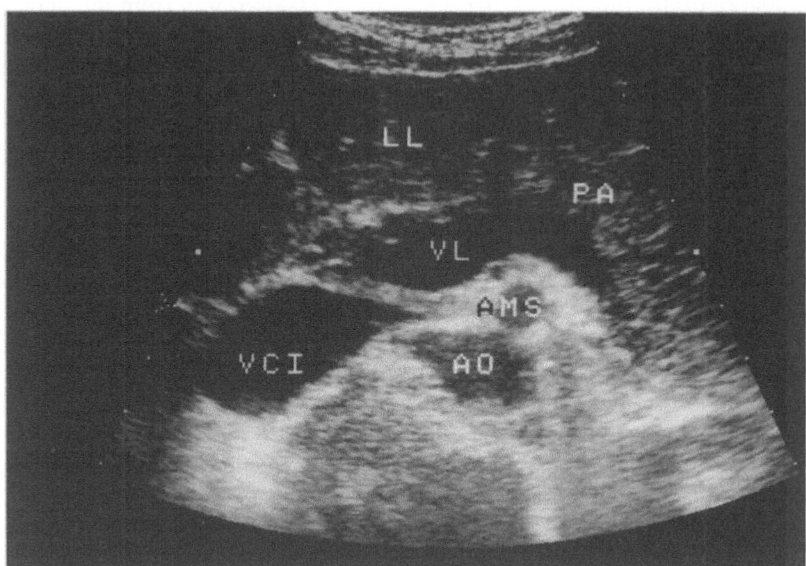

Fig. 6.2. Pancreas. Transverse scan showing the pancreas with its landmarks. *PA*, Pancreas; *VL*, splenic vein; *AMS*, superior mesenteric artery; *VCI*, inferior vena cava; *AO*, aorta; *LL*, left lobe of the liver

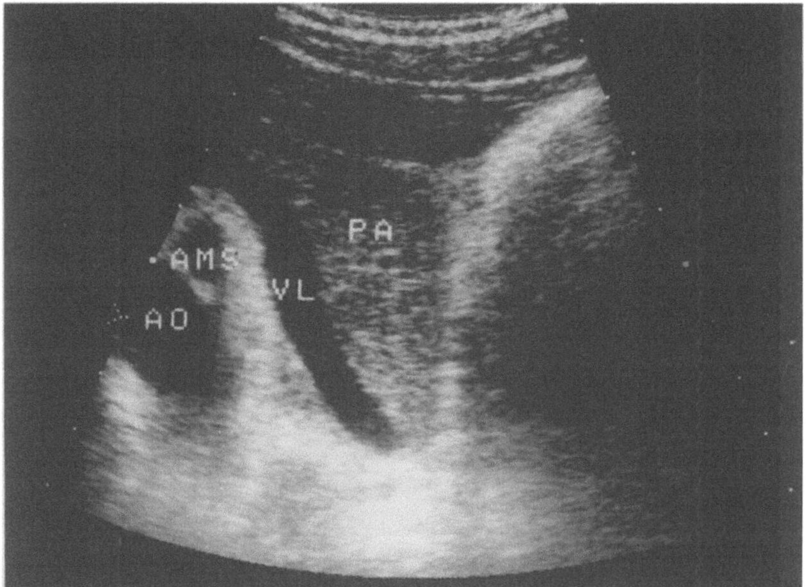

Fig. 6.3. Pancreas. Transverse scan showing the tail of pancreas. Densely echogenic lines with distal acoustic shadowing next to the pancreas due to intestinal gas. *PA*, Pancreas; *VL*, splenic vein; *AMS*, superior mesenteric artery; *AO*, aorta

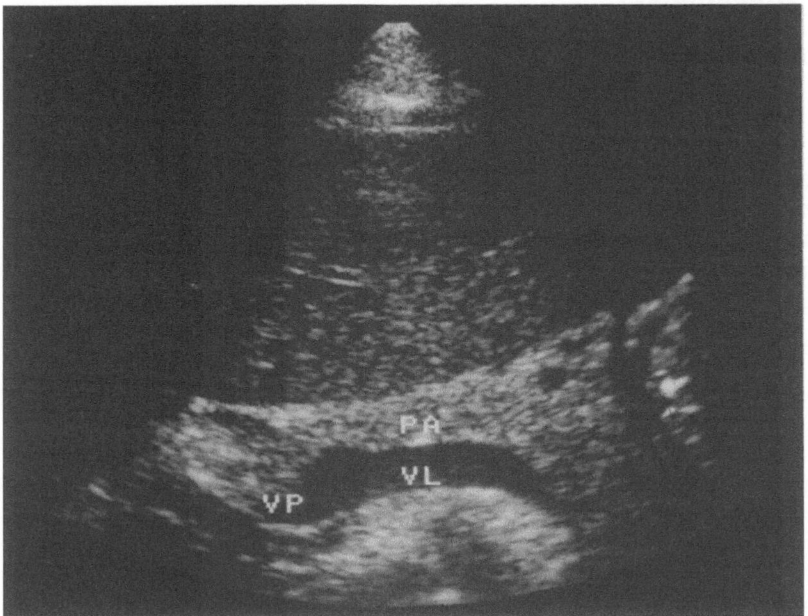

Fig. 6.4. Pancreas. In older people the gland can be much more echogenic than the adjacent liver (lipomatosis of the pancreas). *PA*, Pancreas; *VL*, splenic vein; *VP*, portal vein

Echogenic pancreas in young people:
- Alcohol
- Obesity
- Diabetes
- Steroids

The pancreatic duct may be seen over short segments as an echogenic line or a hypo-echoic tube in the centre of the pancreas.

6.2.2.1 Normal Dimensions

Pancreas:
- Head < 3 cm
- Body < 2.5 cm
- Tail < 2.5 cm
- Pancreatic duct < 2 mm
- Splenic vein < 1 cm

6.2.3 Sonopathology

6.2.3.1 Acute Pancreatitis

Clinical Data

Aetiology:
- Alcohol
- Gallstones
- Trauma
- Mumps
- Viral hepatitis
- Hyperlipidaemia
- Hyperparathyroidism

Abdominal crisis of considerable severity. Tenderness, guarding, nausea, ileus. A severe attack may be marked by bruising in the left flank. Dyspnoea may occur as part of respiratory distress syndrome.

Sonographic Diagnosis

Criteria

→ Enlarged pancreas
  - Focal
  - Generalized
→ Heterogeneous, hypoechoic echopattern
→ Peripancreatic fluid

In mild or early acute pancreatitis, the pancreas may appear normal. 50% of patients with biochemically proven acute pancreatitis have an entirely normal ultrasound appearance. The main role of ultrasound in acute pancreatitis is for the detection or exclusion of complications.

Other findings may include:
- Pancreatic necrosis
- Pancreatic abscess
- Pancreatic pseudocysts
- Pancreatic duct dilatation
- Bile duct dilatation
- Pleural effusion
- Ileus

Sonographic Differential Diagnosis

Pancreatic carcinoma. Focal acute pancreatitis may be mistaken for a fluid collection.

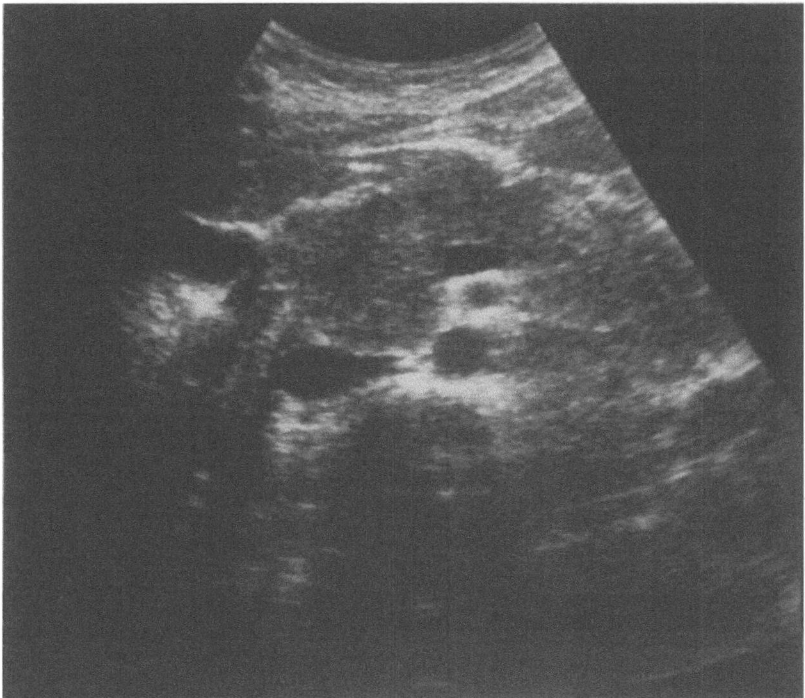

Fig. 6.5. Acute pancreatitis. The whole of the pancreas is of reduced reflectivity and the gland is bulky with an ill-defined margin

6.2.3.2 Pancreatic Necrosis

Clinical Data

Pancreatic necrosis is a complication of acute pancreatitis.

Sonographic Diagnosis

Criterion

→ Fluid collections
  - Within the pancreas
  - In the lesser sac
  - In the peritoneal cavity

Secondary infection of the inflamed pancreas or fluid collections may give rise to abscess formation and the necrotic pancreas may haemorrhage.

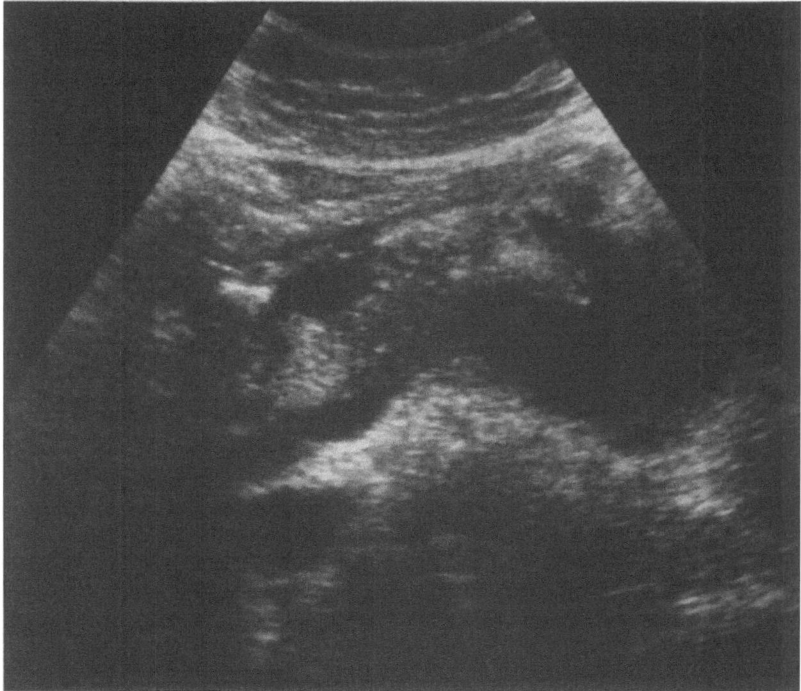

Fig. 6.6. Pancreatic necrosis. Fluid collections occur due to tissue necrosis or fluid exudation. The scan shows extensive anechoic areas peripancreatically

Sonographic Differential Diagnosis

Differential diagnosis:
- ◆ Pancreatic abscess
- ◆ Pancreatic pseudocysts

6.2.3.3 Chronic Pancreatitis

Clinical Data

Aetiology:
- ◆ Alcohol

The disease may be silent for long periods and present with complications such as pancreatic steatorrhoea and diabetes mellitus. However, pain is the characteristic feature and it can be acute and relapsing or chronic and unremitting.

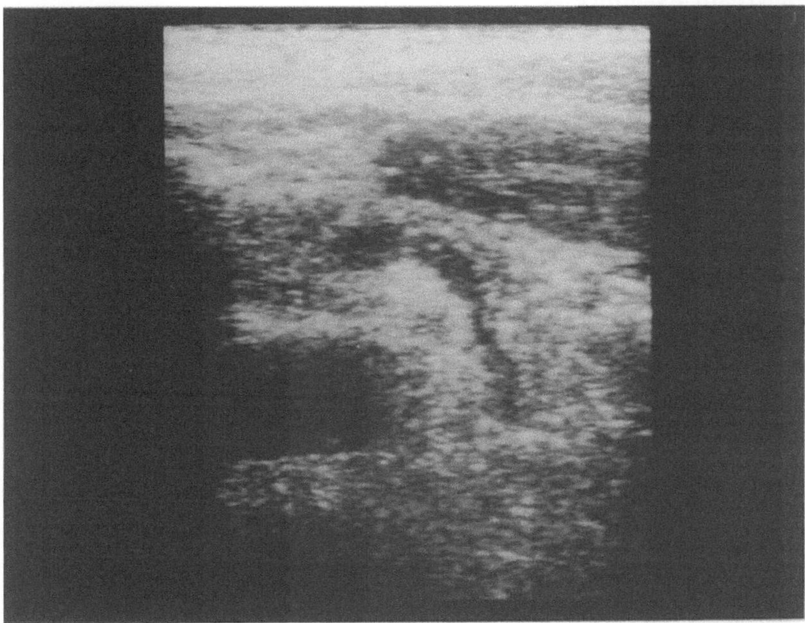

Fig. 6.7. Chronic pancreatitis. The calculi and calcifications within the pancreas are seen as echogenic foci

Sonographic Diagnosis

Criteria

→ Enlarged pancreas
  – Focal
  – Generalized
→ Heterogeneous, hyperechoic echopattern
→ Dilated pancreatic duct
→ Pseudocysts
→ Calcifications

The pancreas may also show a normal appearance. In the late stages of chronic pancreatitis, the gland becomes atrophic.

Sonographic Differential Diagnosis

Focal hypoechoic inflammatory areas may mimic pancreatic carcinoma.

6.2.3.4 Pancreatic Pseudocysts

Clinical Data

Pancreatic pseudocysts should be suspected when the patient continues to complain of pain and the serum amylase remains elevated. A firm rounded swelling in the epigastrium may be felt.

Sonographic Diagnosis

Criteria
→ Oval anechoic lesion
→ Irregular border
→ Distal acoustic enhancement

Internal echoes within a pancreatic pseudocyst are due to clot or necrotic tissue.

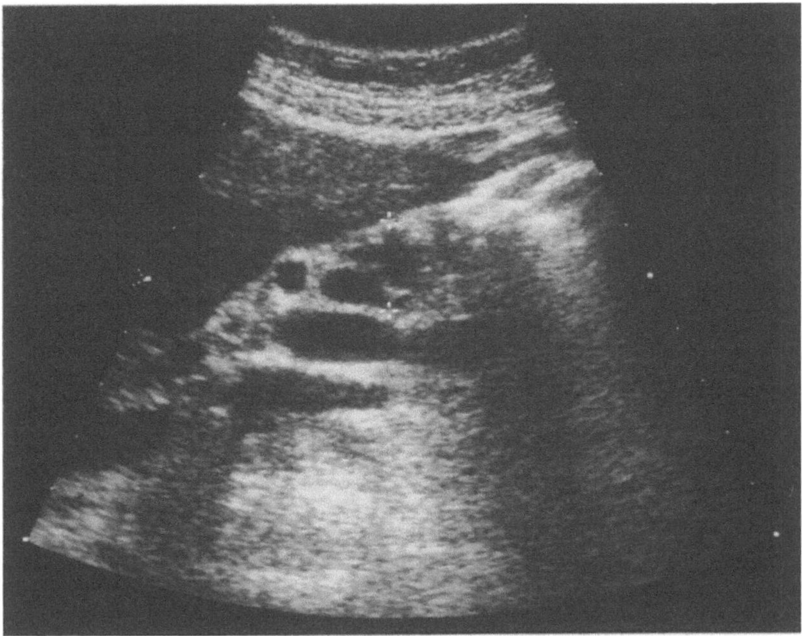

Fig. 6.8. Pancreatic pseudocysts

Sonographic Differential Diagnosis

Differential diagnosis:
◆ Cystic pancreatic tumour
◆ Gallbladder
◆ Duodenum
◆ Vessel
◆ Aortic aneurysm
◆ Splenic cyst
◆ Renal cyst

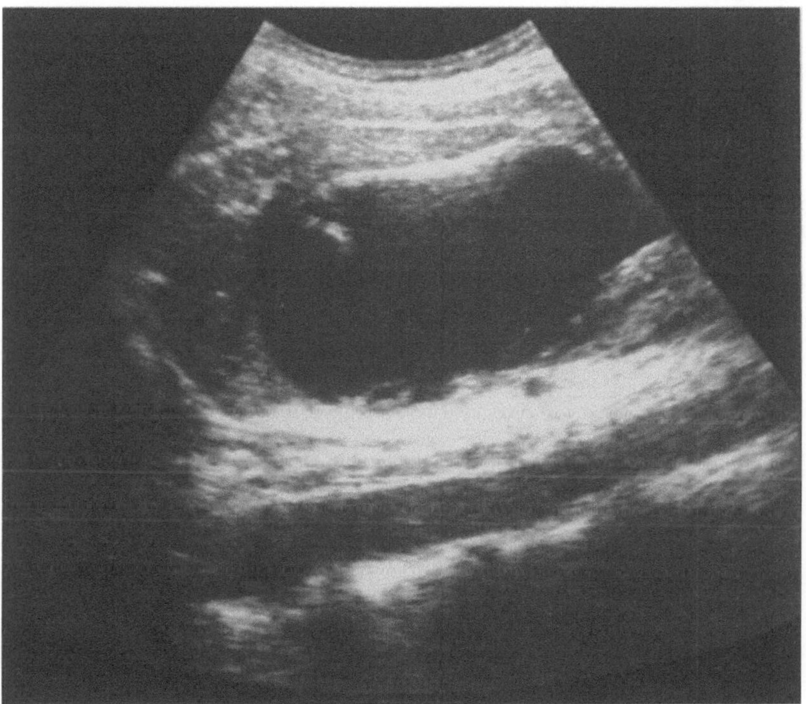

Fig. 6.9. Pancreatic pseudocyst. The scan shows a large fluid-filled space anterior to the aorta

6.2.3.5 Pancreatic Duct Dilatation

Clinical Data

Aetiology:
- ◆ Chronic pancreatitis
- ◆ Pancreatic carcinoma
- ◆ Duodenal diverticulum

Sonographic Diagnosis

Criterion

→ Dilated pancreatic duct

Sonographic Differential Diagnosis

The pancreatic duct calibre increases with age. Duct dilatation tends to be more irregular in pancreatic carcinoma than in acute or chronic pancreatitis.

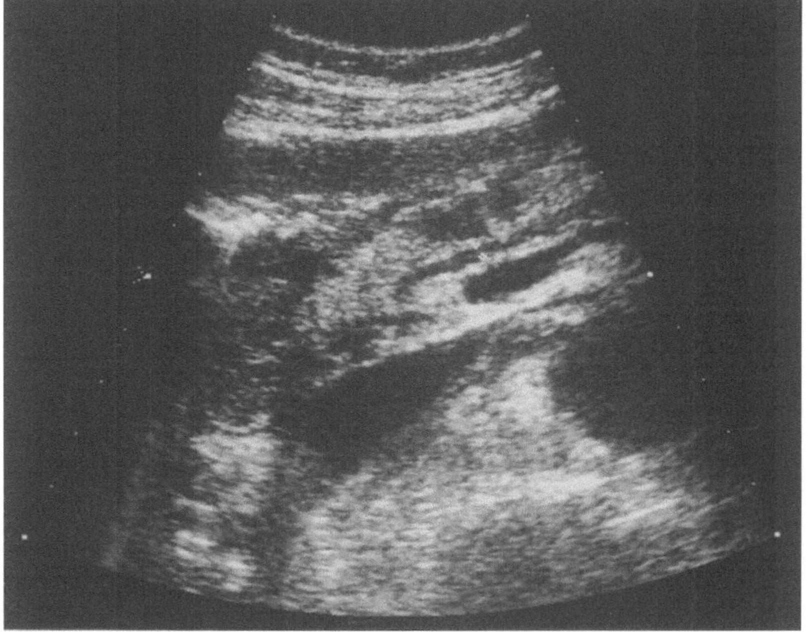

Fig. 6.10. Pancreatic duct dilatation. The dilated pancreatic duct must not be confused with the splenic vein

6.2.3.6 Pancreatic Carcinoma

Clinical Data

The commonest presentation is obstructive jaundice when the lesion is in the head. Cancer in the body or tail causes chronic pancreatic pain, which can defy diagnosis for months until the tumour reaches a large size. Loss of weight.

Sonographic Diagnosis

Criteria

→ Heterogeneous, hypoechoic mass
→ Dilated pancreatic duct
→ Dilated bile duct

Hyperechoic pancreatic carcinomas are very rare. In small carcinomas pancreatic duct dilatation may be the only sonographic abnormality. If a mass is visualized, ultrasonography allows guided biopsy. 70% of carcinomas occur in the head of pancreas.

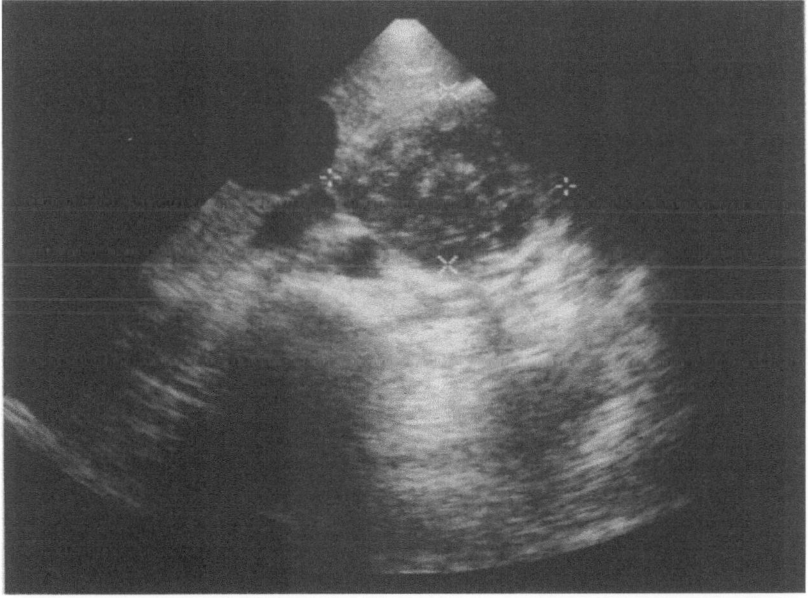

Fig. 6.11. Pancreatic carcinoma. Heterogeneous, hypoechoic mass infiltrating the splenic vein. The mass is well defined and smooth in outline

Other findings may include:
◆ Liver metastases
◆ Lymph node metastases
◆ Portal vein thrombosis
◆ Splenic vein thrombosis
◆ Ascites
◆ Splenomegaly

Sonographic Differential Diagnosis

Differential diagnosis:
◆ Focal pancreatitis
◆ Lymphoma
◆ Pancreatic metastasis

6.2.4 Checklist for Reporting

Pancreas
• **Size**
  – **Head**
  – **Body**
  – **Tail**
• **Contour**
• **Echopattern**
Pancreatic duct
• **Diameter**
Gallbladder
• **Size**
Bile ducts
• **Diameter**
Vessels
• **Portal vein**
• **Splenic vein**
• **Superior mesenteric vein**
• **Superior mesenteric artery**
• **Inferior vena cava**
• **Aorta**
Stomach

Chapter 7 Spleen

7.1 Imaging Modalities

Sonography is the method of choice to image the spleen. Imaging modalities are:

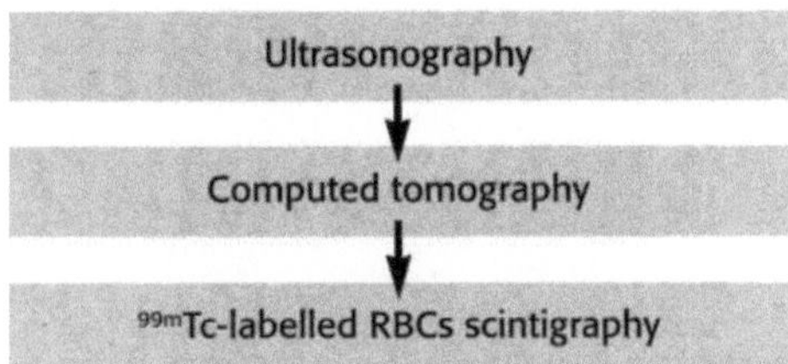

7.2 Ultrasonography

7.2.1 Examination Technique

No special preparation of the patient is needed. The spleen can best be imaged in the left intercostal section. This means that the patient should be lying:

- In the supine position or with the left side slightly raised
- With the left arm behind the head to enlarge the intercostal space
- Deep inspiration and abdominal pressure

If the spleen is very small, it should be examined from posterior. The assessment of the cranial pole is more successful with sector and convex probes than with linear probes.

7.2.2 Sonoanatomy

The spleen is normally kidney-shaped. The size is very variable and may change in a short space of time in response to infection and other stresses. At ultrasound, the spleen has a homogeneous appearance with the same echogenicity as the liver. When normal in size, its position renders it more difficult to image than the liver but if the spleen is enlarged it becomes easy to examine with ultrasound.

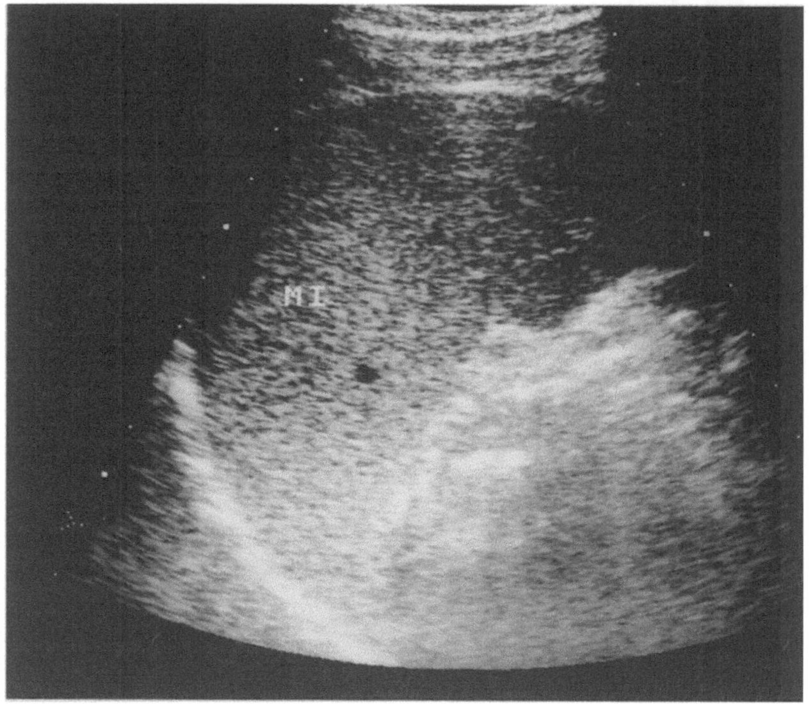

Fig. 7.1. Spleen. The splenic parenchyma is usually more echogenic than the adjacent kidney and similar in appearance to the liver. *MI*, Spleen

Non-visualization of the spleen:
◆ Aplasia
◆ Hypoplasia
◆ Splenectomy
◆ Atrophy

7.2.2.1 Normal Dimensions

Spleen:
◆ Length < 11 cm
◆ Width < 7 cm
◆ Depth < 4 cm

7.2.3 Sonopathology

7.2.3.1 Splenomegaly

Clinical Data

In many tropical countries enlargement of the spleen is endemic. It may be due to malaria or to other parasites. Lymphoproliferative, myeloproliferative, and connective tissue diseases are the most commonly encountered causes in temperate climates. Hepatic cirrhosis or portal or splenic vein thrombosis resulting in congestive splenomegaly is universally distributed.

Sonographic Diagnosis

Criterion

→ Enlarged spleen

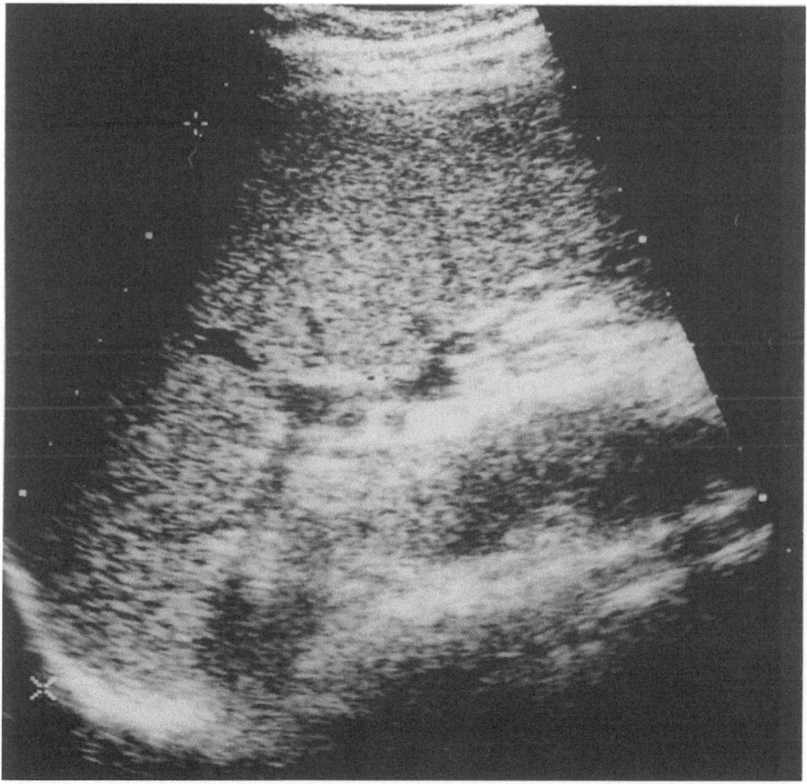

Fig. 7.2. Splenomegaly

Sonographic Differential Diagnosis

Changes in echopattern are non-specific.

7.2.3.2 Splenuncule

Clinical Data

Splenuncule or accessory splenic tissue is found in 20%–30% of post-mortem examinations. These accessory spleens are usually found around the splenic hilum.

Sonographic Diagnosis

Criterion

→ Mass with spleen-like echopattern
  - Solitary or multiple
  - Spherical or oval

Sonographic Differential Diagnosis

Differential diagnosis:
◆ Lymph node
◆ Tumour of the pancreatic tail
◆ Adrenal mass

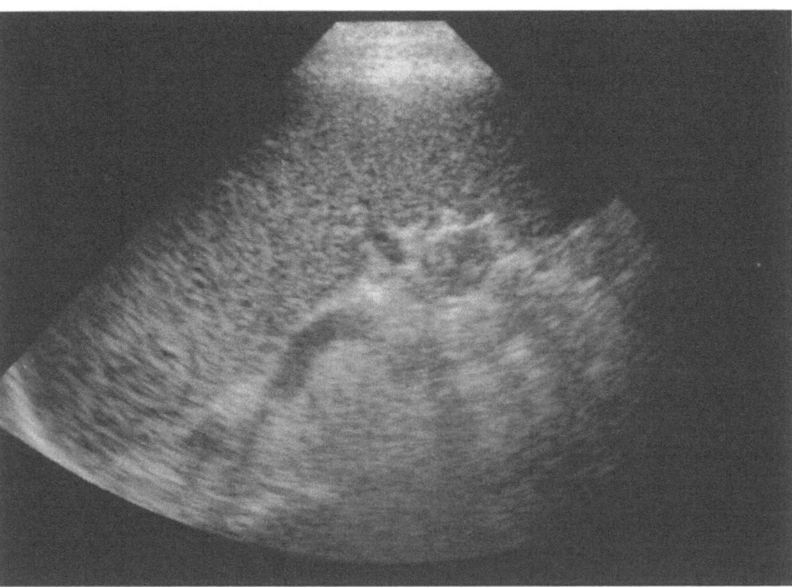

Fig. 7.3. Splenuncule at the splenic hilum. The echopattern of the mass is similar to the spleen

7.2.3.3 Abscess

Clinical Data

Aetiology:
◆ Infection
◆ Trauma

Despite the frequency of septicaemia splenic abscesses are uncommon.

Sonographic Diagnosis

Criteria

→ Anechoic or hypoechoic area
→ Internal debris
→ Gas bubbles

Sonographic Differential Diagnosis

Differential diagnosis:
◆ Cyst
◆ Haematoma
◆ Infarction

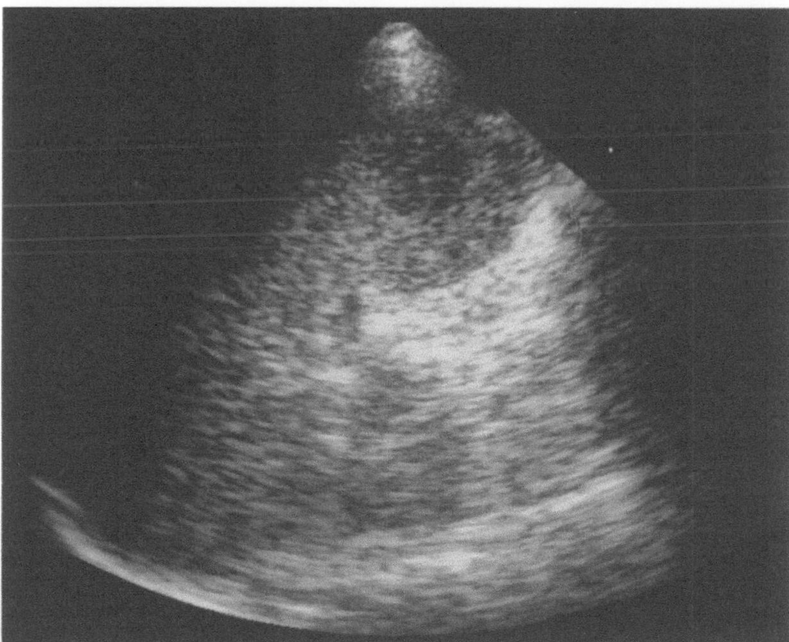

Fig. 7.4. Splenic abscess. No recognizable wall

7.2.3.4 Haematoma

Clinical Data

Pain and tenderness occur in the left upper abdomen and loin, with radiation to the left shoulder tip as the diaphragm is involved. The patient is restless, pale, shocked, and sweating.

Sonographic Diagnosis

Criteria

→ Initially anechoic collections
→ Hyperechoic lesion as the blood clots
→ Later complex appearance

Splenic lacerations are seen as anechoic defects in the margin and parenchyma.

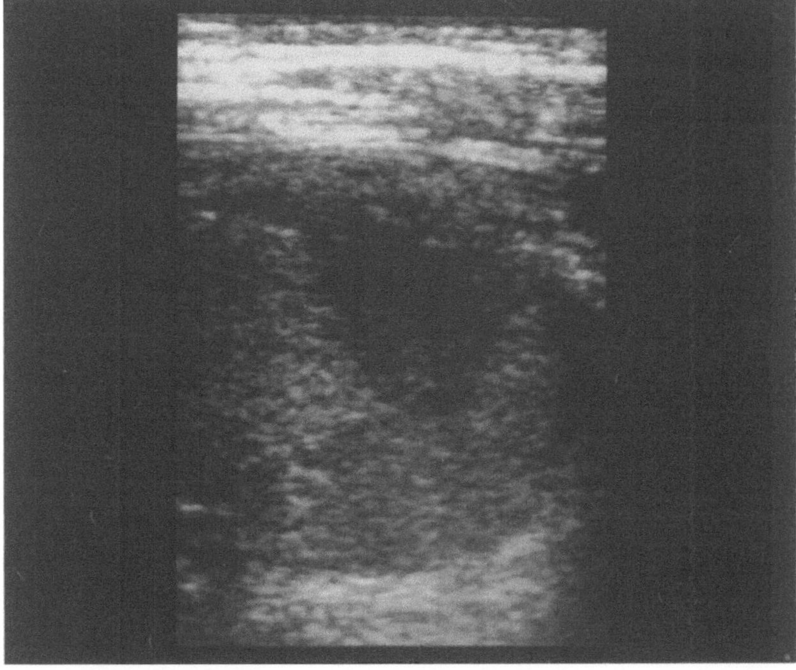

Fig. 7.5. Splenic haematoma

Sonographic Differential Diagnosis

Splenic calcification:
◆ Haematoma
◆ Abscess
◆ Infarction
◆ Tumour
◆ Hydatid cyst
◆ Tuberculosis
◆ Histoplasmosis
◆ Atherosclerosis

7.2.3.5 Infarction

Clinical Data

Aetiology:
◆ Subacute bacterial endocarditis
◆ Leukaemia
◆ Sickle cell anaemia
◆ Atherosclerosis

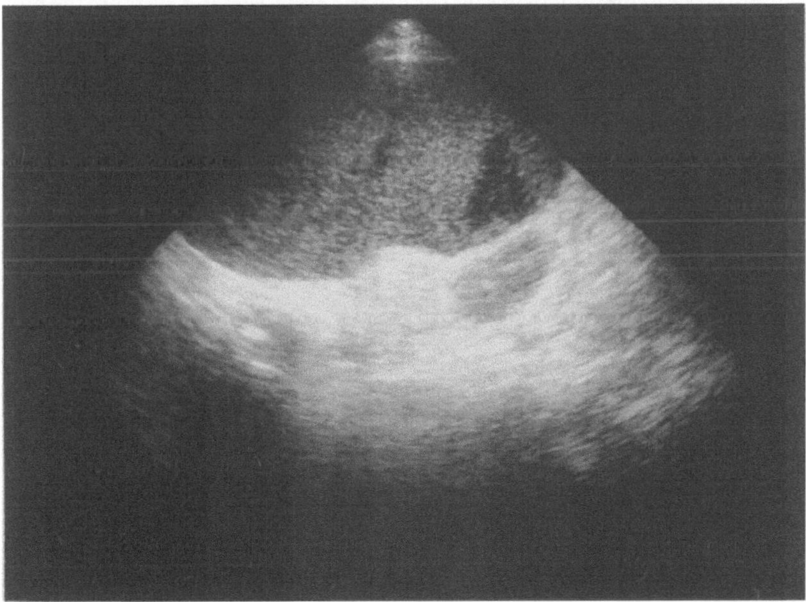

Fig. 7.6. Splenic infarction. The scan shows the characteristic wedge-shaped hypoechoic lesion

Sonographic Diagnosis

Criteria

→ Initially wedge-shaped hypoechoic lesion
→ Later small echogenic scar

Sonographic Differential Diagnosis

Differential diagnosis:
◆ Haematoma
◆ Abscess
◆ Tumour

7.2.3.6 Cysts

Clinical Data

Aetiology:
◆ Congenital
◆ Acquired
  – Trauma
  – Infection

Splenic cysts are far less common than renal or hepatic cysts. Hydatid cysts are the most common infective cysts in the spleen.

Sonographic Diagnosis

Criteria

→ Spherical or oval anechoic lesion
→ Sharp and well-defined border
→ Distal acoustic enhancement
→ Prominent posterior border

Hydatid cysts may show calcification.

Sonographic Differential Diagnosis

Differential diagnosis:
◆ Haematoma
◆ Abscess
◆ Infarction
◆ Necrotic tumour
◆ Renal cyst
◆ Pancreatic pseudocyst

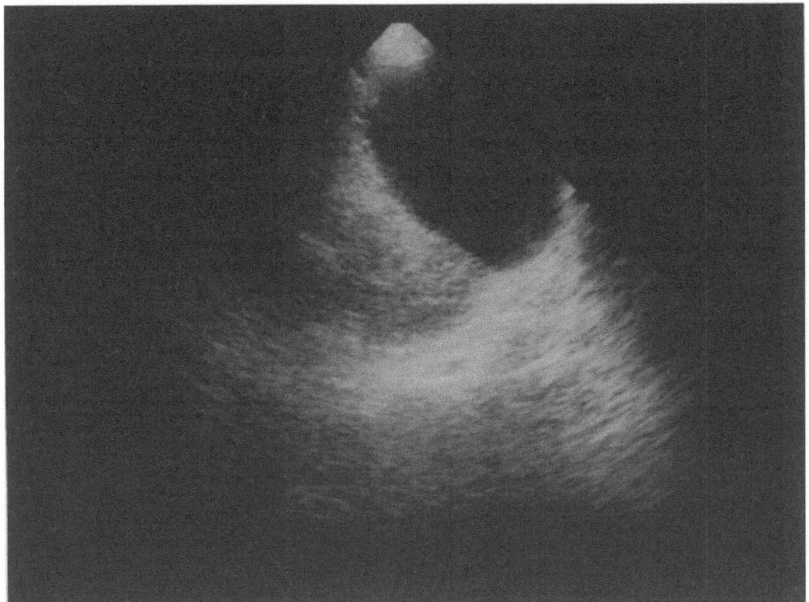

Fig. 7.7. Splenic cyst

7.2.3.7 Lymphoma

Clinical Data

Splenic involvement in lymphoma is rare and is easily missed.

Sonographic Diagnosis

Criteria
→ Enlarged spleen
→ Multiple hypoechoic foci

Sonographic Differential Diagnosis

Differential diagnosis:
◆ Complicated cysts
◆ Metastases
◆ Multiple abscesses

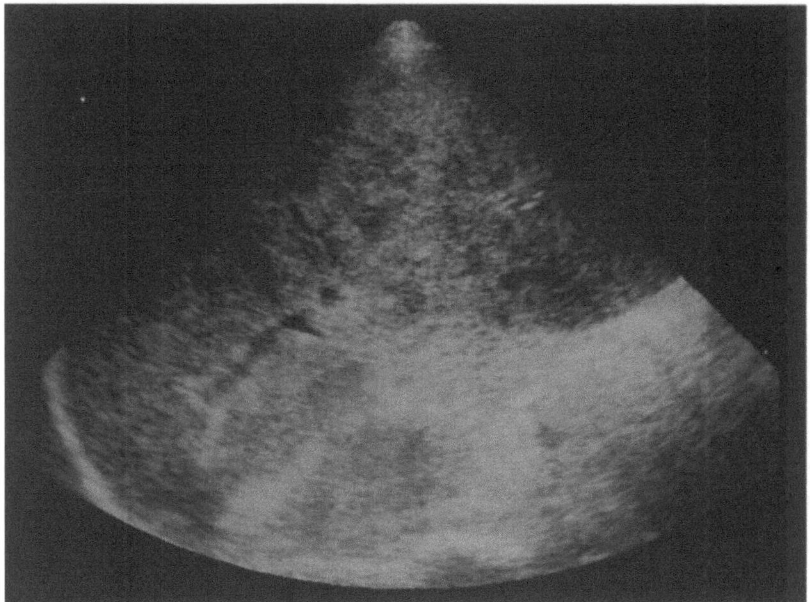

Fig. 7.8. Lymphoma

7.2.3.8 Metastases

Clinical Data

The spleen is an uncommon site of metastatic disease.

Sonographic Diagnosis

Criterion

→ Hypoechoic or hyperechoic lesion

Sonographic Differential Diagnosis

The differential diagnosis includes all solid splenic mass lesions.

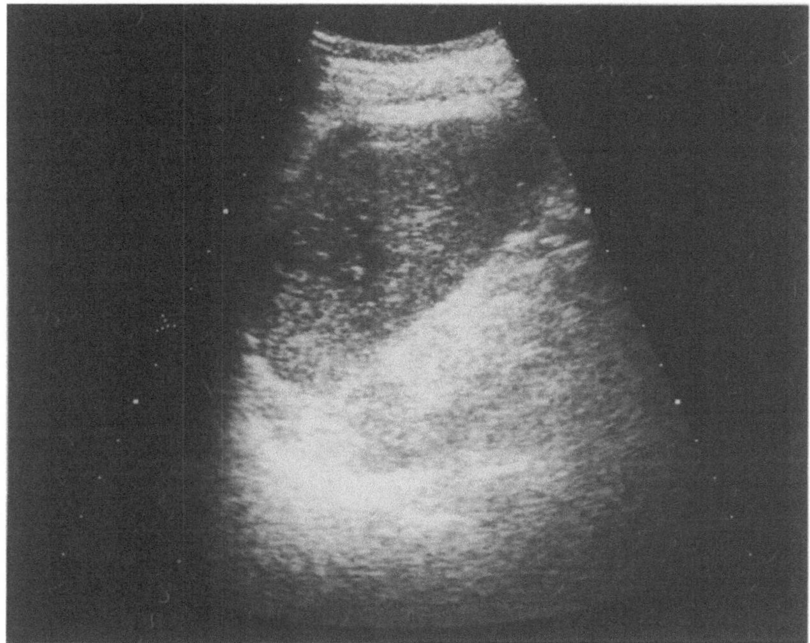

Fig. 7.9. Splenic metastasis. The scan shows a hypoechoic focus with an ill-defined border

7.2.4 **Checklist for Reporting**

Spleen
- **Position**
- **Size**
- **Contour**
- **Echopattern**

Vessels
- **Splenic vein**

Chapter 8 Intestine

8.1 Imaging Modalities

Imaging modalities are:

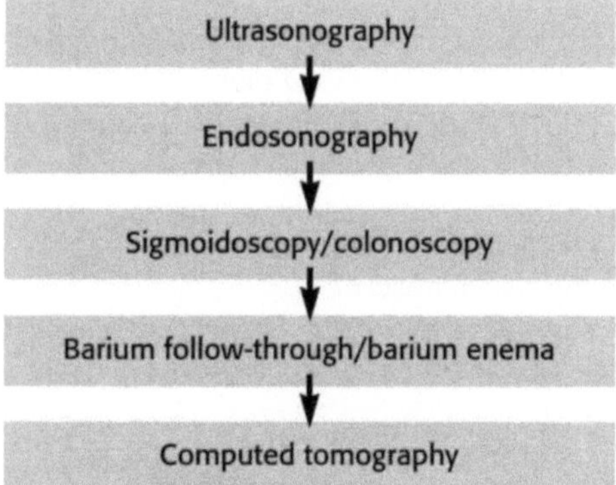

8.2 Ultrasonography

8.2.1 Examination Technique

Due to acoustic shadowing caused by intestinal gas, sonographic examination is less satisfactory for the intestine than for parenchymal organs such as liver, kidneys, and spleen. But by using 5- or 7.5-MHz linear transducers, ultrasonography makes an important contribution to the diagnosis of appendicitis, ileus, Crohn's disease, ulcerative colitis, and intestinal neoplasms.

For the examination of the intestine the patient's stomach must be empty. To assess intestinal peristalsis, the transducer must be maintained in one position for some time.

With pressure on the probe:
◆ Peristalsis can be stimulated
◆ Compressibility of the intestinal wall can be checked
◆ Intestinal gases can be expelled

The large bowel usually contains air and is thus not clearly visualized sonographically in the majority of cases. By means of hydro-colon sonography, however, the colon can be imaged and assessed in its entirety. Prior bowel preparation by means of aperients or washout is most important to rid the intestine of faecal material, which might otherwise mask small lesions and cause confusion by simulating polyps. After intramuscular injection of butylscopolamine the colon is filled with 1000–1500 ml of water per rectum. The spasmolytic serves to suppress the defecation impulse. The overall display of the colon is made with a 3.5-MHz probe, the detailed assessment with 5- and 7.5-MHz probes.

For the preoperative staging of carcinomas of the gastrointestinal tract endosonography plays an important role. Both tumour infiltration and lymphadenopathy can be assessed precisely by means of endosonography.

8.2.2 Sonoanatomy

The small intestine comprises the duodenum, jejunum, and ileum. The duodenum is C-shaped and curves round the head of the pancreas. The combined pancreatic and bile ducts drain into the duodenum at the sphincter of Oddi. The large intestine consists of the caecum, ascending colon, transverse colon, descending colon, sigmoid colon, and rectum.

The intestine is frequently filled with gas giving rise to areas of:
◆ Marked echogenicity
◆ Distal shadowing
◆ Reverberation echoes

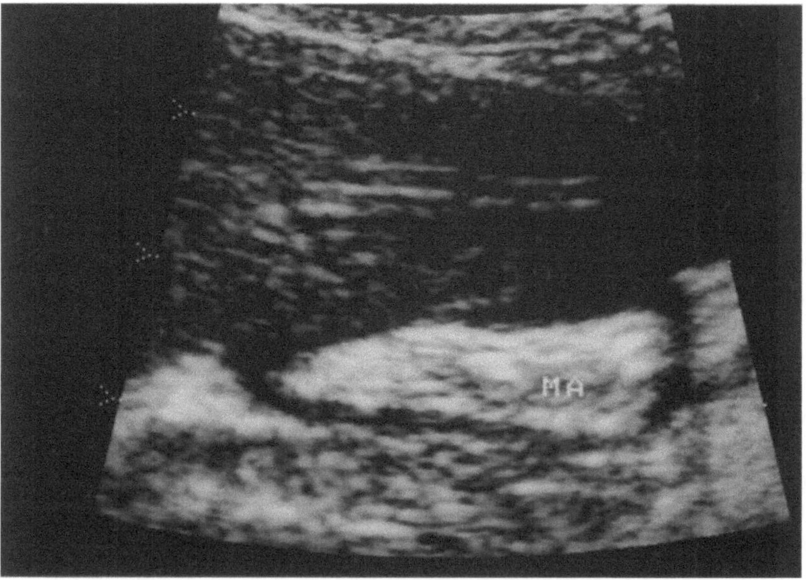

Fig. 8.1. Stomach. Transverse scan showing the antrum of the stomach (magnification). Note the ring or bull's eye appearance. *MA,* Stomach

Normal loops are compliant and are easily deformed during examination. They alter configuration during waves of peristalsis.

Intra-operative scanning of the bowel wall with a high frequency probe:
- Inner hyperechoic layer: mucosa
- Inner hypoechoic layer: muscularis mucosae
- Central hyperechoic layer: submucosa
- Outer hypoechoic layer: muscularis propria
- Outer hyperechoic layer: serosa

8.2.2.1 Normal Dimensions

Intestine:
- Small intestine
  - Diameter < 3 cm
  - Wall thickness < 3 mm
- Large intestine
  - Diameter < 6 cm
  - Wall thickness < 3 mm

8.2.3 Sonopathology

8.2.3.1 Appendicitis

Clinical Data

The diagnosis of appendicitis rests entirely upon the history and clinical examination. Pain is the most constant feature, beginning in the midepigastrium and moving to the right lower quadrant where it is persistent. Anorexia and nausea follow the onset of pain. The temperature is usually marginally raised. The right leg may be flexed as a result of irritation of the psoas muscle. There is tenderness and muscle guarding at McBurney's point. Rebound tenderness is a sign of peritoneal inflammation.

Sonographic Diagnosis

Criteria
- → Visualization of the appendix
- → Wall thickening
- → Dilated lumen
- → No peristalsis
- → No compressibility
- → Tenderness
- → Faecoliths
- → Echogenic foci
- → Acoustic shadowing

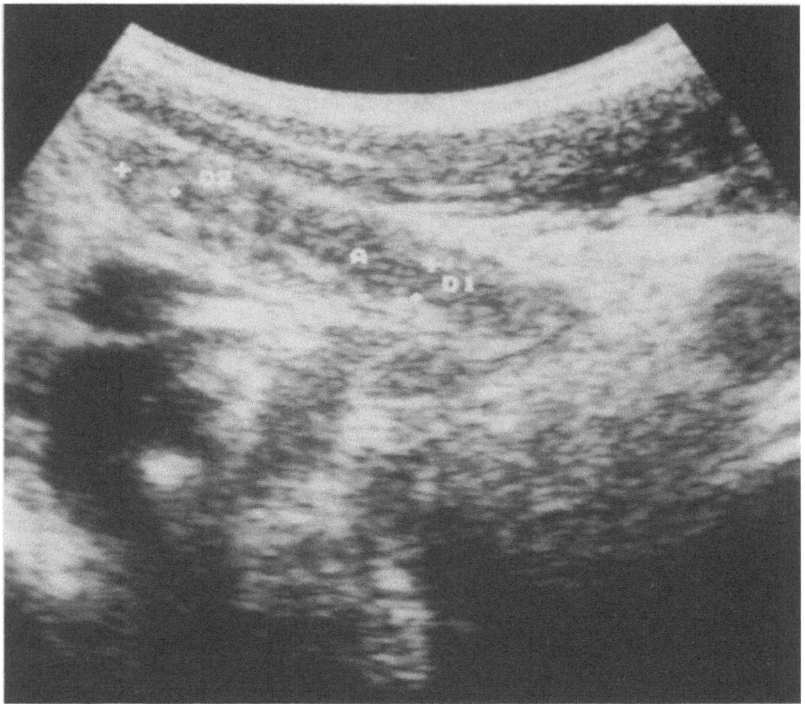

Fig. 8.2. Appendicitis. In the longitudinal scan, the appendix has a tubular structure

Other findings include fluid around the appendix, abscess formation, and lymphadenopathy.

Ultrasonography may confirm the diagnosis of appendicitis in patients whose symptoms are not typical. The clinical complications of appendicitis – appendix abscess, portal vein thrombosis, and liver abscess – can be assessed sonographically.

Sonographic Differential Diagnosis

Normal bowel loops.

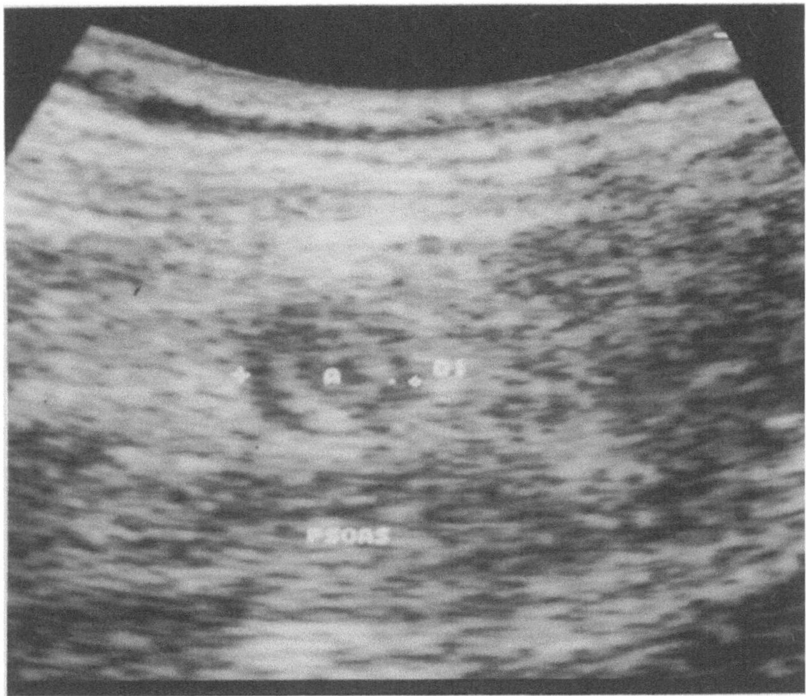

Fig. 8.3. Appendicitis. Note the typical target appearance of bowel in the transverse scan

8.2.3.2 Ileus

Clinical Data

Aetiology:
- ◆ Mechanical
  - Obstructed hernia
  - Adhesions
  - Foreign body
  - Carcinoma
  - Benign strictures
  - Volvulus
  - Pyloric stenosis
  - Intussusception
- ◆ Paralytic
  - Postoperative ileus
  - Peritonitis
  - Electrolyte imbalance
  - Pancreatitis
  - Retroperitoneal haematoma

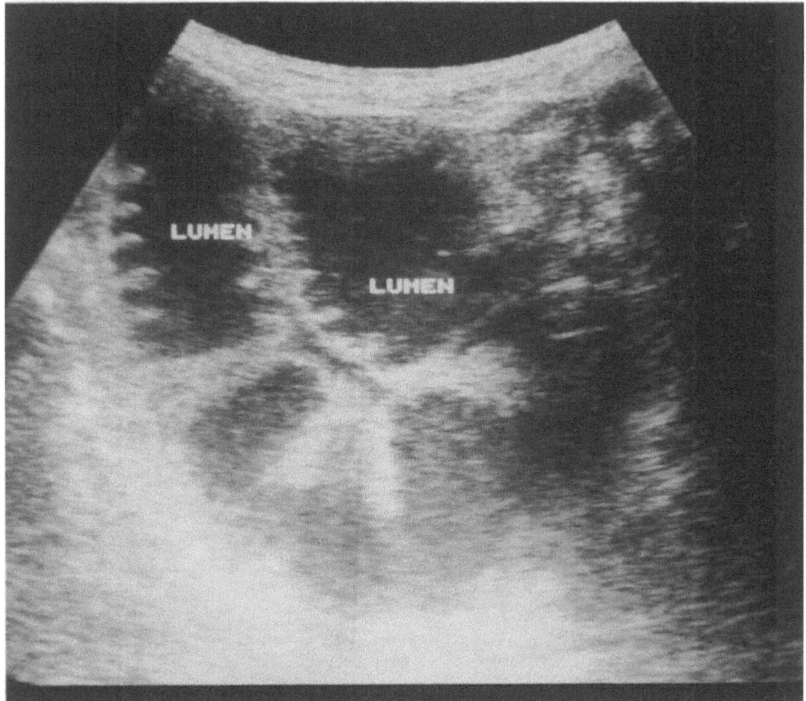

Fig. 8.4. Ileus

The symptoms and signs of mechanical ileus are vomiting, dehydration, abdominal distension, and absolute constipation. Pain may be present or absent, colicky or continuous, and depends entirely upon the cause and type of obstruction.

The symptoms and signs of paralytic ileus are effortless vomiting and abdominal distension. Dehydration and constipation are variable.

Sonographic Diagnosis

Criteria

→ Distended bowel loops
→ Fluid-filled bowel
→ Variable peristalsis

The colon is peripherally situated in the abdomen whilst the small bowel is more centrally placed.

Sonographic Differential Diagnosis

The sonographic findings are pathognomonic.

8.2.3.3 Inflammatory Bowel Diseases

Clinical Data

The clinical features of Crohn's disease are in the main abdominal pain and bowel disturbance, with predominant diarrhoea. Loss of weight, failure to grow.

The typical symptoms of ulcerative colitis are blood-stained diarrhoea and crampy abdominal discomfort relieved by defecation. Pain is seldom severe.

Sonographic Diagnosis

Criteria

→ Focal or generalized bowel wall thickening
→ Rigid loops
→ Abscess formation

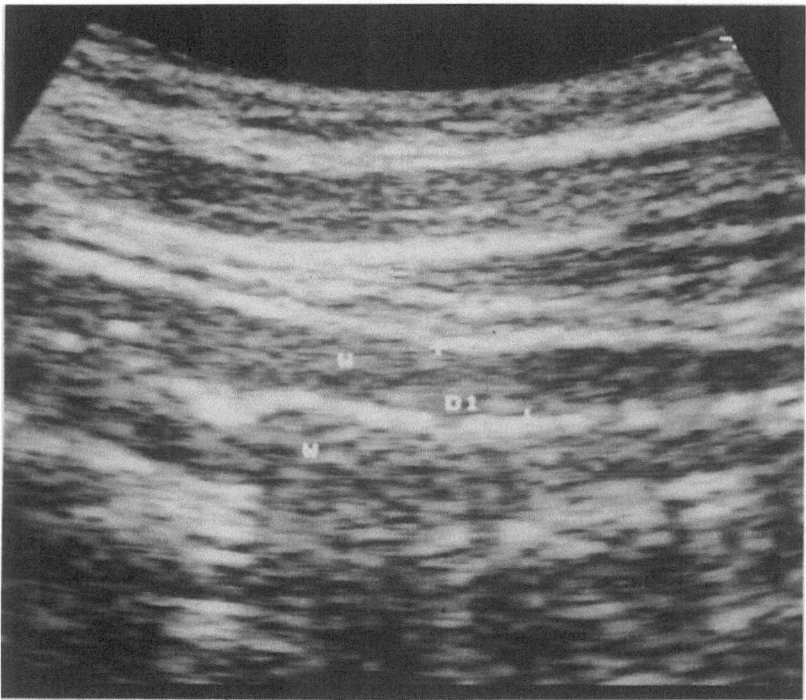

Fig. 8.5. Crohn's disease. Crohn's disease and ulcerative colitis are the commonest causes of chronic large bowel inflammation. Bowel wall thickening is the most important sonographic feature although this finding is non-specific

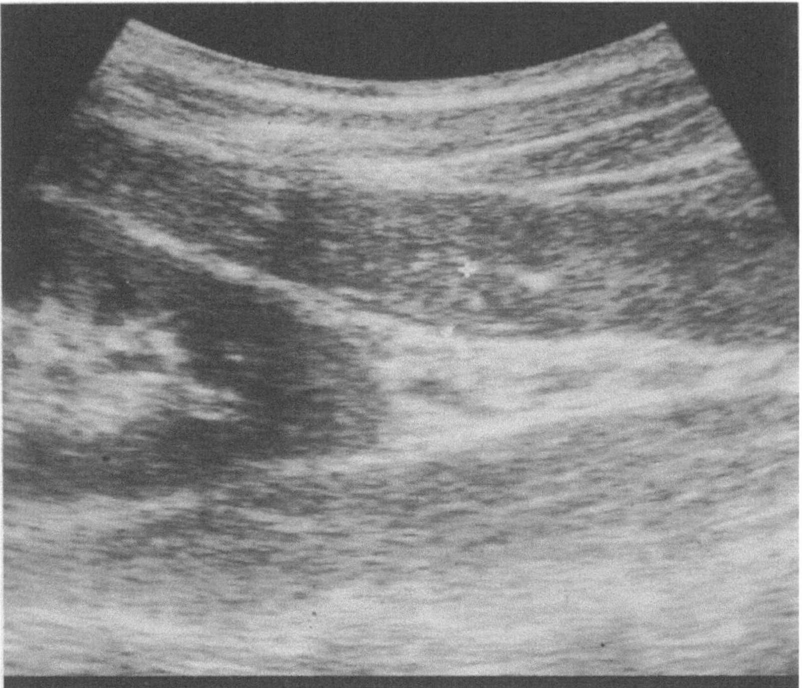

Fig. 8.6. Crohn's disease

Sonographic Differential Diagnosis

Bowel wall thickening:
- ◆ Inflammatory bowel diseases
- ◆ Carcinoma of the colon
- ◆ Diverticular mass
- ◆ Intussusception
- ◆ Lymphoma

8.2.3.4 Carcinoma of the Colon

Clinical Data

The onset of symptoms is almost always slow and usually insidious. Altered bowel habit, rectal bleeding, passage of mucus. Loss of well-being. There may be a palpable abdominal or rectal mass.

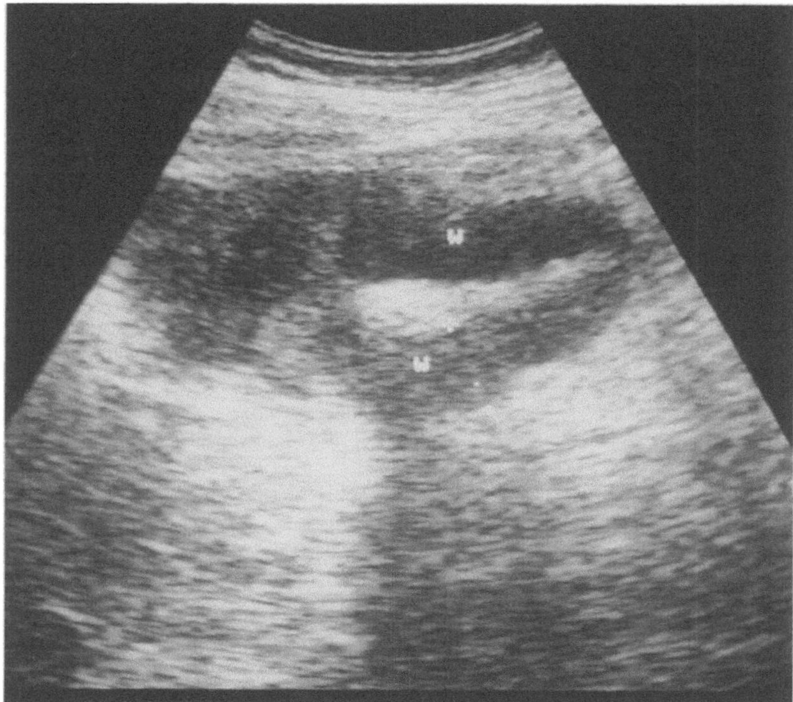

Fig. 8.7. Carcinoma of the colon. The thickened wall of this bowel lesion resembles renal parenchyma and the gas-containing lumen mimics the renal sinus (pseudo-kidney sign)

Sonographic Diagnosis

Criteria

→ Mass or target appearance
→ Focal bowel wall thickening
→ Infiltrative growth

The mass may lie within the bowel lumen or replace the bowel wall.

Sonographic Differential Diagnosis

Small bowel tumours are frequently not visualized sonographically.

8.2.4 Checklist for Reporting

Intestine
- **Wall thickness**
- **Wall layers**
- **Peristalsis**
- **Gas**
- **Atypical target appearance**
- **Palpation**
- **Tenderness**
- **Configuration**

Chapter 9 Kidneys

9.1 Imaging Modalities

Sonography is the method of choice to image the kidneys. Imaging modalities are:

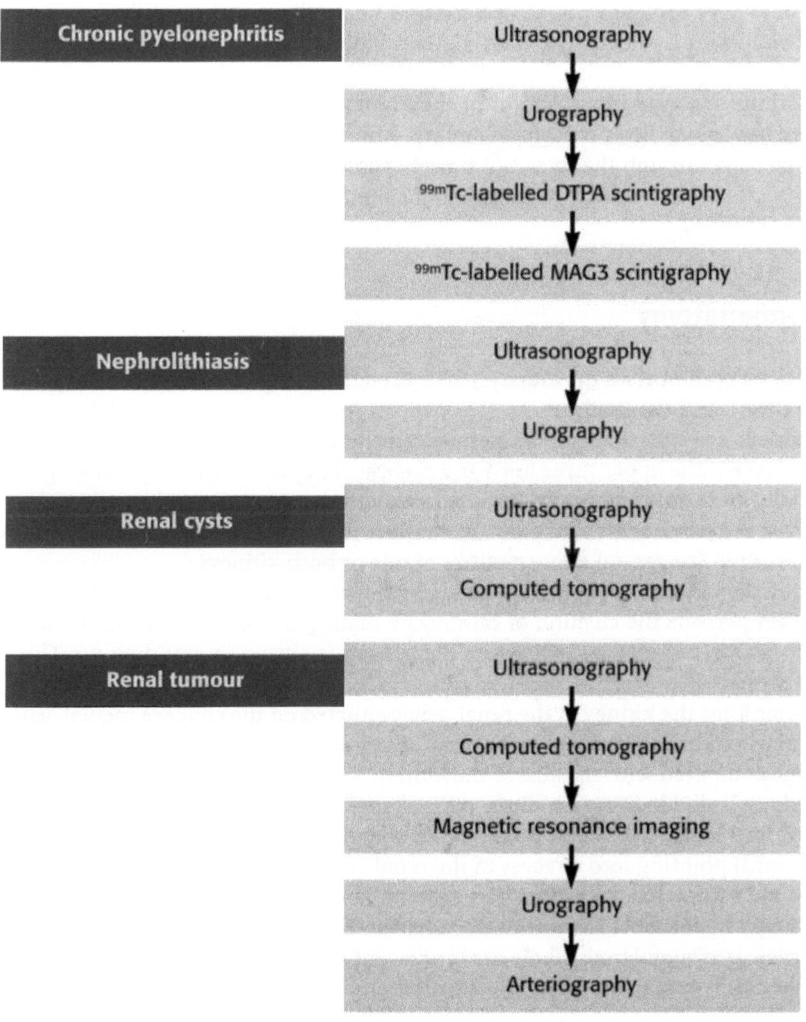

9.2 Ultrasonography

9.2.1 Examination Technique

Special preparation of the patient is unnecessary. The examination takes place using a 3.5-MHz convex transducer, and for the detailed assessment a 5-MHz transducer. The kidneys are scanned in the supine position or:

◆ With the right side slightly raised for the right kidney
◆ With the left side slightly raised for the left kidney

Examination from posterior with the patient in the prone position can also be recommended. Both longitudinal and transverse sections must be performed. Transverse sections through the kidneys show the renal hilum and the renal vessels. Sections taken obliquely may give the appearance of variation in renal parenchymal thickness and, therefore, should be avoided. The contralateral kidney should always be scanned for comparison.

Successful ultrasound examination of the kidneys is influenced by the size of the patient and how much fat is present. When examining from the front, the right kidney is often well seen through the liver, but bowel usually masks the left kidney. It should not be assumed that an atypical structure in the renal bed is a kidney; this might prove to be a bowel loop.

9.2.2 Sonoanatomy

The urinary tract comprises the kidneys, their ureters joining them to the urinary bladder in the pelvis, and the urethra.

The kidneys are situated against the posterior body wall behind the retroperitoneum at the level of the upper three lumbar vertebrae. They are bean-shaped, being concave medially and convex laterally. During foetal development the embryonic kidneys migrate from the pelvis to this location. Any failure in normal development and migration may result in congenital abnormalities of one or both kidneys.

Normally the kidneys are held in position by the perinephric fat, a surrounding pad of fat. In thin persons the cushion of fat may be inadequate, and one or both kidneys may fall forwards and downwards when the person is sitting or standing up. This is known as ptosis.

The ureter joins the kidney at the renal pelvis situated on the concave medial aspect of the kidney in its hilum along with the renal artery and vein. The blood vessels are relatively large compared with the size of the kidney.

The kidney is divided into an outer cortical and an inner medullary portion, and subdivided into lobes. Each lobe is conical in shape, its base being the cortex and its apex (pyramid) pointing into a recess in the renal pelvis known as a calyx.

Ultrasound shows that the kidneys are smooth in outline. In the adult, the renal cortex is normally hypoechoic relative to the adjacent liver or spleen, and the renal pyramids are seen as triangular anechoic areas adjacent to the renal sinus. The corticomedullary junction is demarcated by the echogenic arcuate arteries. The parenchyma sur-

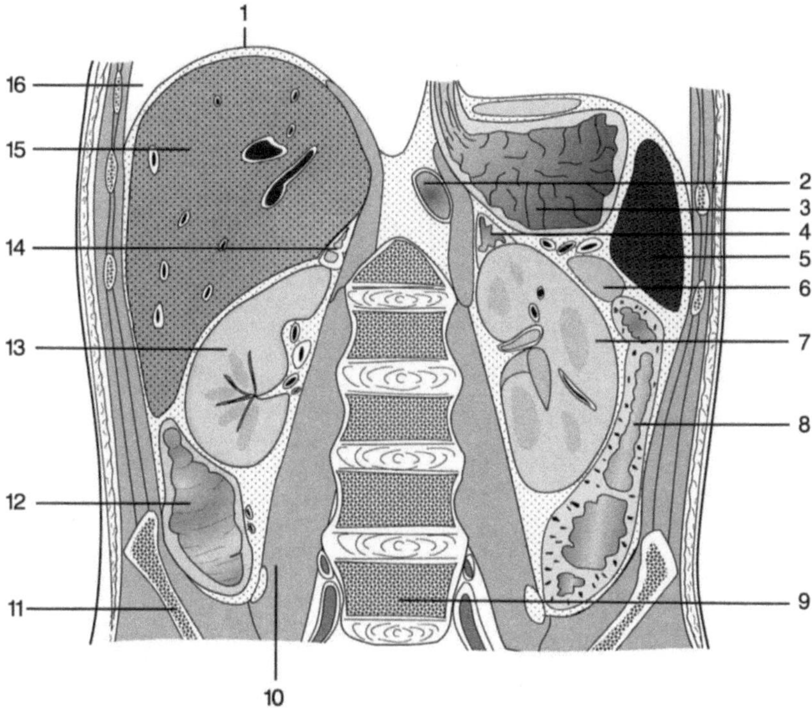

Fig. 9.1. Renal region. *1*, Diaphragm; *2*, aorta; *3*, stomach; *4*, left adrenal; *5*, spleen; *6*, pancreas; *7*, left kidney; *8*, descending colon; *9*, vertebral body; *10*, psoas muscle; *11*, ala of the ilium; *12*, caecum and ascending colon; *13*, right kidney; *14*, right adrenal; *15*, liver; *16*, costodiaphragmatic recess

rounds a central hyperechoic region, known as the renal sinus or central echo complex, consisting of:

◆ Collecting system
◆ Connective tissue
◆ Blood vessels

Columnar hypertrophy may give rise to a projection of cortex between the pyramids which may indent the central echo complex and simulate a neoplasm. This condition, however, shows no distortion of the renal contour.

Normal renal lobulation:
◆ Foetal lobulation
◆ Dromedary hump
◆ Anterior indentation

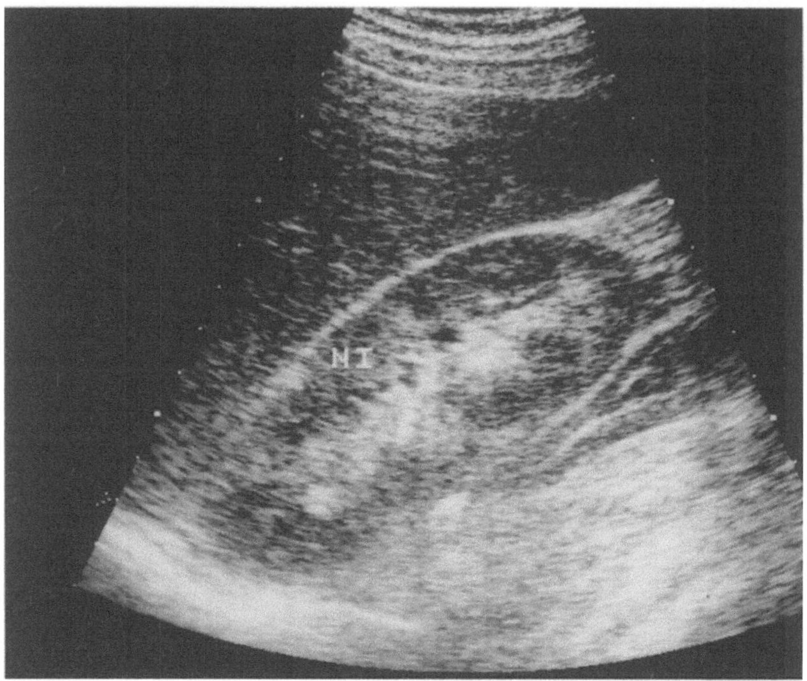

Fig. 9.2. Kidney. Longitudinal scan showing the hypoechoic renal cortex and the echogenic renal sinus or central echo complex. *NI*, Kidney

Non-visualization of the kidneys:
◆ Bowel
◆ Agenesis
◆ Aplasia
◆ Hypoplasia
◆ Ectopia
◆ Malformation
◆ Atrophy

Ectopic kidneys usually lie in the pelvis due to failure of ascent.

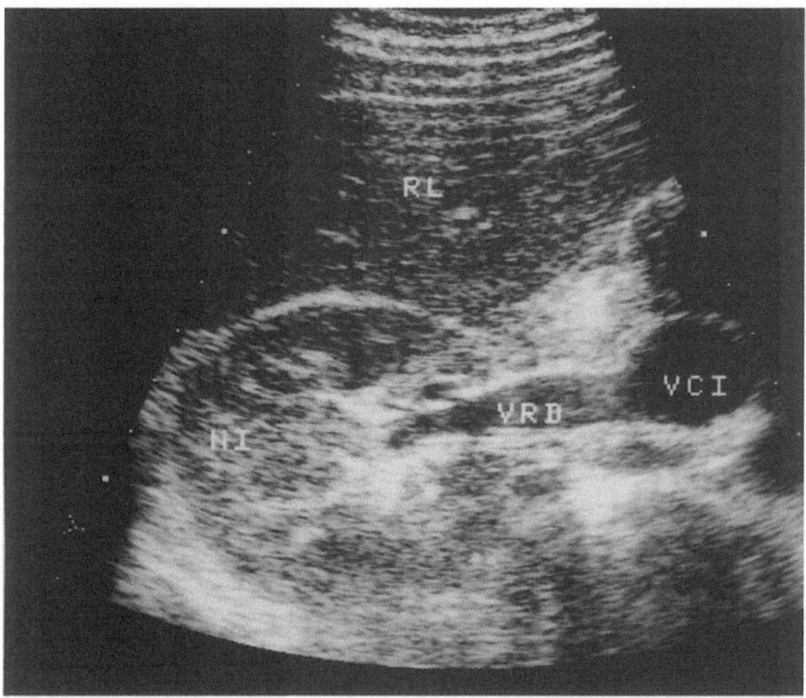

Fig. 9.3. Kidney. Transverse scan. The kidney is bean-shaped with a central concavity or hilum on its medial border which receives – from anterior to posterior – the renal vein, renal artery, and ureter. *NI*, Kidney; *VRD*, right renal vein; *VCI*, inferior vena cava; *RL*, right lobe of the liver

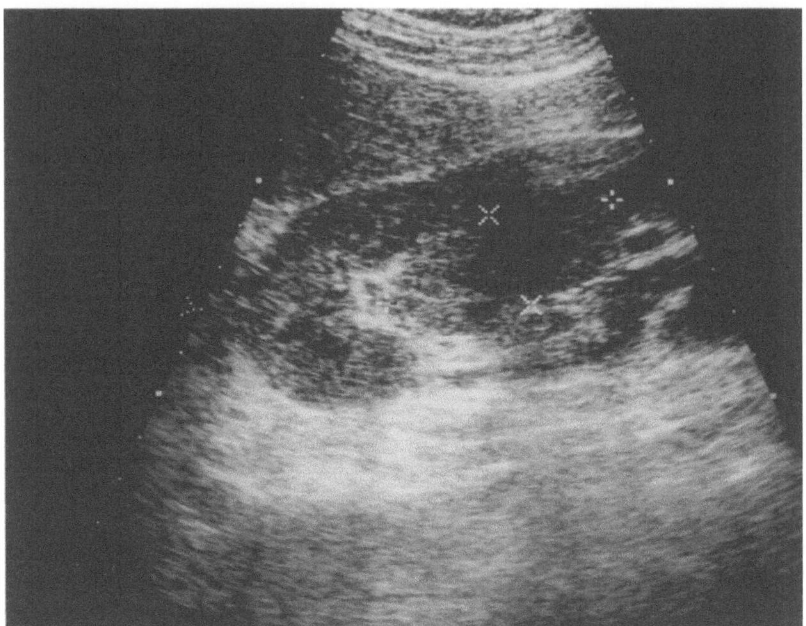

Fig. 9.4. Columnar hypertrophy

9.2.2.1 Normal Dimensions

Kidneys:
- Length < 12 cm
- Width < 6 cm
- Depth < 5 cm
- Parenchyma 1.5–2.5 cm
- Parenchyma pelvis ratio
  - 30 years: approximately 1.7:1
  - 30–60 years: 1.2–1.6:1
  - 60 years: approximately 1.1:1
- Mobility on respiration 3–6 cm

The renal size is related to age, weight, and body surface area. The left kidney is usually slightly longer than the right kidney but the difference in size should be a maximum of 1.5 cm. After drinking, the renal pelvis can be widened up to 2 cm.

9.2.3 Sonopathology

9.2.3.1 Malformations

Clinical Data

The commonest renal malformation is persistence of foetal lobulation; it is of no significance. Other malformations include:

- Unilateral agenesis
- Hypoplastic kidney
- Ectopic kidney
- Horseshoe kidney
- Pancake kidney

Approximately 10% of patients have renal abnormalities. This high incidence is explained by the complex embryology of the region.

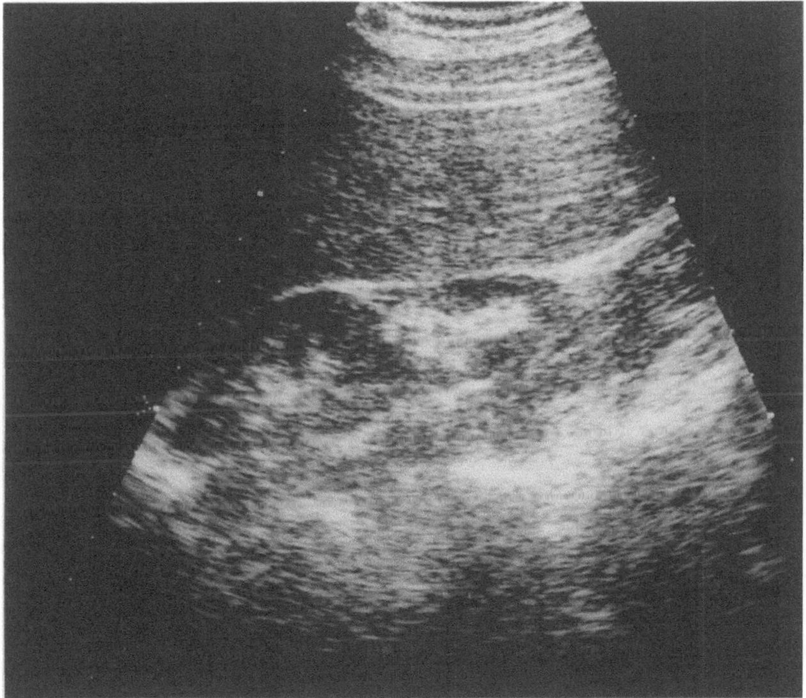

Fig. 9.5. Renal duplication. Division of the collecting system echoes into two groups

Sonographic Diagnosis

Criteria

→ Enlarged kidney
→ Division of the central echo complex

Duplications of the renal collecting system and ureter are the most common anomalies of the urinary tract.

Sonographic Differential Diagnosis

This appearance may be mimicked by oblique sections through a normal kidney or columnar hypertrophy.

9.2.3.2 Chronic Pyelonephritis

Clinical Data

The onset of acute pyelonephritis is abrupt with loin pain, shivering, fever, and malaise. There may or may not be frequency and dysuria. Examination shows tenderness in the affected loin. Acute pyelonephritis is a serious disorder because it can lead to chronic pyelonephritis particularly if recurrent attacks occur and, if bilateral, can cause end-stage renal failure, preceded by hypertension and proteinuria.

Sonographic Diagnosis

Criteria

→ Shrunken, hyperechoic kidney
→ Parenchymal thinning
→ Dilated collecting system
→ Calyceal blunting

In acute pyelonephritis, the kidney usually appears normal.

End-stage renal disease usually results in the kidney being reduced to a small, ovoid, featureless and rather bright structure in which the collecting system echoes may be poorly seen.

Sonographic Differential Diagnosis

Differential diagnosis:
◆ Chronic glomerulonephritis
◆ Hypertension
◆ Focal infarction

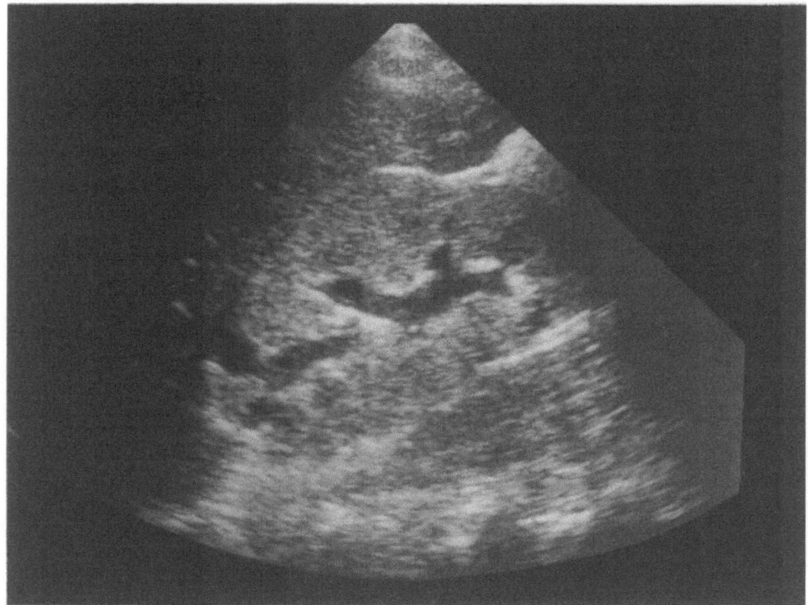

Fig. 9.6. Chronic pyelonephritis. The appearance is non-specific

9.2.3.3 Atrophy

Clinical Data

Small, shrunken kidneys are found in many renal disorders such as chronic glomerulo-nephritis.

Sonographic Diagnosis

Criteria

→ Shrunken kidney
→ Loss of cortico-medullary differentiation
→ Irregular margin

Sonographic Differential Diagnosis

Small kidney:
◆ Unilateral
  – Chronic pyelonephritis
  – Renal artery stenosis
  – Renal vein thrombosis

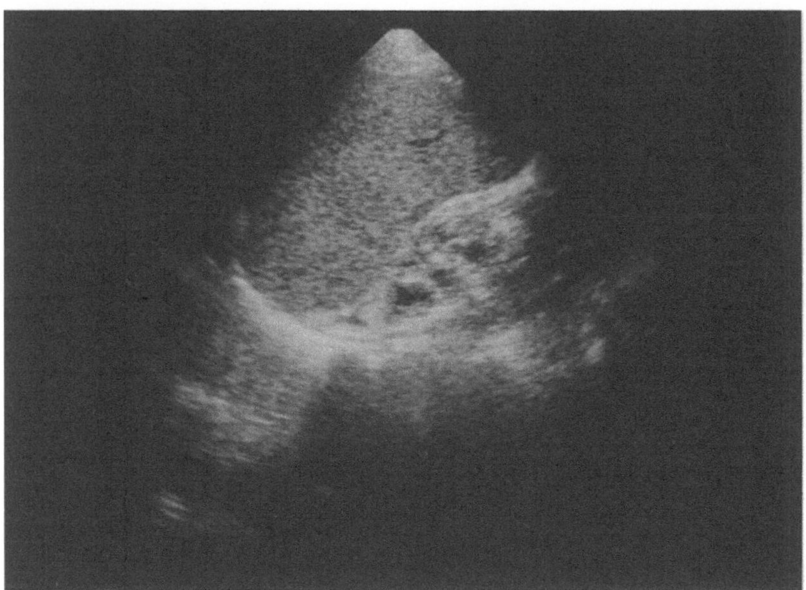

Fig. 9.7. Renal atrophy. The kidney is very small with extreme thinning of the parenchyma and alteration of the echotexture

◆ Bilateral
  – Chronic glomerulonephritis
  – Hypertension
  – Diabetes mellitus

Any long-standing renal parenchymal disease may result in bilateral small kidneys.

9.2.3.4 Papillary Necrosis

Clinical Data

Aetiology:
◆ Infection
◆ Urinary obstruction
◆ Analgesic abuse
◆ Nephrotoxic drugs
◆ Diabetes

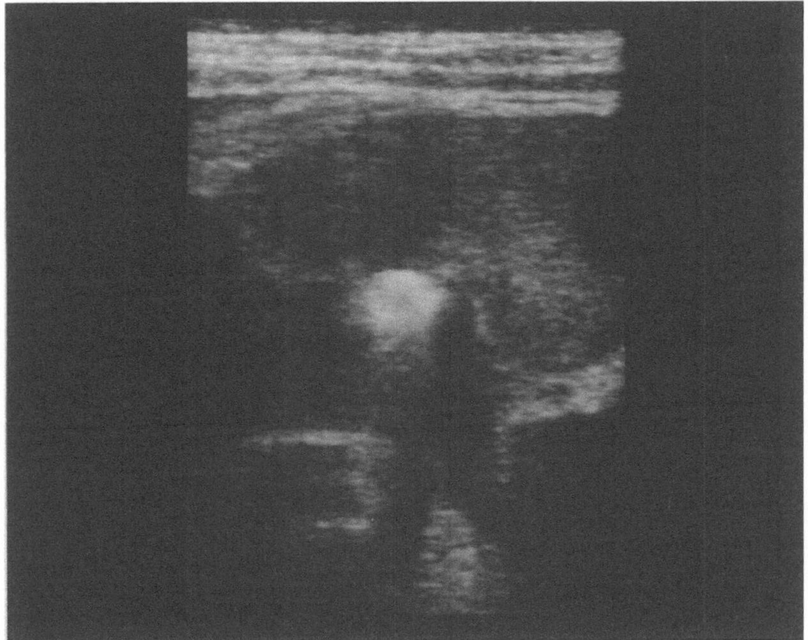

Fig. 9.8. Renal papillary necrosis. The scan shows a calcified sloughed papilla

Sonographic Diagnosis

Criteria

→ Initially normal appearance
→ Later juxtacalyceal cavities
→ Hydronephrosis

Sloughed papillae may calcify and thus mimic nephrolithiasis.

Sonographic Differential Diagnosis

Differential diagnosis:
◆ Focal infarct
◆ Pyelonephric scar
◆ Tuberculous scar

9.2.3.5 Nephrocalcinosis

Clinical Data

Nephrocalcinosis may occur in any case of hypercalcaemia or hypercalcuria.

Sonographic Diagnosis

Criteria

→ Densely hyperechoic medullary pyramids
→ Occasionally distal acoustic shadowing

Medullary nephrocalcinosis is found in hyperparathyroidism, bone involvement in extensive malignancy, and vitamin D excess, whereas cortical nephrocalcinosis is seen in chronic glomerulonephritis, renal cortical necrosis, and Alport's disease.

Sonographic Differential Diagnosis

Renal pyramidal fibrosis usually forms part of a generalized parenchymal abnormality and may have the same appearance.

Hyperechoic renal parenchyma:
◆ Glomerulonephritis
◆ Acute renal failure
◆ Interstitial nephritis
◆ Diabetic nephropathy
◆ Tumour infiltration

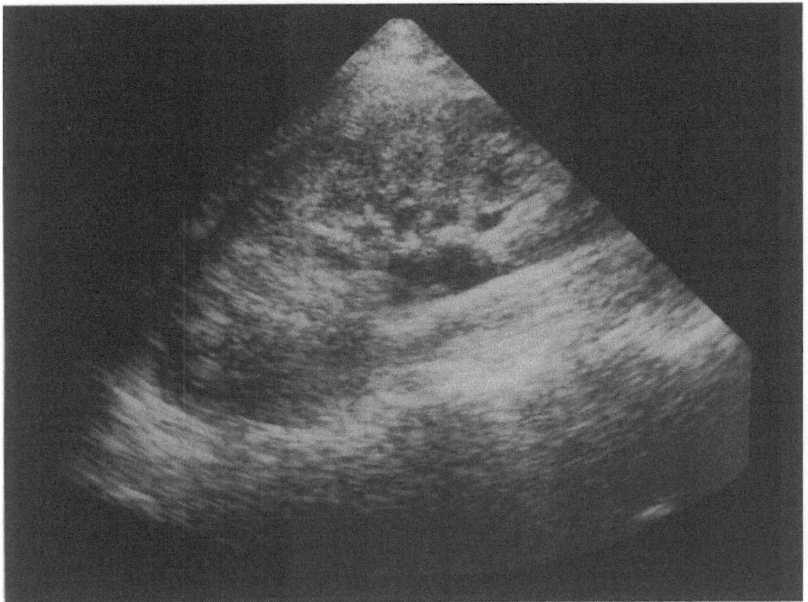

Fig. 9.9. Medullary nephrocalcinosis

9.2.3.6 Nephrolithiasis

Clinical Data

Pain and haematuria are the most prominent symptoms, though neither is invariable. Often the first indication of the presence of a calculus is an attack of renal colic due to the passage of a stone into or down the ureter. Frequency usually accompanies colic. If infection supervenes, the symptoms and signs of pyelitis or even pyonephrosis or perinephric abscess may occur. Stones which fill the renal pelvis and calyces (staghorn calculi) may be quite painless.

Sonographic Diagnosis

Criteria

→ Echogenic focus
→ Distal acoustic shadowing

Small calculi are easily lost in the central echo complex if the collecting system is not dilated.

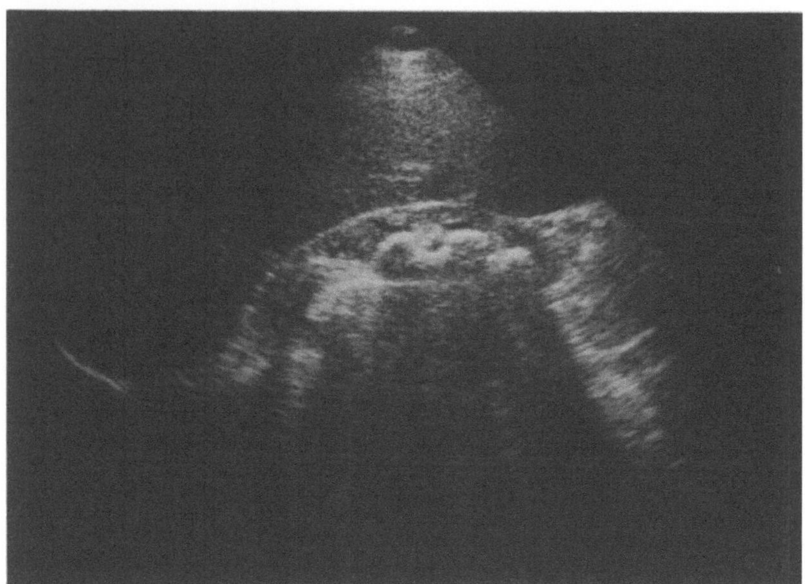

Fig. 9.10. Nephrolithiasis. Curvilinear echogenic lines with distal acoustic shadowing due to multiple calculi

Sonographic Differential Diagnosis

Differential diagnosis:
- Calcified renal tumour
- Calcified renal artery
- Nephrocalcinosis
- Arcuate artery
- Gas
- Stent
- Drain

9.2.3.7 Hydronephrosis

Clinical Data

Obstruction to the outflow of urine from the kidney leads to distension first of the renal pelvis, then the calyces. Later, thinning of the renal parenchyma leads to reduction of renal function. The kidney may be converted into a functionless sac in which infection and stone formation are common sequels. Bilateral hydronephrosis may lead to renal failure and death unless the cause can be treated.

Sonographic Diagnosis

Criteria

→ Stage I
  - Dilatation of the renal collecting system
  - No parenchymal thinning
→ Stage II
  - Dilatation of the renal collecting system
  - Parenchymal thinning
→ Stage III
  - Bag of water
  - Loss of parenchyma

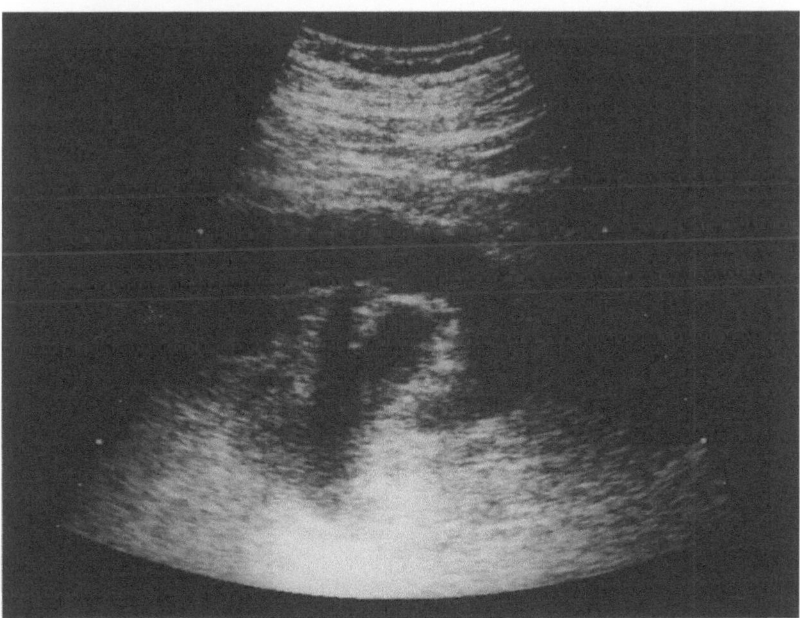

Fig. 9.11. Hydronephrosis, stage I

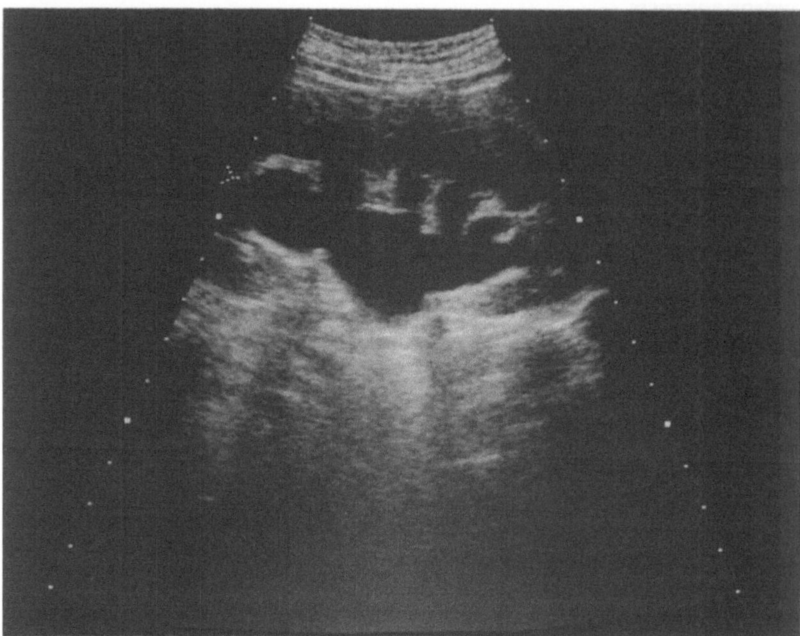

Fig. 9.12. Hydronephrosis, stage II. The enlarged renal pelvis can be seen to communicate with the distended calyces

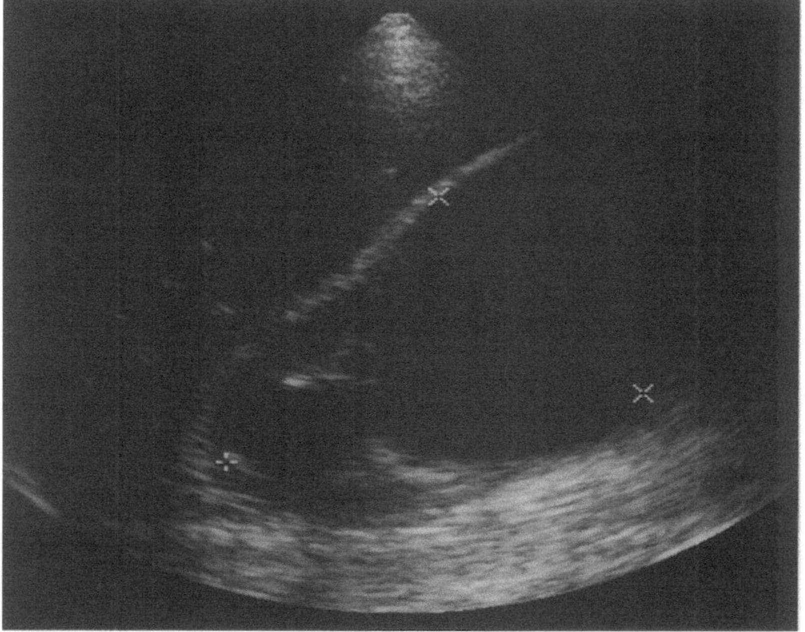

Fig. 9.13: Hydronephrosis, stage III

Visualization of the collecting system depends upon the rate of urine formation and the rate of urine drainage. Slight dilatation is a common normal finding during diuresis or when the bladder is full. The dilatation usually resolves when the bladder is emptied.

Sonographic Differential Diagnosis

Differential diagnosis:
- Diuresis
- Lucent pyramids
- Renal cysts
- Polycystic kidneys
- Necrotic tumour
- Haematoma

Perirenal fluid collections:
- Ascites
- Urinoma
- Seroma
- Haematoma
- Abscess

9.2.3.8 Cysts

Clinical Data

Renal cysts are common incidental findings. They are found in 50% of adults over 50 years and may reach a great size. Although they are usually asymptomatic, they may sometimes cause aching pain.

Apart from severe renal impairment in childhood, most people with polycystic kidneys are unaware of them until adult life. Common presentations are large swellings, haematuria, hypertension, and renal failure.

Sonographic Diagnosis

Criteria

→ Spherical or oval anechoic lesion
→ Sharp and well-defined border
→ Distal acoustic enhancement
→ Prominent posterior border

When the cyst arises in a parapelvic location it may compress part of the renal collecting system. If cysts have been complicated by haemorrhage or infection, they may have an irregular margin, internal echoes, and septa. Such an appearance, however, may also be due to intracystic or necrotic tumour.

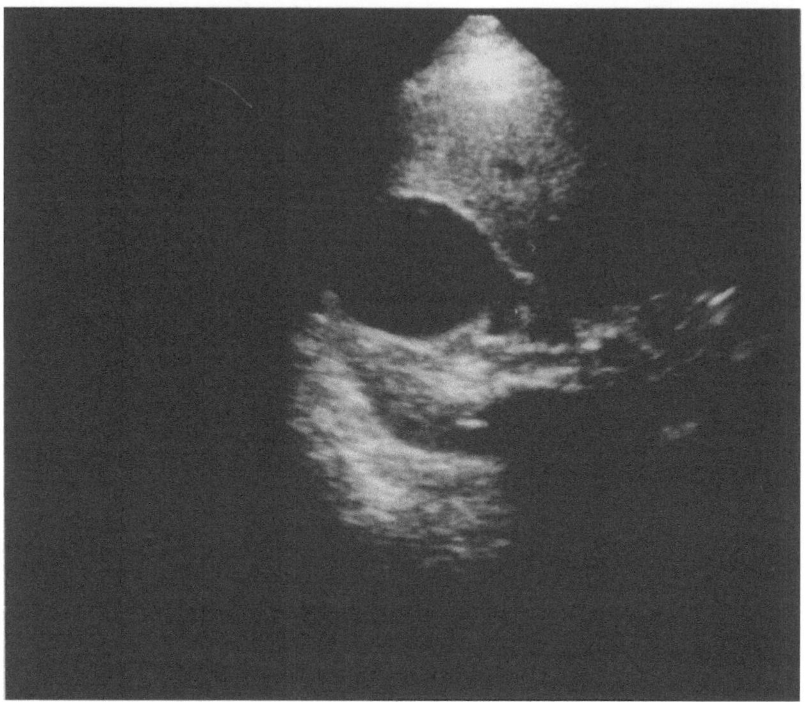

Fig. 9.14. Renal cyst. Clearly defined echofree cyst lying in the upper pole of the kidney

Polycystic disease:
- Enlarged kidneys
- Irregular contour
- Multiple cysts of differing sizes

Sonographic Differential Diagnosis

Small cysts appear anechoic only when they are in the focal zone of the ultrasound beam. If the appearances are typically those of a simple cyst, then no further examinations are necessary.

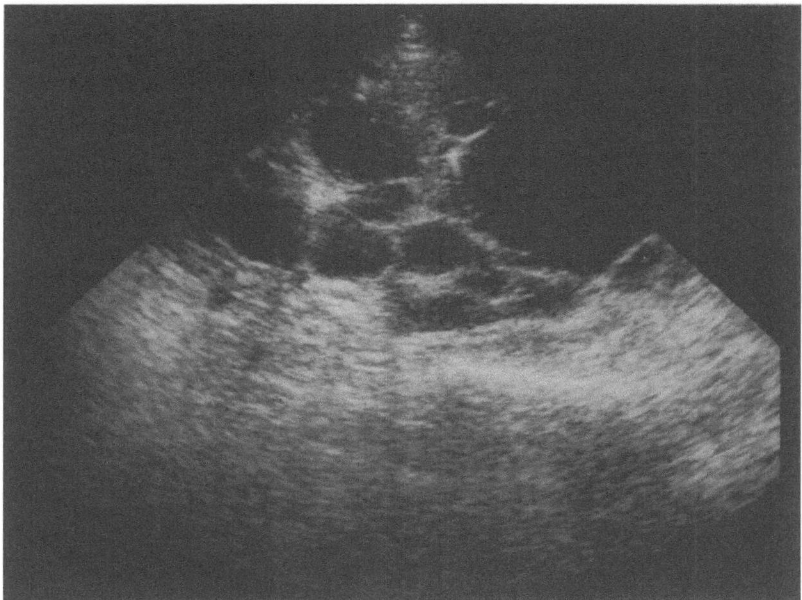

Fig. 9.15. Polycystic kidney. Only islands of renal tissue may be seen between the cysts

9.2.3.9 Angiomyolipoma

Clinical Data

Angiomyolipomas are relatively benign tumours containing blood vessels, muscle, and fat. They may be associated with tuberous sclerosis and are frequently multiple. Angiomyolipomas rarely cause symptoms.

Sonographic Diagnosis

Criterion

→ Well-defined, hyperechoic mass

Sonographic Differential Diagnosis

Hyperechoic renal cell carcinoma.

CT scanning reveals the high fat content of the lesion and also permits a correct specific diagnosis to be made.

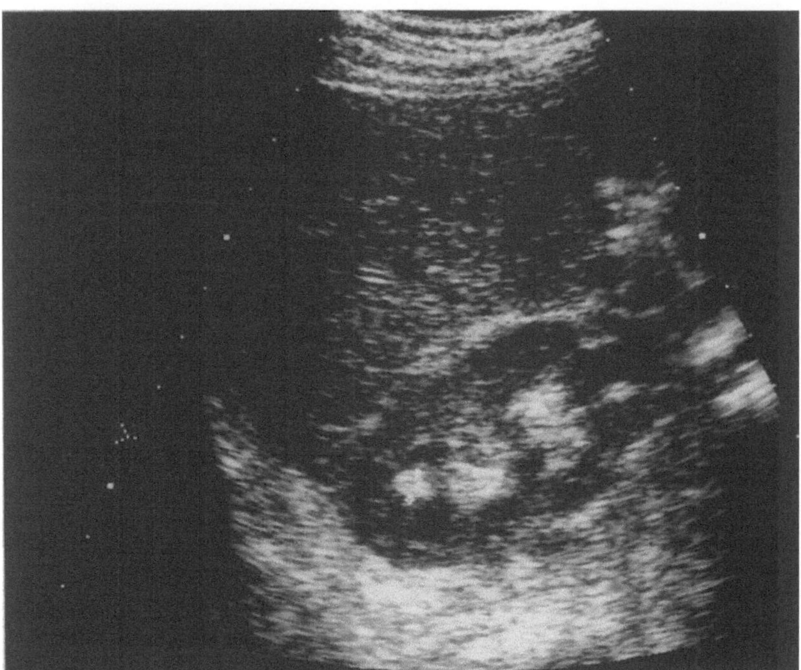

Fig. 9.16. Angiomyolipoma. The lesion is clearly defined, highly reflective but does not exhibit distal acoustic shadowing

9.2.3.10 Nephroblastoma (Wilms' Tumour)

Clinical Data

Nephroblastoma of the kidney is one of the few malignant tumours of children. Common symptoms are haematuria, enlargement of the abdomen, and fever. The tumour grows rapidly and may become very large.

Sonographic Diagnosis

Criteria

→ Well-circumscribed solid mass
→ Variable echogenicity

Any solid renal mass in a young child should be assumed to be a Wilms' tumour until proven otherwise.

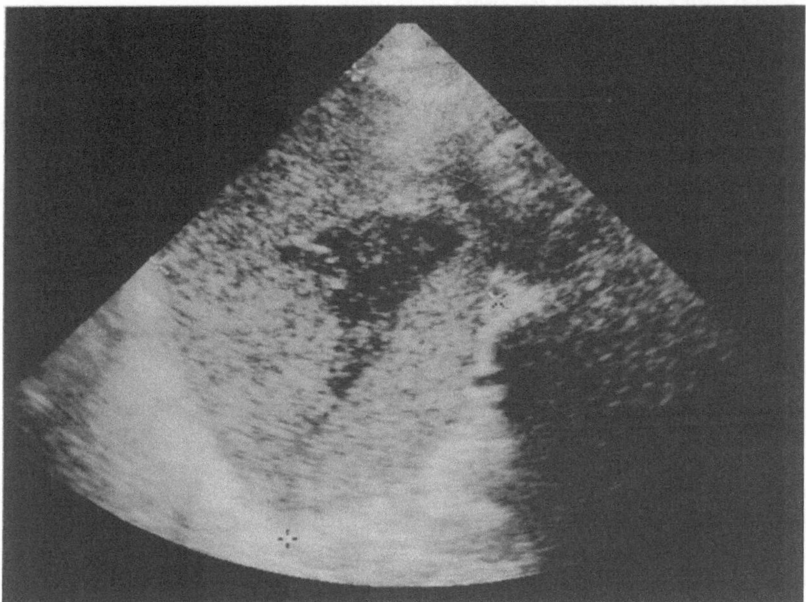

Fig. 9.17. Wilms' tumour. The anechoic area in the centre of the mass is due to necrosis

Sonographic Differential Diagnosis

Pararenal mass:
- ◆ Right side
  - – Adrenal
  - – Liver
- ◆ Left side
  - – Adrenal
  - – Spleen
  - - Pancreas
- ◆ Bilateral
  - – Adrenal
  - – Lymph nodes

9.2.3.11 Renal Cell Carcinoma (Grawitz' Tumour)

Clinical Data

Renal cell carcinoma is the commonest malignant tumour of the kidney. Adults aged 50 years or over are most commonly affected, men more often than women. Painless haematuria is a common presenting symptom and clots may give rise to colic. Pain in the loin also occurs. The sudden appearance of a left-sided varicocele may be a mode of presentation. Renal cell carcinoma commonly causes fever. Anaemia, loss of weight, and malaise are often associated.

Sonographic Diagnosis

Criteria

→ Hypo-, iso- or hyperechoic mass
→ Distorted renal architecture
→ Extension of tumour into the renal vein and the inferior vena cava

In adults, the commonest cause of renal vein thrombosis is tumour extension. The thrombus may be visible within the renal vein and colour Doppler shows reduced or absent flow.

Renal metastases are usually hypoechoic masses. They occur particularly frequently in carcinoma of the lung, breast, stomach, and in melanoma.

Sonographic Differential Diagnosis

Differential diagnosis:
◆ Columnar hypertrophy
◆ Complicated cyst
◆ Abscess
◆ Haematoma

A solid mass should be assumed to be a tumour until proven otherwise. Biopsy is often required to make a firm diagnosis.

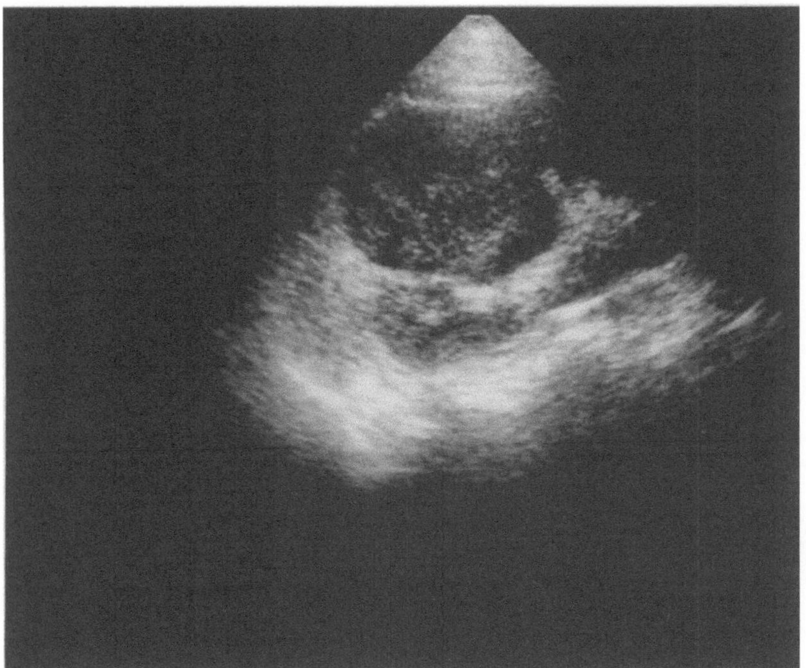

Fig. 9.18. Renal cell carcinoma

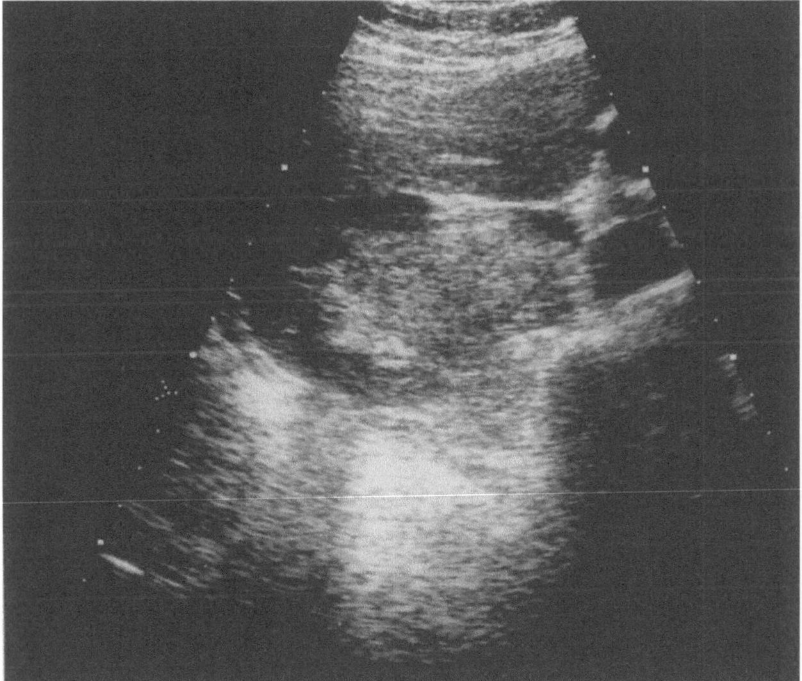

Fig. 9.19. Urothelial carcinoma. The scan shows a hypoechoic mass in the renal collecting system

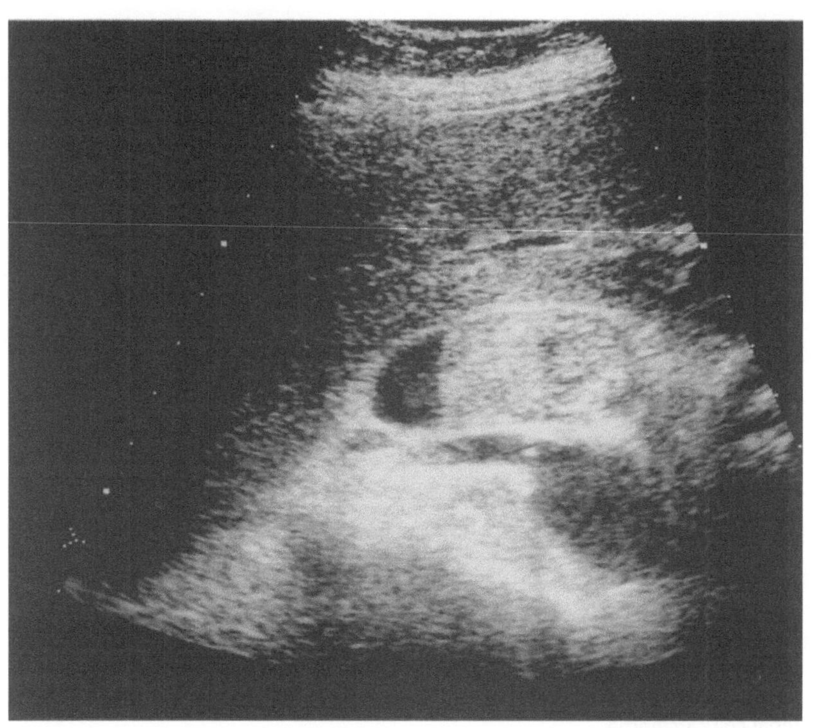

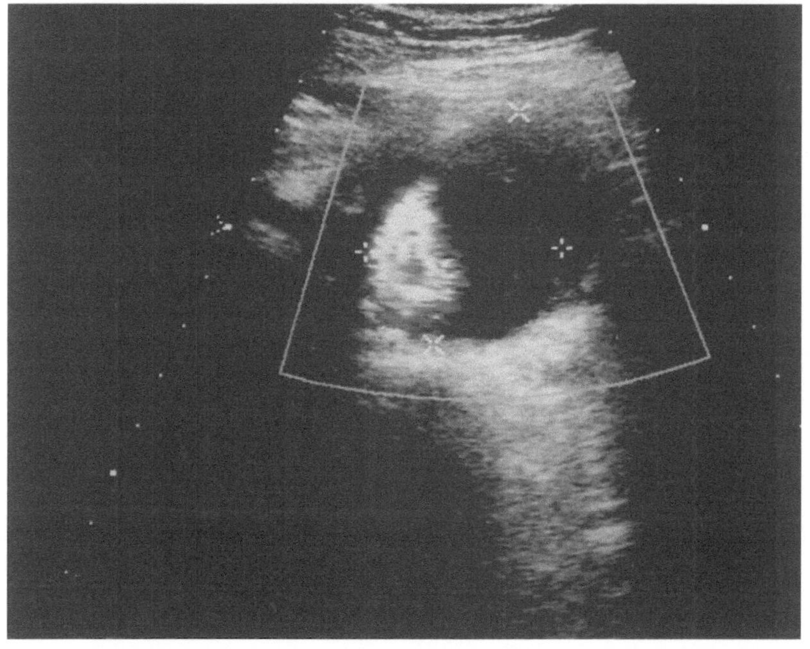

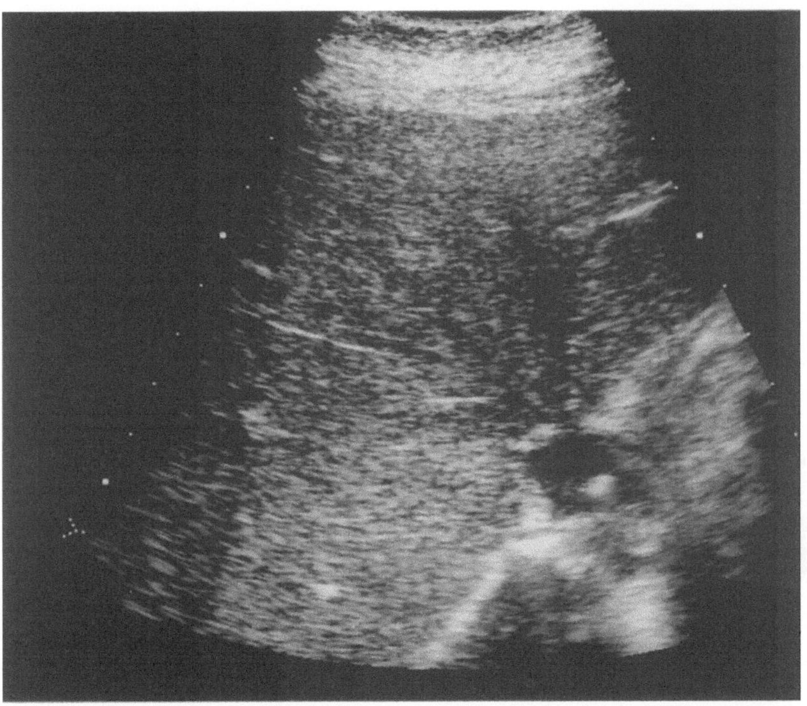

Fig. 9.20 a–c. Tumour thrombus. Extension of the carcinoma through the renal vein into the inferior vena cava. **a** The bright echoes indicate the tumour thrombus. **b** Colour Doppler appearance. **c** Tip of the tumour thrombus floating in the inferior vena cava

9.2.4 Checklist for Reporting

Kidneys
- **Position**
- **Mobility**
- **Size**
- **Contour**
- **Echopattern**
  - **Parenchyma**
  - **Central echo complex**

Vessels
- **Renal artery**
- **Renal vein**
- **Inferior vena cava**

Perinephric space

Chapter 10 Adrenals

10.1 Imaging Modalities

Imaging modalities are:

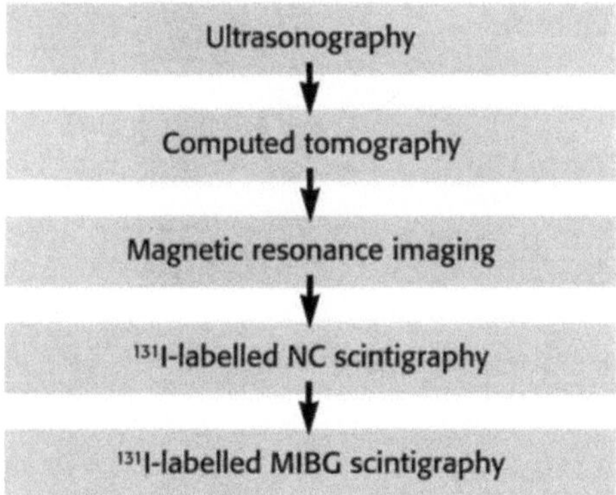

10.2 Ultrasonography

10.2.1 Examination Technique

The normal adrenal glands of adults cannot be imaged reliably, however good the examination technique may be. This applies particularly to the left adrenal, located posterior to the gas containing stomach. With newborn babies, in contrast, the adrenals are physiologically hyperplastic and can be scanned readily. Hypoechoic cortex and hyperechoic medulla are easily distinguishable.

The right adrenal should be examined in subcostal sections, the left adrenal in intercostal sections. Supine position of the patient is preferable. Sometimes the image can be improved by maximum inspiration or a scoliosis position. Landmarks of the adrenals are the cranial poles of the kidneys.

10.2.2 Sonoanatomy

Each adrenal gland lies in the perinephric space and is firmly attached to Gerota's fascia by fibrous bands. The right gland is triangular or pyramidal in shape, the left being crescentic or semilunar.

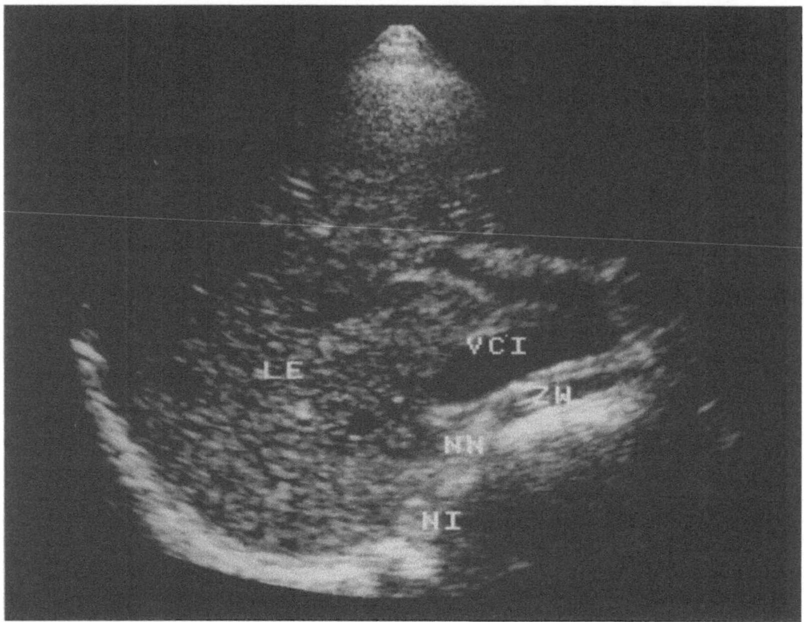

Fig. 10.1. Adrenal gland. The scan shows the right adrenal lying in front of the right crus of diaphragm behind the inferior vena cava and bare area of liver at the upper pole of the right kidney. *NN*, adrenal gland; *ZW*, diaphragm; *VCI*, inferior vena cava; *LE*, liver; *NI*, kidney

Anatomical relationships:
- ◆ Right adrenal
  - – Right kidney
  - – Liver
  - – Inferior vena cava
- ◆ Left adrenal
  - – Left kidney
  - – Tail of pancreas
  - – Aorta

Normal adrenal glands are rarely visible. They may appear as hypoechoic structures relative to the surrounding fat. The right crus of diaphragm may be mistaken for the adrenal gland surrounded by perirenal fat.

10.2.2.1 Normal Dimensions

Adrenals:
- ◆ Length < 5 cm
- ◆ Width < 3 cm
- ◆ Depth < 1 cm

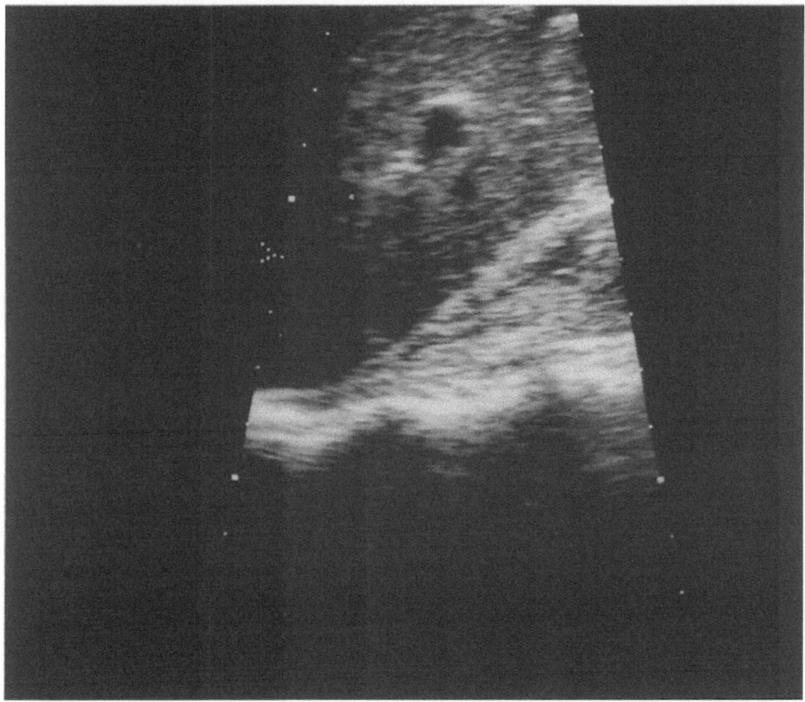

Fig. 10.2. Adrenal gland. The right adrenal shown on this scan is triangular in shape (magnification)

10.2.3 Sonopathology

10.2.3.1 Cysts

Clinical Data

Adrenal cysts are usually asymptomatic and thus of little clinical relevance.

Sonographic Diagnosis

Criteria

→ Spherical or oval anechoic lesion
→ Sharp and well-defined border
→ Distal acoustic enhancement
→ Prominent posterior border

Small cysts may not be detectable as reverberation echoes may make them appear solid.

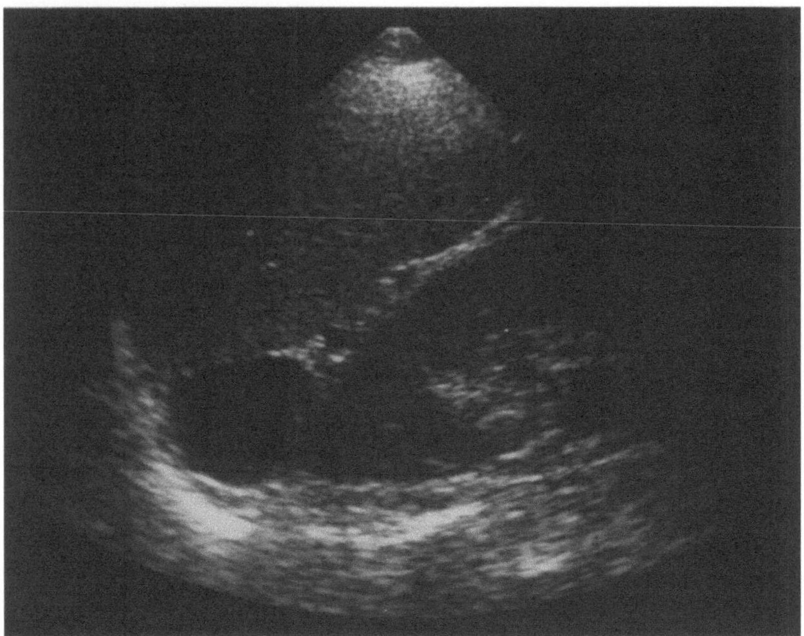

Fig. 10.3. Adrenal cyst

Sonographic Differential Diagnosis

If the cyst wall is irregular, tumour necrosis should be considered in differential diagnosis.

10.2.3.2 Hyperplasia

Clinical Data

Patients may present with Cushing's syndrome, adrenogenital syndrome, or Conn's syndrome.

Sonographic Diagnosis

Criteria

→ Hypoechoic mass
→ Well-defined margin

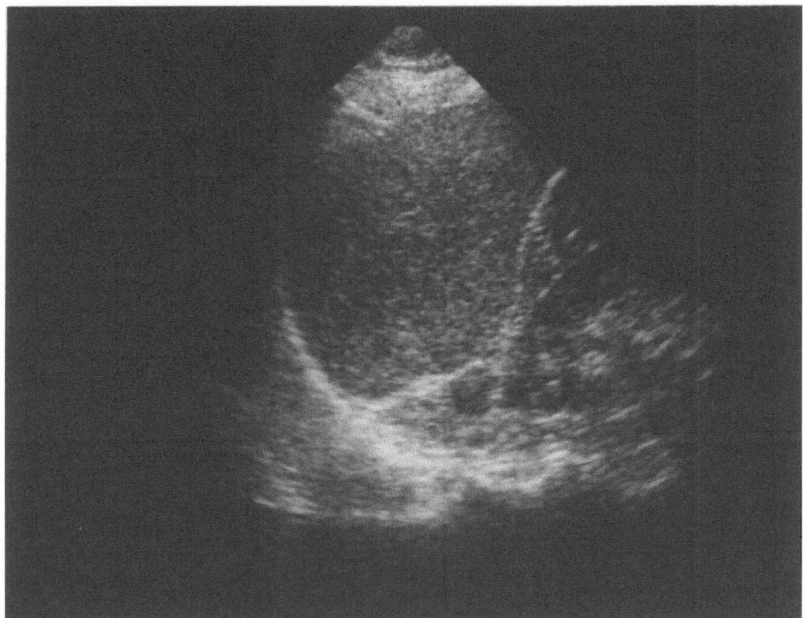

Fig. 10.4. Adrenal hyperplasia

Sonographic Differential Diagnosis

Adrenal hyperplasia occurs almost always bilaterally, an adrenal adenoma is unilateral.

Bilateral adrenal masses:
- Metastases
- Hyperplasia
- Haematomas
- Cysts

10.2.3.3 Phaeochromocytoma

Clinical Data

Hypertension, headaches. There occurs sometimes a characteristic picture of paroxysmal hypertension, with concurrent headaches, nose bleeds, or pulmonary oedema. Palpitations with or without tachycardia are common. Increased perspiration is a frequent complaint. Tremor, weakness, weight loss, anorexia, and constipation occur.

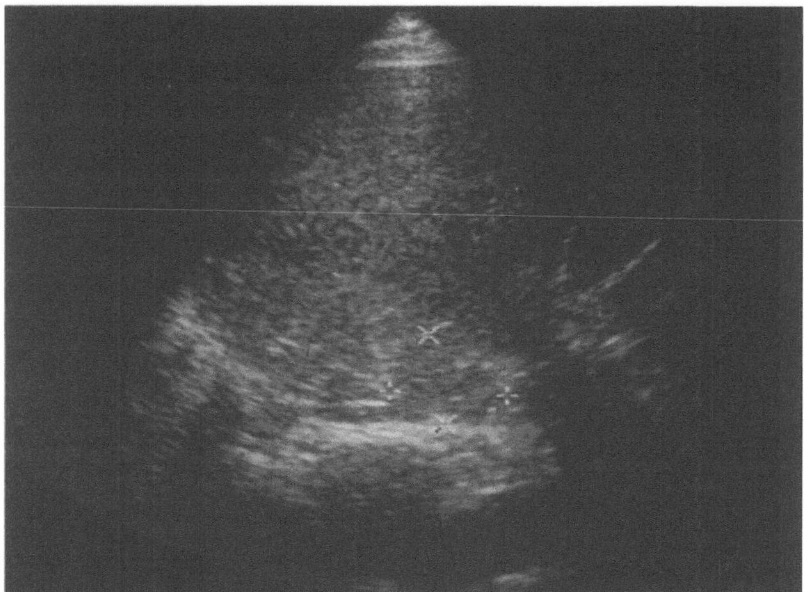

Fig. 10.5. Phaeochromocytoma. This relatively small mass shows a homogeneous and hypo-echoic echopattern

Sonographic Diagnosis

Criterion

→ Hypoechoic or complex mass

In large phaeochromocytomas, the echopattern is usually heterogeneous due to cystic, necrotic, and calcified areas.

Phaeochromocytomas are 10% extra-adrenal, 10% are malignant, and 10% bilateral.

Sonographic Differential Diagnosis

The differential diagnosis includes all solid adrenal masses.

10.2.3.4 Neuroblastoma

Clinical Data

Neuroblastoma is a common solid tumour of childhood arising mainly in the adrenal gland, but also from any portion of the extra-adrenal sympathetic chain, including the retroperitoneum or chest. A palpable abdominal mass or evidence of a metastatic lesion to liver, lung or bone may be the initial presentation.

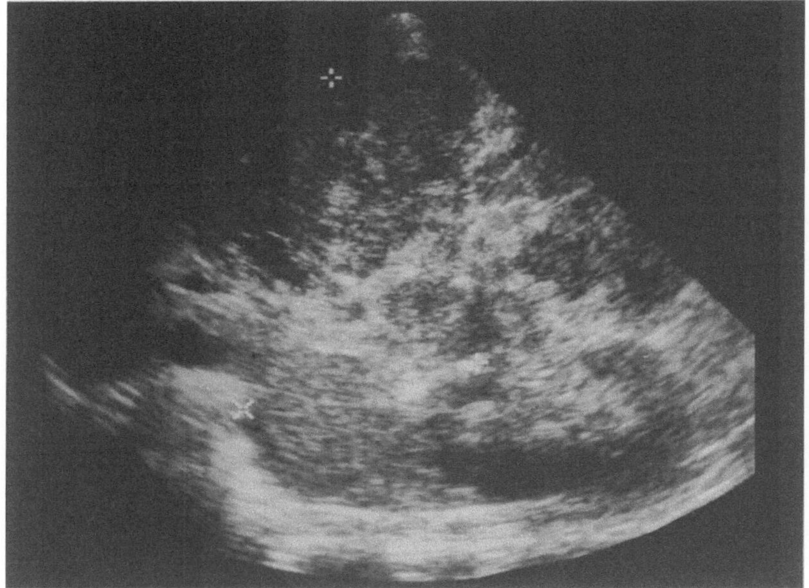

Fig. 10.6. Neuroblastoma. The scan shows a large complex mass with solid and cystic areas

Sonographic Diagnosis

Criteria

→ Large heterogeneous mass
→ Frequently calcific foci

Sonographic Differential Diagnosis

The most important differential diagnosis is nephroblastoma (Wilms' tumour).

10.2.3.5 Metastases

Clinical Data

Aetiology:
◆ Carcinoma of the lung
◆ Carcinoma of the stomach
◆ Lymphoma
◆ Melanoma
◆ Carcinoma of the pancreas
◆ Carcinoma of the kidney

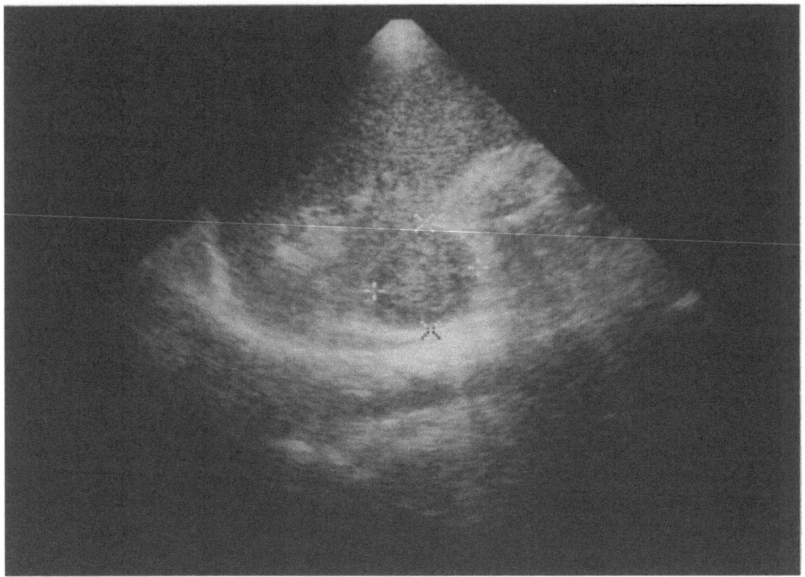

Fig. 10.7. Adrenal metastasis. Note the solid appearance and the well defined margin of this rather small metastasis

Sonographic Diagnosis

Criterion

→ Hypoechoic, frequently bilateral mass

Metastases are the commonest malignant adrenal lesions. Adrenal carcinoma occurs less frequently and is usually very large at diagnosis.

Sonographic Differential Diagnosis

Differential diagnosis:
- Carcinoma
- Hyperplasia
- Adenoma

10.2.4 Checklist for Reporting

Adrenals
- Size
- Echopattern

Chapter 11 Retroperitoneum

11.1 Imaging Modalities

Imaging modalities are:

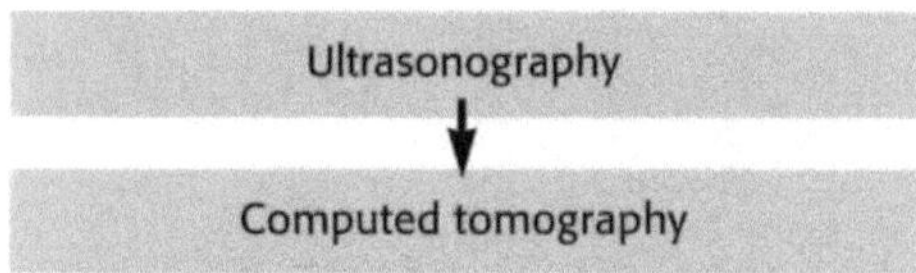

11.2 Ultrasonography

11.2.1 Examination Technique

The retroperitoneum is best examined in the morning as it is easily obscured by over-lying bowel gas. The majority of gas within the bowel is swallowed air and this is at a minimum when the patient awakes. The stomach should be empty. 3.5-MHz convex and sector probes are used. The abdominal wall should be compressed by the transducer to expel intestinal gases. The large abdominal vessels and their branches are scanned in longitudinal and transverse sections. Oblique sections exaggerate the vascular dimensions. For the diagnosis of iliac lymphadenopathy, the bladder should be full.

Obesity and overlying intestinal gases may significantly impair the sonographic imaging of the retroperitoneum.

11.2.2 Sonoanatomy

Retroperitoneal fat, which is hyperechoic, surrounds the various retroperitoneal structures, which are seen as relatively anechoic areas. The aorta and the inferior vena cava, as expected, are easily identified. Only enlarged lymph nodes are identifiable.

Aortic branches:
- Coeliac trunk
  - Common hepatic artery
  - Splenic artery
- Superior mesenteric artery
- Renal arteries
- Common iliac arteries

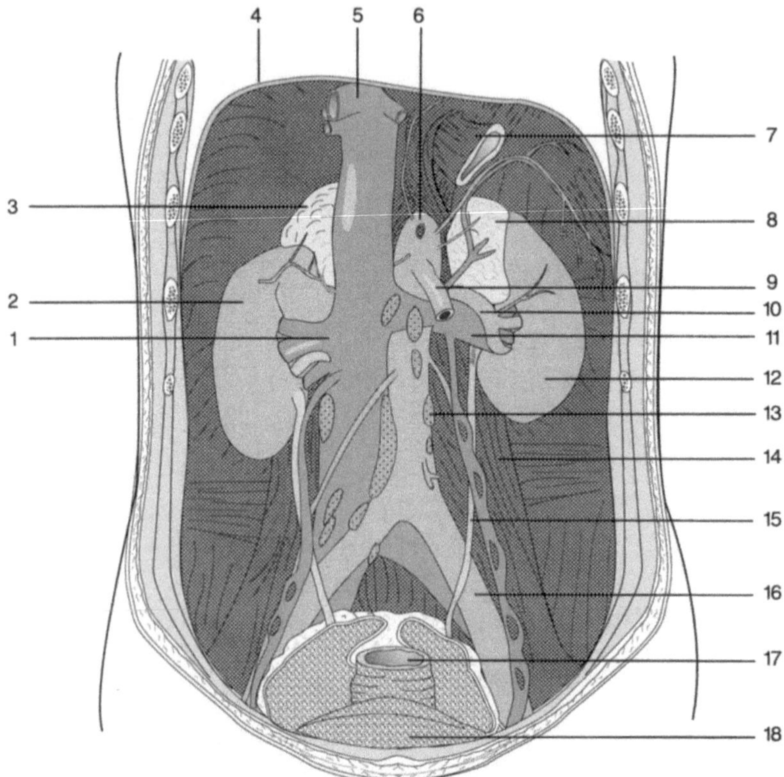

Fig. 11.1. Retroperitoneal region. *1*, Right renal vein; *2*, right kidney; *3*, right adrenal; *4*, diaphragm; *5*, inferior vena cava; *6*, aorta; *7*, oesophagus; *8*, left adrenal; *9*, superior mesenteric artery; *10*, left renal artery; *11*, left renal vein; *12*, left kidney; *13*, lymph node; *14*, psoas muscle; *15*, ureter; *16*, common iliac artery; *17*, rectum; *18*, bladder

The left gastric artery and the inferior mesenteric artery are rarely visible.

The inferior vena cava forms at the level of the fifth lumbar vertebral body. The right renal artery is seen passing behind the inferior vena cava just before it enters the liver. Inferior vena cava distension varies with:

◆ Cardiac cycle
◆ Respiration
◆ Position

Distension occurs in right-heart failure and fluid overload.

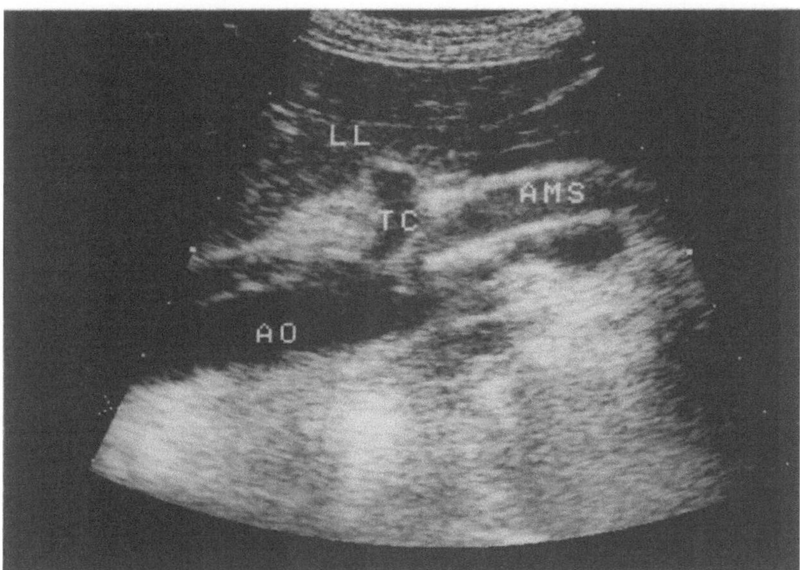

Fig. 11.2. Retroperitoneum. Longitudinal scan of the coeliac trunk. *TC*, Coeliac trunk; *AMS*, superior mesenteric artery; *AO*, aorta; *LL*, left lobe of the liver

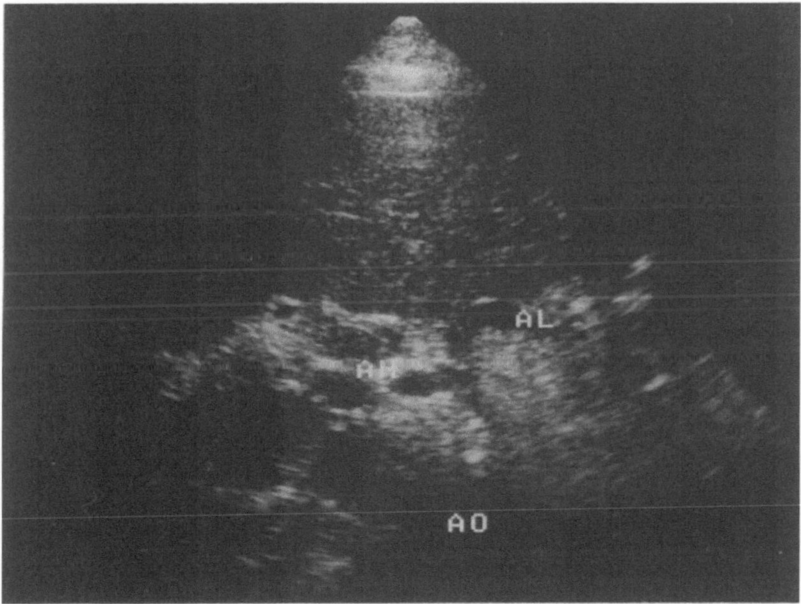

Fig. 11.3. Retroperitoneum. Transverse scan of the coeliac trunk. *AH*, Hepatic artery; *AL*, splenic artery; *AO*, aorta

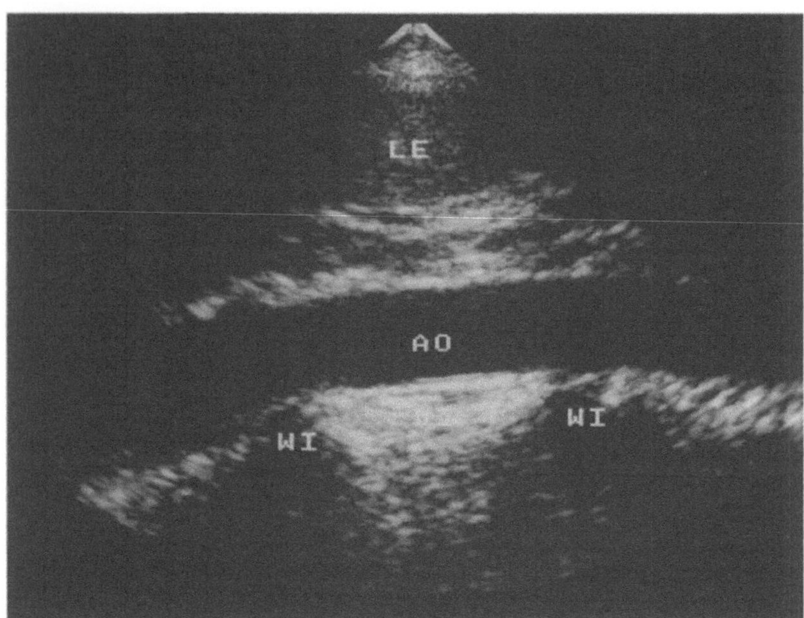

Fig. 11.4. Retroperitoneum. Longitudinal scan of the aorta. *AO*, Aorta; *LE*, liver; *WI*, vertebral body; *DI*, intervertebral disc

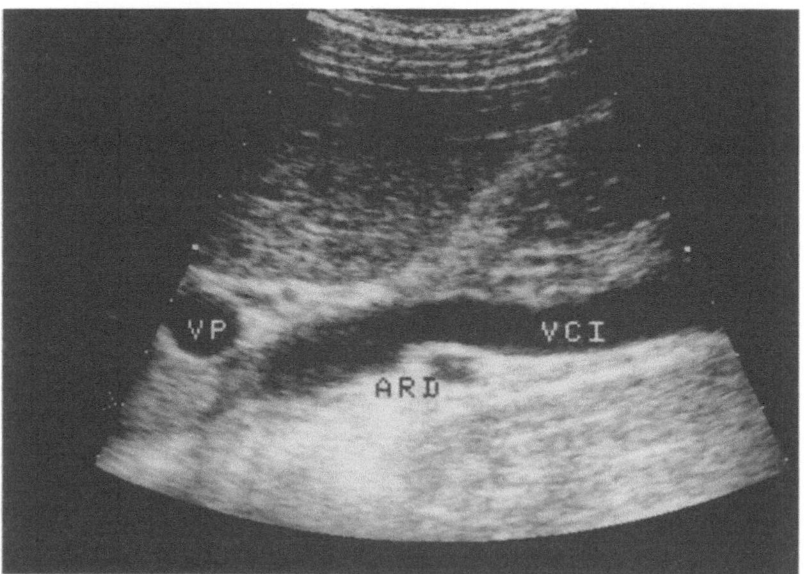

Fig. 11.5. Retroperitoneum. Longitudinal scan of the inferior vena cava. The inferior vena cava shows posterior indentation due to the right renal artery. *VCI*, Inferior vena cava; *ARD*, right renal artery; *VP*, portal vein

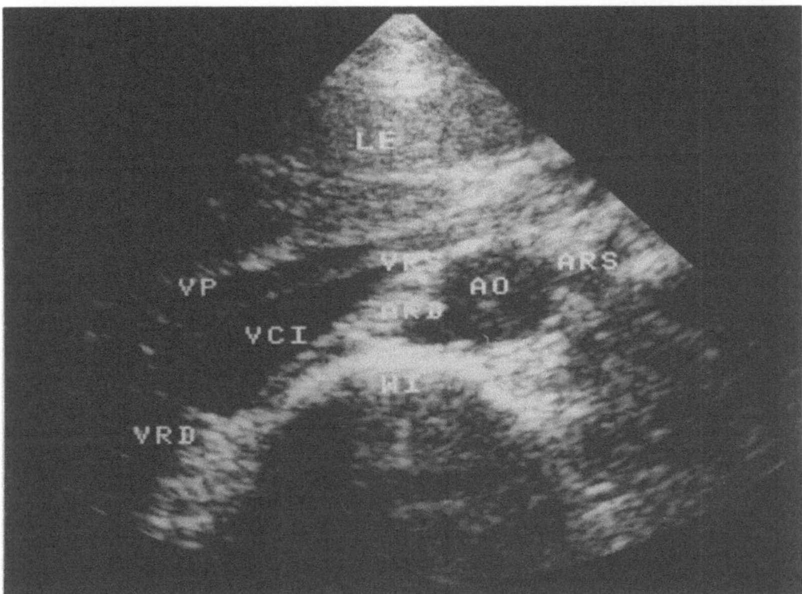

Fig. 11.6. Retroperitoneum. Transverse scan. *AO*, Aorta; *ARD*, right renal artery; *ARS*, left renal artery; *VCI*, inferior vena cava; *VRD*, right renal vein; *VRS*, left renal vein; *VP*, portal vein; *LE*, liver; *WI*, vertebral body

11.2.2.1 Normal Dimensions

Retroperitoneum:
- ◆ Aorta
  - Cranial < 2.5 cm
  - Caudal < 2 cm
- ◆ Inferior vena cava < 2.5 cm
- ◆ Superior mesenteric artery < 0.5 cm
- ◆ Aortomesenteric angle < 30°
- ◆ Aortovertebral distance < 0.5 cm
- ◆ Lymph nodes < 1 cm

11.2.3 Sonopathology

11.2.3.1 Clips

Clinical Data

Clips are mainly seen after lymphadenectomy.

Sonographic Diagnosis

Criterion

→ Echogenic foreign body with reverberation artefacts

Sonographic Differential Diagnosis

Typical appearance.

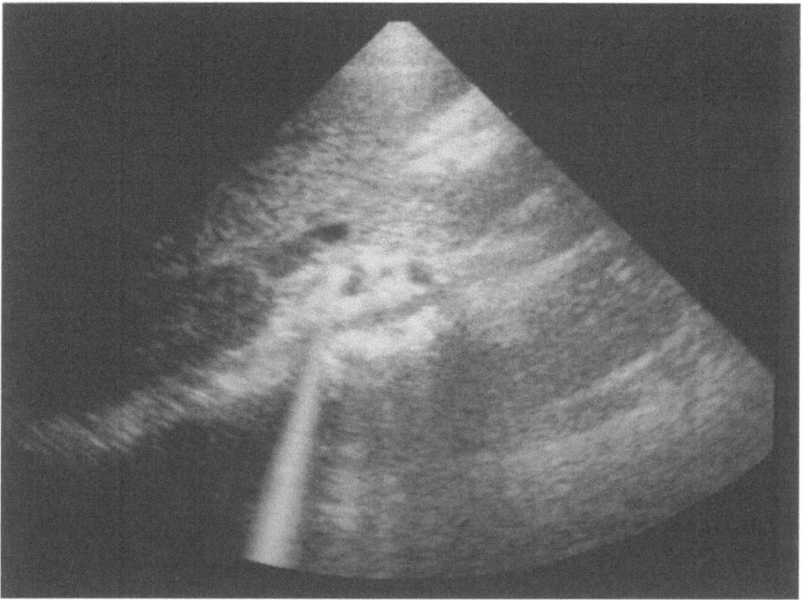

Fig. 11.7. Surgical clips

11.2.3.2 Atherosclerosis of the Aorta

Clinical Data

Atherosclerosis of the aorta is usually asymptomatic unless occlusion occurs, plaques encroach on the ostia of one or more major branches, or embolization occurs. Symptoms and signs relate to the organ and tissues in which clinically significant ischaemia occurs, and several characteristic syndromes may be seen.

Sonographic Diagnosis

Criteria

→ Echogenic aortic wall
→ Distal acoustic shadowing
→ Changing diameter

Sonographic Differential Diagnosis

Imaging in multiple planes is particularly important if the aorta is tortuous.

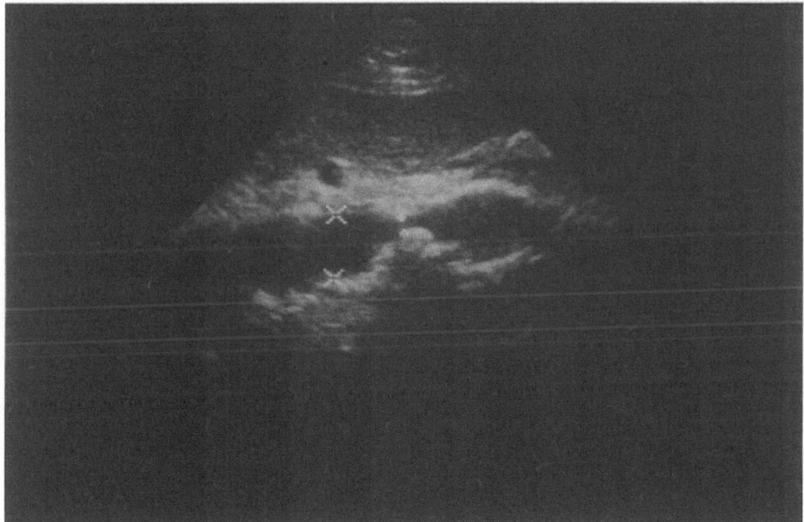

Fig. 11.8. Atherosclerosis of the aorta

11.2.3.3 Atherosclerosis of the Aortic Branches

Clinical Data

The risk factors of arteriosclerosis are:
- ◆ Hypertension
- ◆ Smoking
- ◆ Hyperlipidaemia
- ◆ Diabetes
- ◆ Hyperuricaemia
- ◆ Obesity

Sonographic Diagnosis

Criteria

- → Echogenic vessel wall
- → Distal acoustic shadowing
- → Changing diameter

Sonographic Differential Diagnosis

Typical findings.

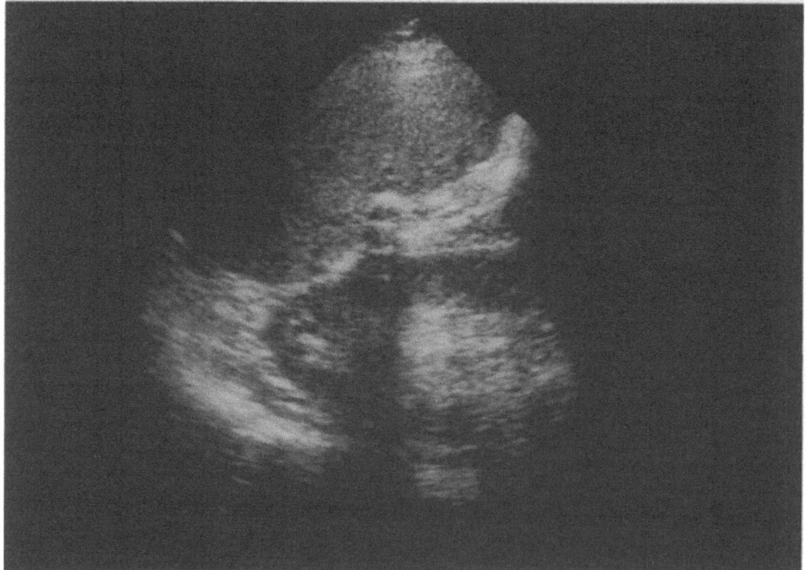

Fig. 11.9. Atherosclerosis of the splenic artery

11.2.3.4 Aortic Aneurysm

Clinical Data

Atherosclerosis is almost always the cause of aneurysms of the abdominal aorta which are sited just distal to the renal arteries. Aortic aneurysms frequently extend into the iliac arteries. Pain may be due to pressure on vertebrae or nerves or may warn of impending rupture. Rupture may cause sudden death. Renal colic, anuria, and haematuria may follow involvement of the renal vessels. Backache is a common premonitory symptom.

Sonographic Diagnosis

Criteria

→ Aortic diameter > 3.5 cm
→ Anechoic lumen
→ Hypoechoic clot

In aortic dilatation, the diameter is 2–3.5 cm.

Ultrasonography allows the assessment of:
◆ Aneurysm diameter
◆ Aneurysm configuration
◆ Wall thickness of the aneurysm
◆ Clot within the aneurysm
◆ Dissection of the aneurysm

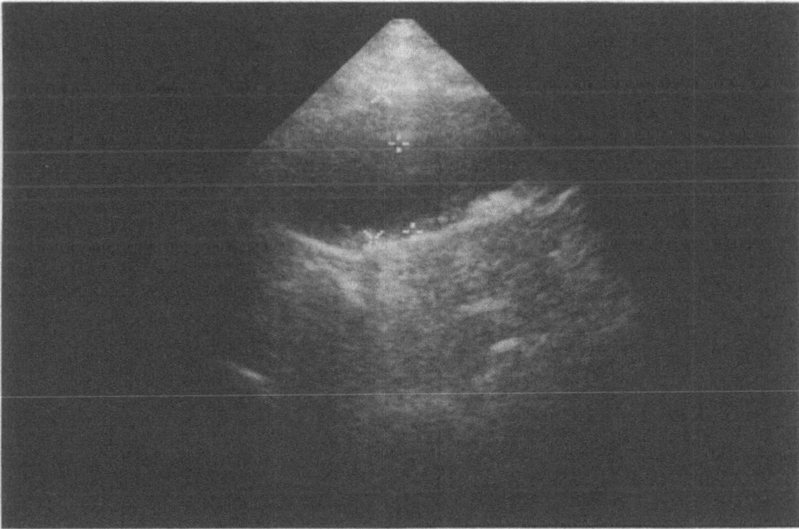

Fig. 11.10. Aortic aneurysm

Sonographic Differential Diagnosis

Differential diagnosis:
◆ Bowel loops
◆ Lymph nodes
◆ Horseshoe kidney
◆ Retroperitoneal fibrosis
◆ Loculated ascites

11.2.3.5 Lymphadenopathy

Clinical Data

Aetiology:
◆ Tumour infiltration
◆ Lymphoma
◆ Inflammatory disease

Sonographic Diagnosis

Criteria

→ Usually hypoechoic masses
→ Displaced vessels

Retroperitoneal lymph nodes of normal size cannot be distinguished from the surrounding connective and fatty tissue.

Sonographic Differential Diagnosis

Lymphoma in particular gives rise to large hypoechoic or even anechoic lymph nodes.

Inferior vena cava obstruction may be caused by retroperitoneal tumours, lymphadenopathy, and retroperitoneal fibrosis. Loss of calibre change with respiration.

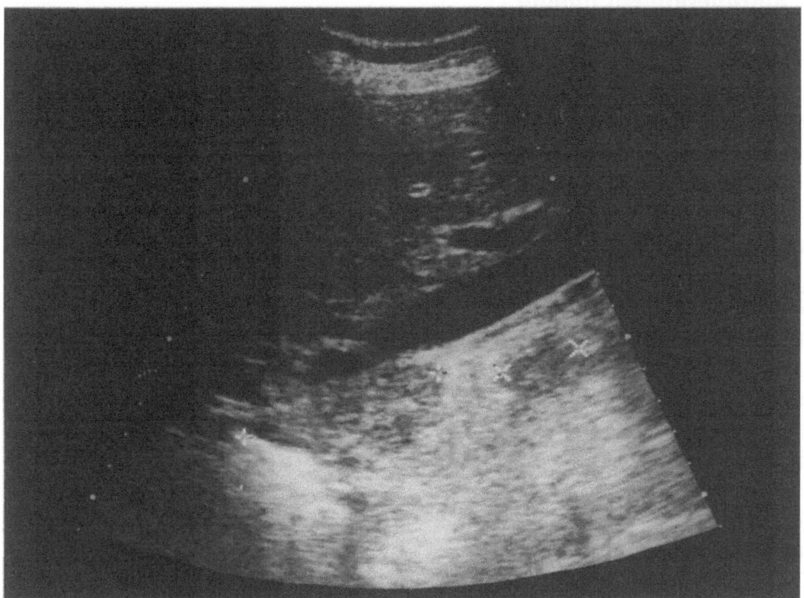

Fig. 11.11. Lymphadenopathy. The scan shows multiple retroperitoneal lymph nodes

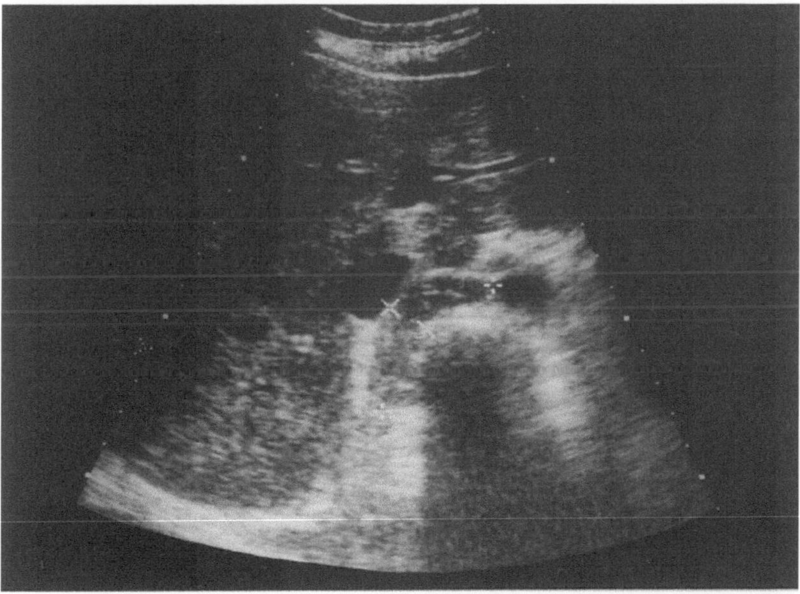

Fig. 11.12. Lymphadenopathy. Oval lymph node distorting and elevating the inferior vena cava

11.2.3.6 Retroperitoneal Tumour

Clinical Data

A retroperitoneal tumour may lead to obstruction of the ureters and, consequently, to renal hydronephrosis and failure.

Sonographic Diagnosis

Criteria

→ Inhomogeneous, usually hypoechoic mass
→ Encasement, displacement, compression, and infiltration of the retroperitoneal vessels

Anechoic areas within the mass may be due to necrotic tissue.

Sonographic Differential Diagnosis

The main diagnostic problem is to determine the origin of the mass.

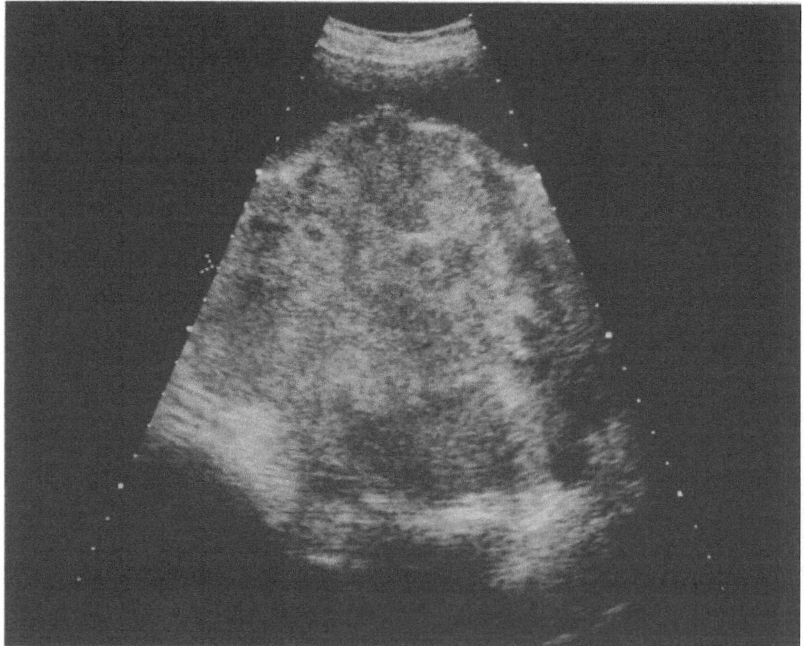

Fig. 11.13. Retroperitoneal tumour. Rhabdomyosarcoma

11.2.4 Checklist for Reporting

Vessels
- **Aorta**
- **Inferior vena cava**

Lymph nodes
- **Para-aortic**
- **Paracaval**
- **Parailiac**
- **Perihepatic**
- **Perisplenic**
- **Perinephric**
  - **Position**
  - **Number**
  - **Size**
  - **Contour**
  - **Echopattern**

Kidneys

Adrenals

Psoas muscle

Chapter ⑫ Bladder

12.1 Imaging Modalities

Imaging modalities are:

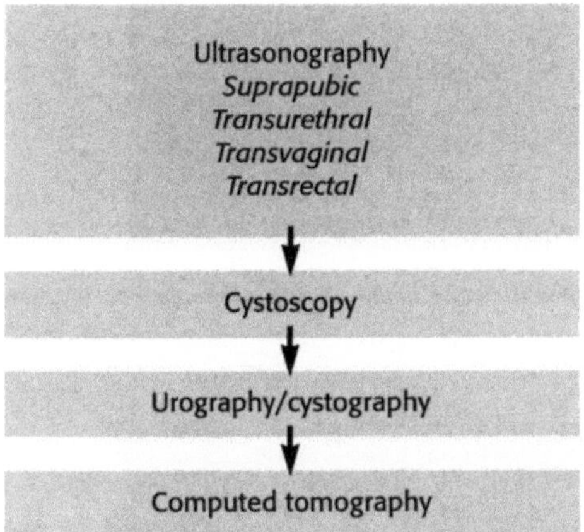

12.2 Ultrasonography

12.2.1 Examination Technique

The urinary bladder must be full. The patient should be in the supine position. Longitudinal and transverse sections are performed whilst the transducer is placed above the symphysis pubis. The bladder must be examined before and after micturition. The bladder volume after micturition should be determined.

12.2.2 Sonoanatomy

Normal ureters are not usually visualized. When dilated the ureter may be seen as a tubular fluid-filled structure.

The urinary bladder is examined in the distended state. It is seen as an anechoic structure in the anterior pelvis. The walls should be sharply defined and barely perceptible.

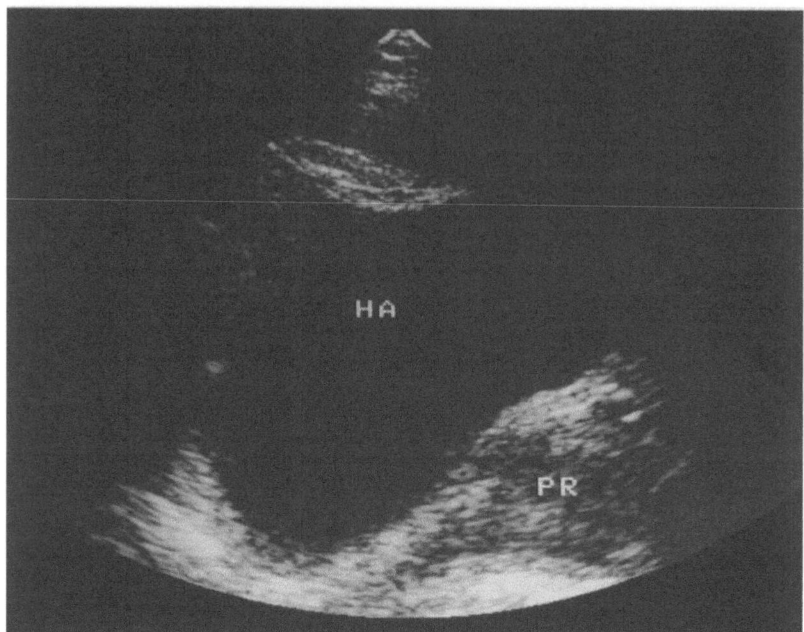

Fig. 12.1. Urinary bladder. Longitudinal scan. The prostate is seen lying inferiorly. *HA*, Bladder; *PR*, prostate

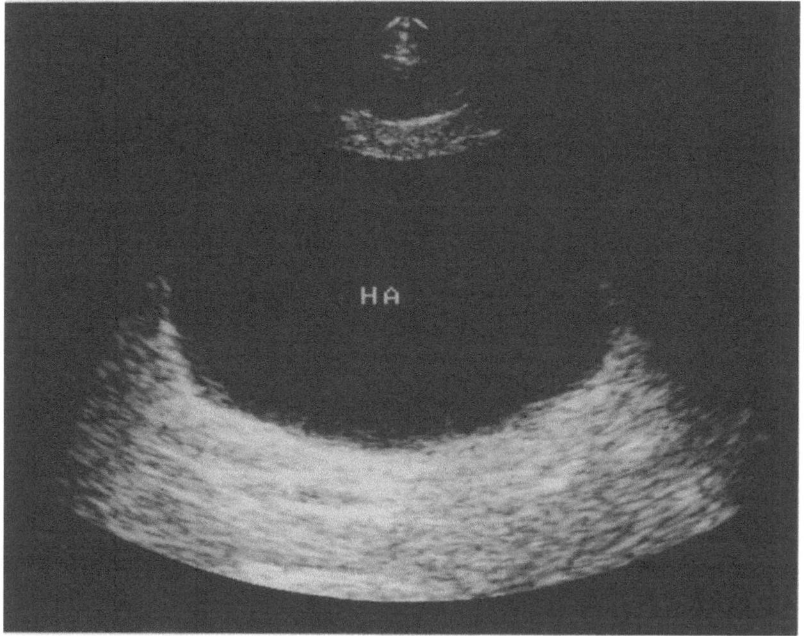

Fig. 12.2. Urinary bladder. Transverse scan. Note the symmetrical outline of the bladder. *HA*, Bladder

12.2.2.1 Normal Dimensions

Bladder:
- Wall thickness
  - When the bladder is not distended < 6 mm
  - When the bladder is distended < 3 mm
- Volume
  - Men before micturition < 750 ml
  - Women before micturition < 550 ml
  - After micturition < 50 ml

12.2.3 Sonopathology

12.2.3.1 Megaureter

Clinical Data

Classification:
- Primary
- Secondary
  - Reflux
  - Obstruction

The patient presents with a urinary tract infection or even with renal failure.

Sonographic Diagnosis

Criterion

→ Dilatation of the ureter

Sonographic Differential Diagnosis

The main differential diagnosis is a ureterocele, i.e. a dilatation of the distal ureter which has herniated through the bladder wall into the bladder lumen.

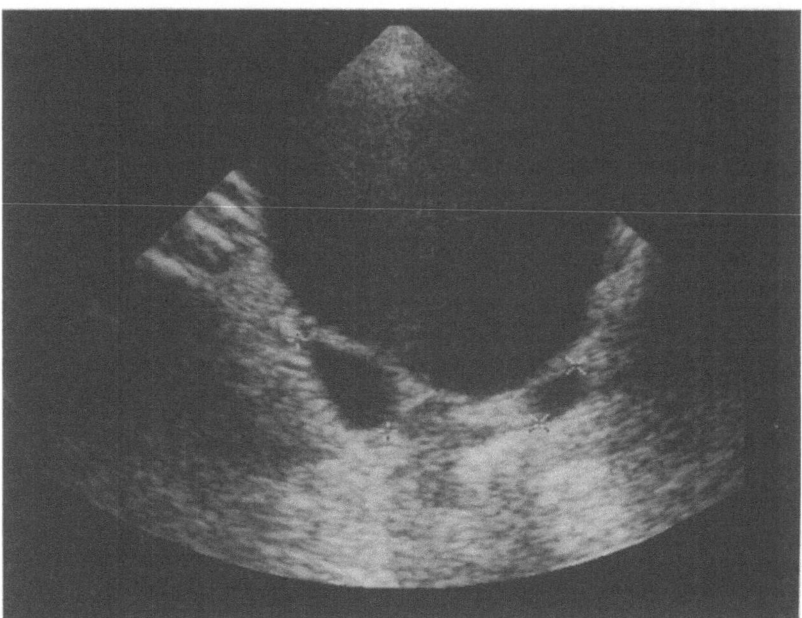

Fig. 12.3. Bilateral megaureter

12.2.3.2 Ureterolithiasis

Clinical Data

Colic, haematuria, frequency, and fever are common, particularly as a calculus passes down the ureter.

Sonographic Diagnosis

Criteria

→ Echogenic structure
→ Acoustic shadowing

Sonographic Differential Diagnosis

Calculi in the bladder are usually due to chronic incomplete bladder emptying and urine stasis.

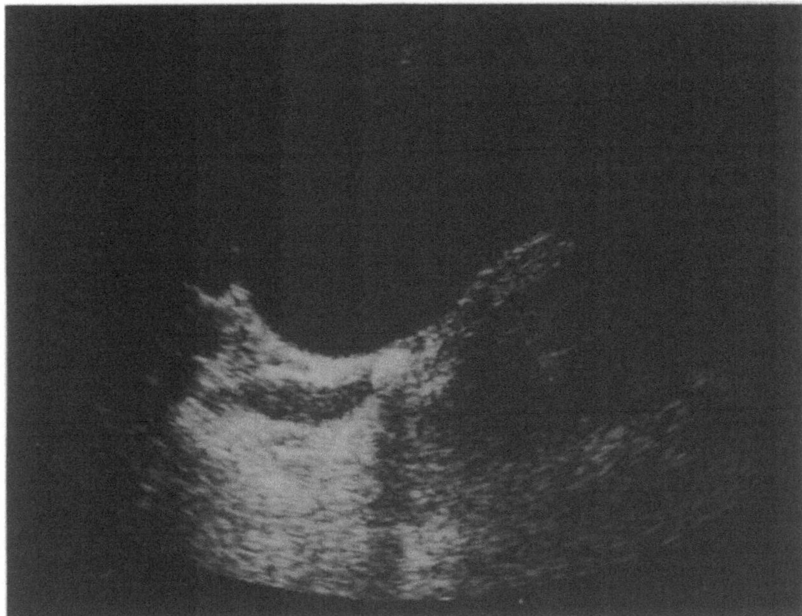

Fig. 12.4. Ureterolithiasis

12.2.3.3 Cystitis

Clinical Data

The patient complains of rapid onset of a severe burning discomfort on micturition, frequency, the passage of small volumes of cloudy urine and perhaps some blood. Fever, generalized aching, malaise.

Sonographic Diagnosis

Criterion

→ Bladder wall thickening

Sonographic Differential Diagnosis

The bladder wall thickness depends upon the degree of distension.

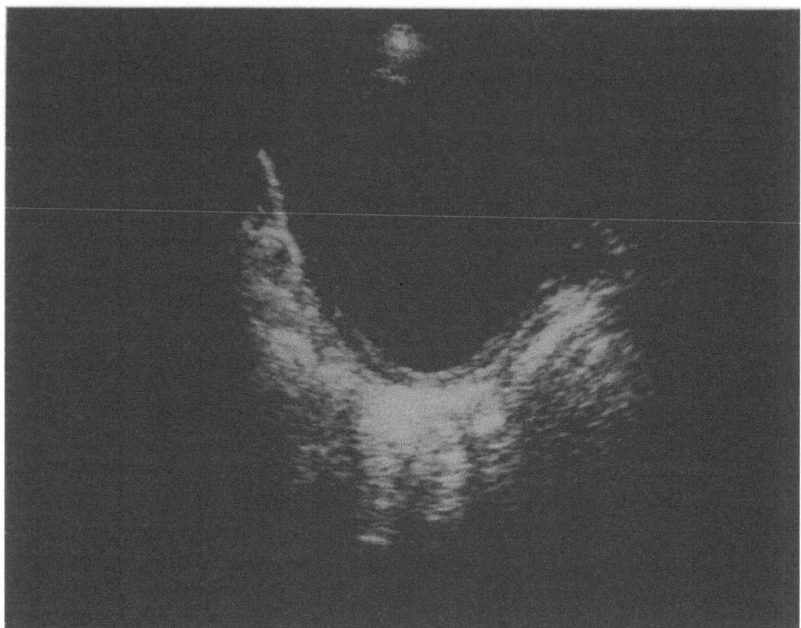

Fig. 12.5. Cystitis

12.2.3.4 Diverticula

Clinical Data

Classification:
◆ Congenital
◆ Acquired
  – Bladder outflow obstruction
  – Neurogenic bladder

Diverticula may be the source of recurrent urinary tract infection, hydronephrosis, calculi, and carcinoma of the bladder. Symptoms of diverticula are usually referable to the causative pathology.

Sonographic Diagnosis

Criteria
→ Anechoic structure around the bladder
→ Increase in size during micturition

Diverticula may contain clot, debris, calculi or tumour.

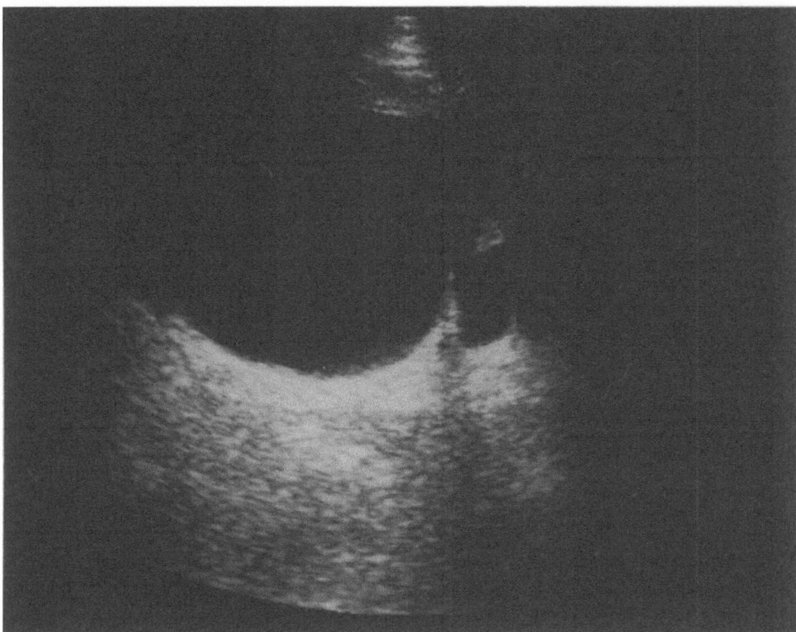

Fig. 12.6. Bladder diverticulum

Sonographic Differential Diagnosis

Cystic structures in the lower abdomen:
- Bladder diverticulum
- Megaureter
- Ureterocele
- Ovarian cyst
- Haematoma
- Abscess
- Lymph node
- Loculated ascites

Perivesical fluid is found in pelvic ascites, haematoma, abscess, urinoma, and after ovulation.

12.2.3.5 Carcinoma

Clinical Data

Haematuria is the classical symptom. Suprapubic or perineal pain may be a feature of the more extensive infiltrating lesions. Occasionally, patients present with symptoms and signs of widespread metastases.

Sonographic Diagnosis

Criteria

→ Usually hyperechoic mass protruding into the bladder lumen
→ Irregular border
→ Wall deformity
→ Loss of continuity of normal bladder wall echoes

The tumour may extend into the perivesical fat.

Sonographic Differential Diagnosis

Intraluminal bladder masses:
◆ Bladder carcinoma
◆ Prostatic hyperplasia
◆ Prostatic carcinoma
◆ Foreign body
◆ Catheter
◆ Clot
◆ Stone
◆ Polyp

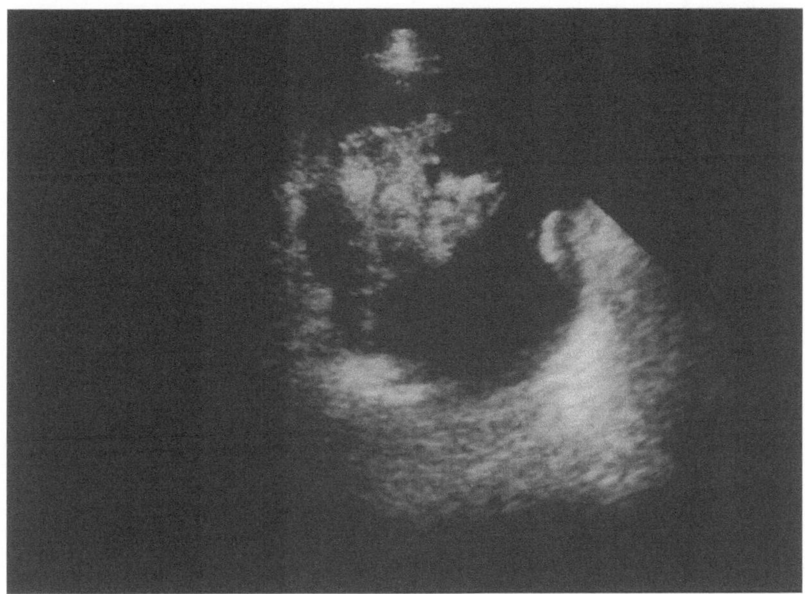

Fig. 12.7. Bladder carcinoma. Note the cauliflower-like growth pattern of this neoplasm

12.2.4 Checklist for Reporting

Bladder
- **Volume**
  - **Before micturition**
  - **After micturition**
- **Shape**
- **Wall thickness**
- **Echopattern**

Chapter **13** **Prostate**

13.1 Imaging Modalities

Sonography is the method of choice to image the prostate. Imaging modalities are:

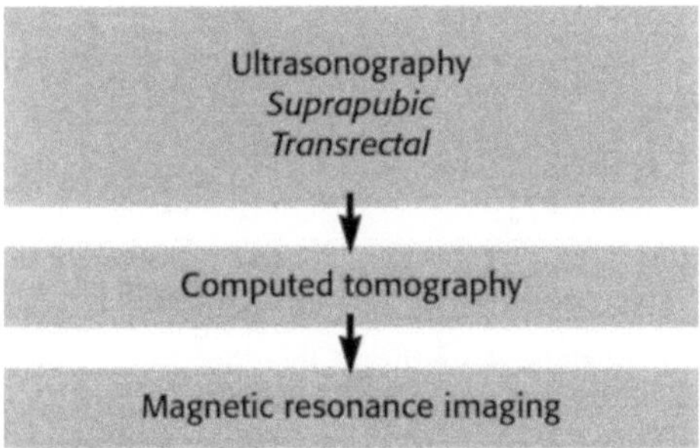

13.2 Ultrasonography

13.2.1 Examination Technique

The bladder should be full as it serves as an acoustic window for the examination of the prostate and the seminal vesicles. The patient is examined in a supine position.

The image quality of transrectal sonography is superior to that of suprapubic sonography because the transducers used in former have a higher frequency, making better resolution possible. Transrectal sonography with simultaneous prostatic biopsy allows accurate tissue diagnosis of prostatic lesions. It also plays an important role in staging carcinomas of the prostate.

13.2.2 Sonoanatomy

The prostate has
◆ A heterogeneous, slightly hyperechoic central zone
◆ A homogeneous, slightly hypoechoic peripheral zone

The seminal vesicles can be visualized behind and slightly above the prostate. They have a tubular shape and are usually hypoechoic.

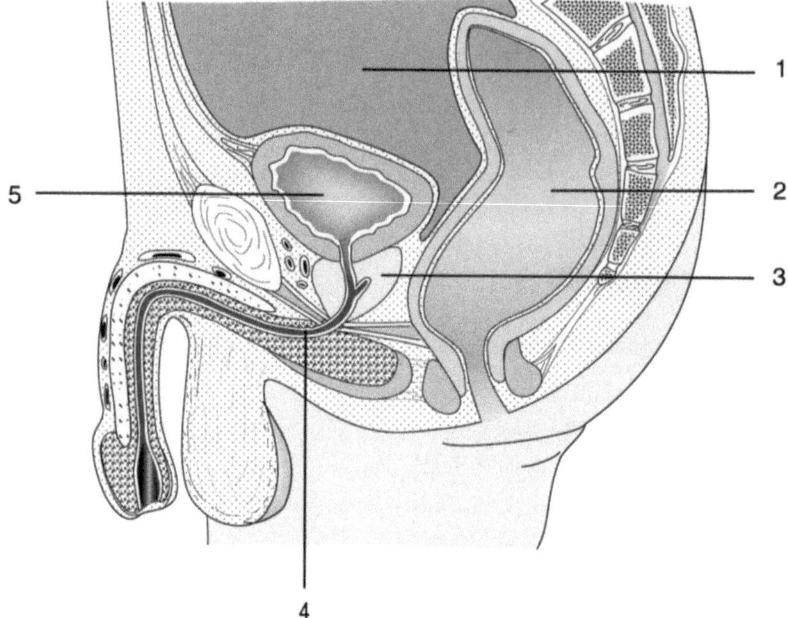

Fig. 13.1. Male pelvis. *1*, Abdomen; *2*, rectum; *3*, prostate; *4*, urethra; *5*, bladder

13.2.2.1 Normal Dimensions

Prostate and seminal vesicles:
◆ Prostate
 – Length < 3 cm
 – Width < 5 cm
 – Depth < 2.5 cm
◆ Seminal vesicles
 – Length < 5 cm
 – Width < 2 cm
 – Depth < 2 cm

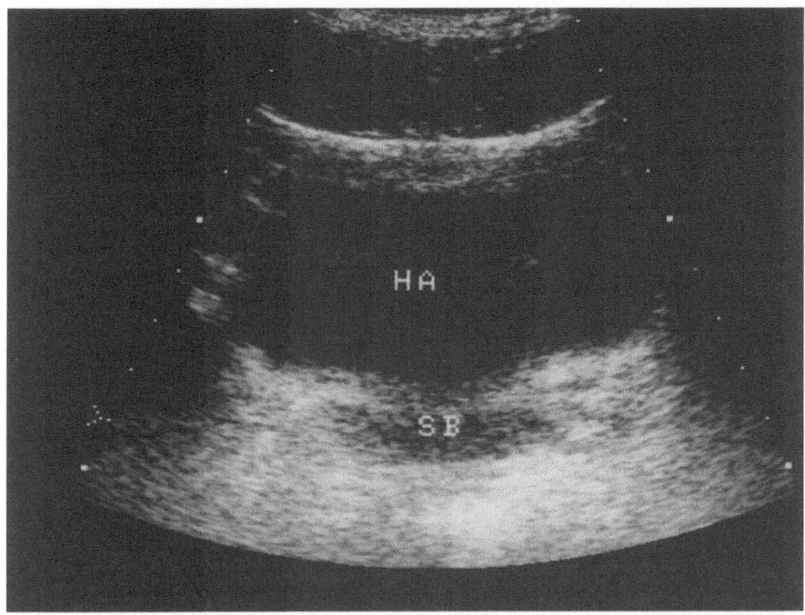

Fig. 13.2. Seminal vesicles. Transverse scan. *SB*, Seminal vesicles; *HA*, bladder

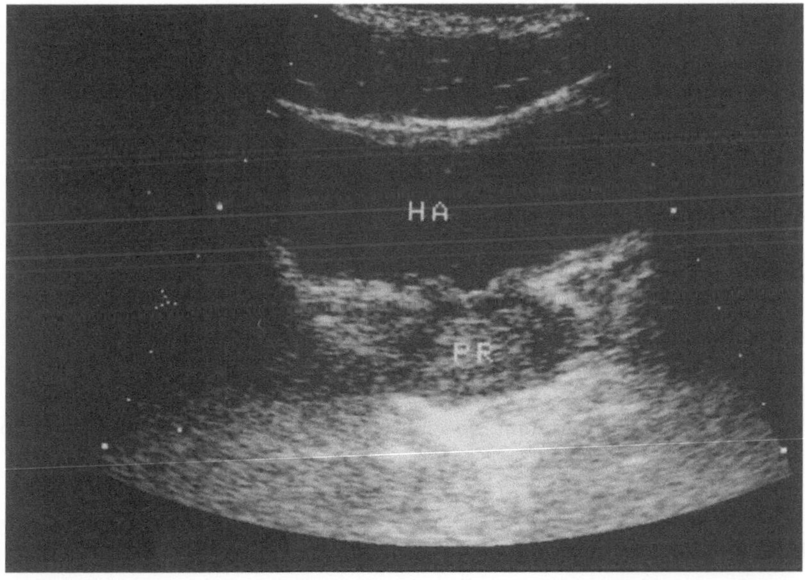

Fig. 13.3. Prostate. Transverse scan. *PR*, Prostate; *HA*, bladder

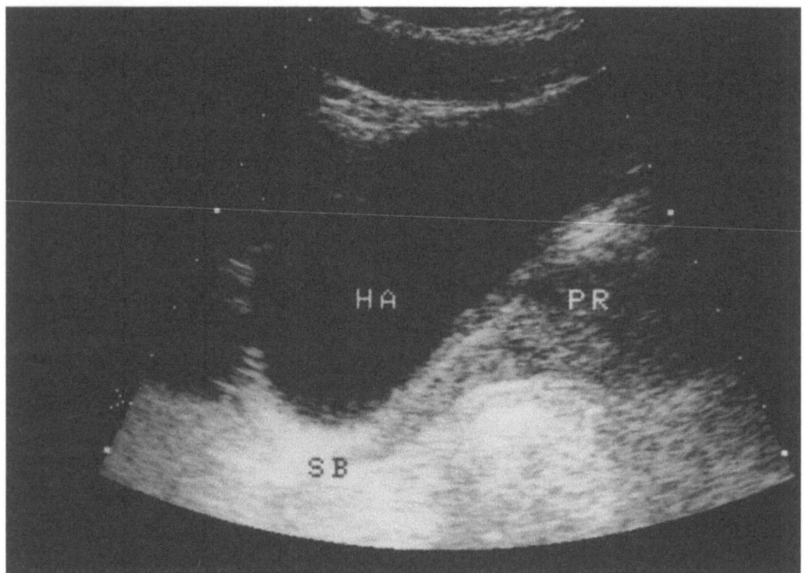

Fig. 13.4. Seminal vesicles and prostate. Longitudinal scan. *SB*, Seminal vesicles; *PR*, prostate; *HA*, bladder

13.2.3 Sonopathology

13.2.3.1 Hyperplasia

Clinical Data

The classical features are frequency, hesitancy, poor flow of urine, urgency, and nocturia.

Sonographic Diagnosis

Criteria

→ Arising in the central zone
→ Symmetrical enlargement
→ Homogeneous, isoechoic or hypoechoic echopattern

Prostatitis, stone formation, and infarction may give rise to an inhomogeneous echopattern.

Sonographic Differential Diagnosis

The most important differential diagnosis is prostatic carcinoma.

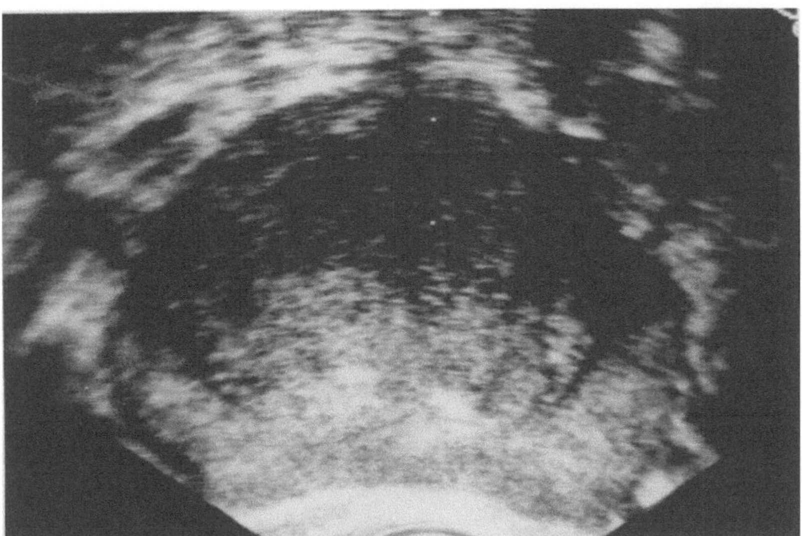

Fig. 13.5. Prostatic hyperplasia. Transrectal sonography

13.2.3.2 Carcinoma

Clinical Data

The symptoms are identical with those of prostatic obstruction due to benign hyperplasia. Hard, irregular gland. Pain from bone metastases may be a prominent feature, and, indeed, may predate obstructive symptoms.

Sonographic Diagnosis

Criteria

→ Arising in the peripheral zone
→ Asymmetrical enlargement
→ Inhomogeneous, hypoechoic echopattern

Sonographic Differential Diagnosis

Differential diagnosis:
◆ Prostatic hyperplasia
◆ Prostatitis
◆ Prostatic infarction

Predominantly hyperechoic masses are rarely malignant.

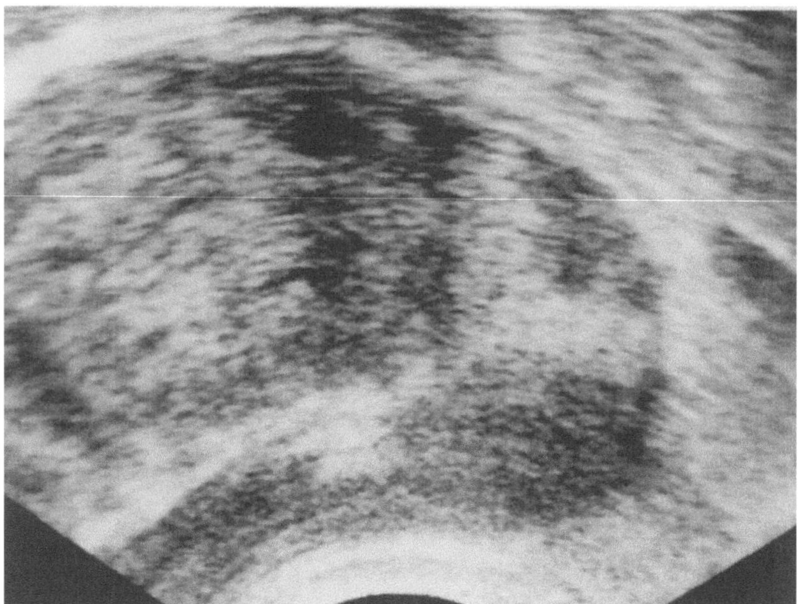

Fig. 13.6. Prostatic carcinoma. Transrectal sonography

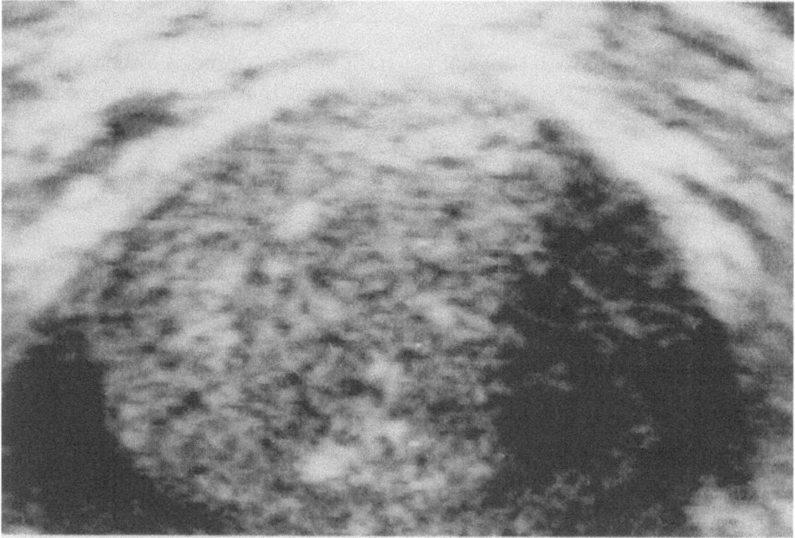

Fig. 13.7. Prostatic carcinoma. Transrectal sonography

13.2.4 Checklist for Reporting

Prostate
- Size
- Capsular continuity
- Gland outline
- Echopattern

Seminal vesicles
- Size
- Symmetry

Chapter 14 Scrotum

14.1 Imaging Modalities

Sonography is the method of choice to image the scrotum. Imaging modalities, are:

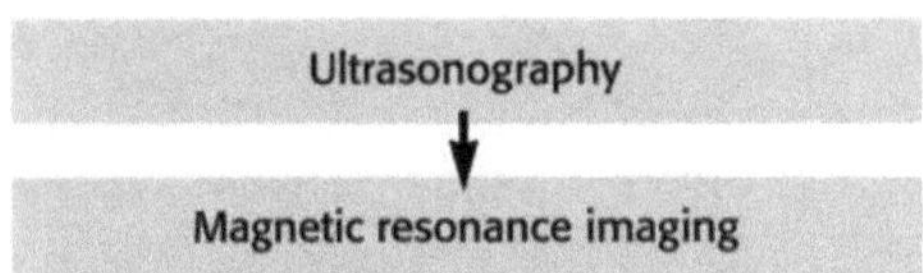

14.2 Ultrasonography

14.2.1 Examination Technique

The patient is scanned in the supine position. The examination is made with a 7.5-MHz linear probe in longitudinal and transverse sections. Both testicles should always be examined, their internal structure in particular.

14.2.2 Sonoanatomy

In the longitudinal plane the testicle has an ovoid and in the transverse plane a round shape. The contour is smooth, the echotexture homogeneous. A small volume of fluid between the visceral and parietal layers of the tunica vaginalis is normal.

The epididymis can be differentiated from the testis by two parallel echogenic lines; it has a coarse echopattern. The head of the epididymis is hyperechoic relative to the testis.

14.2.2.1 Normal Dimensions

Testicles:
- Length < 4 cm
- Width < 3 cm
- Depth < 3 cm

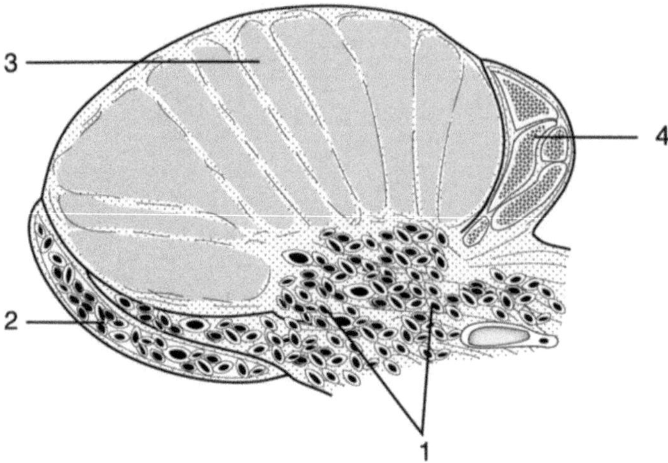

Fig. 14.1. Male genital organs. *1*, Pampiniform plexus; *2*, tail of epididymis; *3*, testicle; *4*, head of epididymis

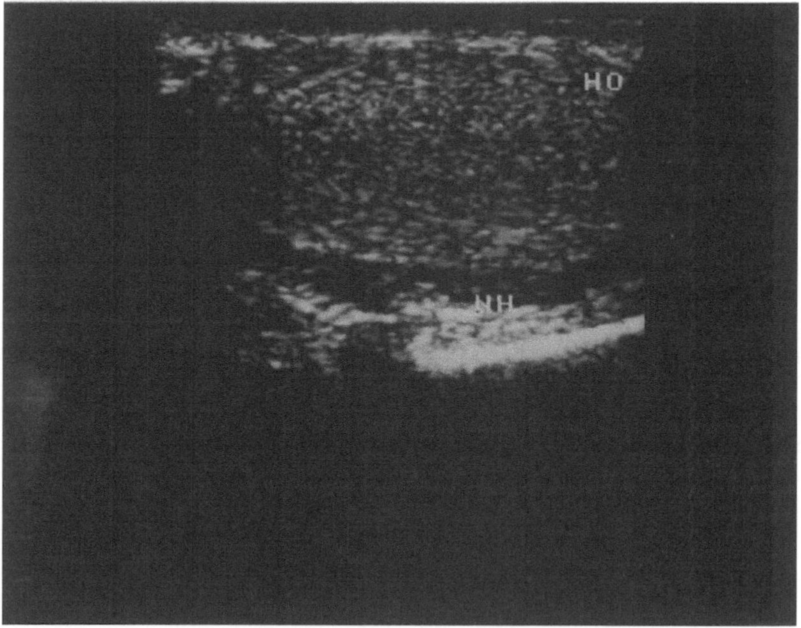

Fig. 14.2. Testicle and epididymis. *HO*, Testicle; *NH*, epididymis

14.2.3 Sonopathology

14.2.3.1 Hydrocele

Clinical Data

Aetiology:
- Epididymitis
- Orchitis
- Testicular torsion
- Testicular tumour

A hydrocele is elastic, fluctuant, and translucent. The scrotum enlarges slowly without pain or tenderness unless haemorrhage or infection has occurred.

Sonographic Diagnosis

Criteria

→ Anechoic, occasionally septate fluid collection around the testicle
→ Abnormally hyperechoic testicle relative to the fluid

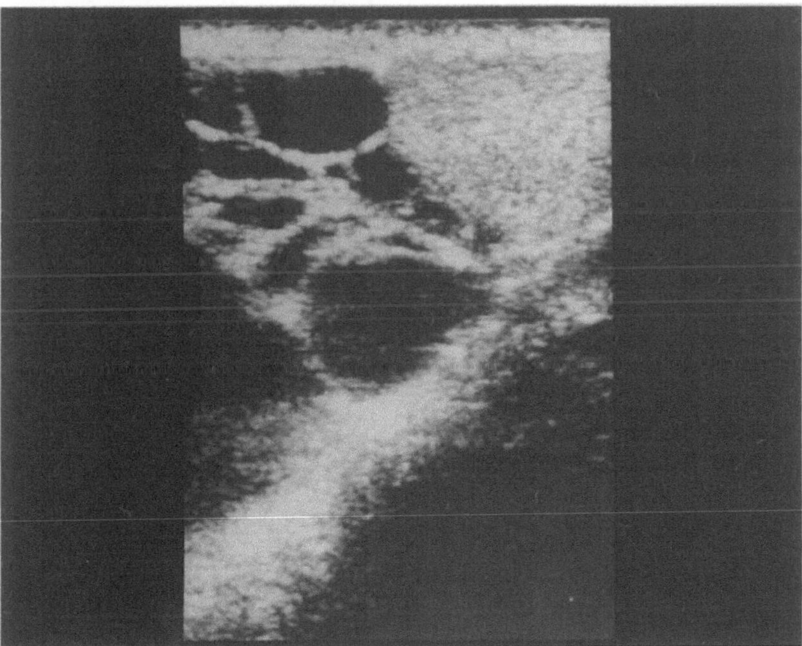

Fig. 14.3. Septate hydrocele

Sonographic Differential Diagnosis

Differential diagnosis:
◆ Scrotal hernia
◆ Haematocele
◆ Paratesticular abscess

14.2.3.2 Varicocele

Clinical Data

A varicocele is a collection of large veins, usually occurring in the left scrotum and feeling like a bag of worms. It is present in the upright position and should empty in the supine position. Very rarely, acute development of a varicocele may be a sign of malignant disease in the left kidney with obstruction of the spermatic vein on that side.

Sonographic Diagnosis

Criteria

→ Tortuous dilated veins arising from the pampiniform venous plexus
→ Augmentation during Valsalva's manoeuvre

Vessel size increases if the patient is examined when standing and performing a Valsalva's manoeuvre. As a left-sided varicocele can be secondary to renal carcinoma, the kidneys should be scanned as well.

Sonographic Differential Diagnosis

The appearance of multiple anechoic channels is typical.

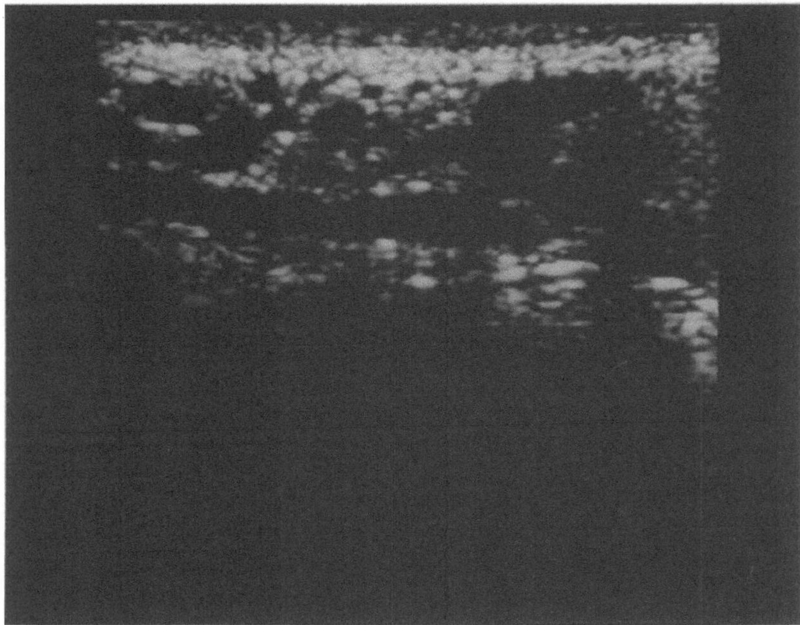

Fig. 14.4. Varicocele

14.2.3.3 Epididymitis

Clinical Data

Aetiology:
◆ Prostatitis
◆ Urethritis
◆ Gonorrhoea
◆ Catheter
◆ Surgery

The epididymis becomes very swollen and tender in acute inflammation. The scrotum may be reddened and oedematous.

The signs of epididymitis are closely similar to those of an acute torsion of the testis.

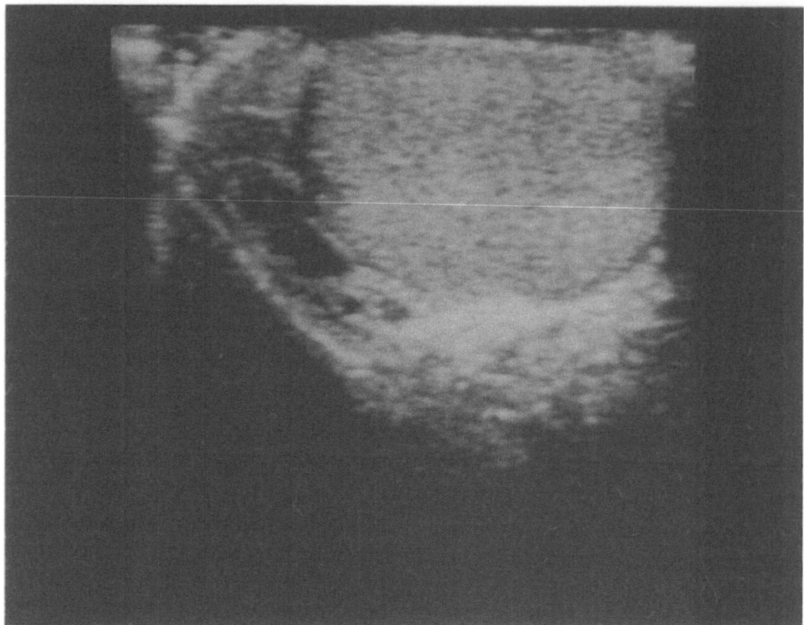

Fig. 14.5. Epididymitis. The testicle is not affected

Sonographic Diagnosis

Criteria

→ Enlarged, hypoechoic epididymis
→ Peritesticular fluid collection
→ Tenderness

Orchitis gives rise to an enlarged, hypoechoic testicle.

Sonographic Differential Diagnosis

The most important differential diagnosis is testicular torsion. In testicular torsion, colour Doppler shows decreased or absent flow in the testicular artery, whereas the flow is increased in epididymitis.

14.2.3.4 Haematoma

Clinical Data

Bleeding usually follows tapping of a hydrocele or an injury to the testis. In the acute phase there may be severe pain and tenderness.

Sonographic Diagnosis

Criterion

→ Complex mass appearance
  – Anechoic blood
  – Hyperechoic clot

Sonographic Differential Diagnosis

The history of a testicular trauma is important for the differential diagnosis.

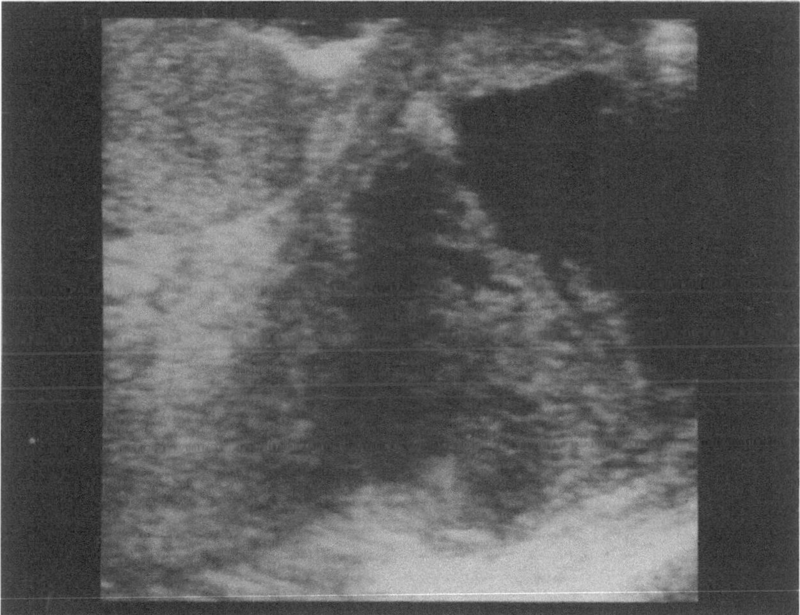

Fig. 14.6. Testicular haematoma. The testicle can be visualized despite the presence of haematoma

14.2.3.5 Seminoma

Clinical Data

The testis becomes enlarged, hard, insensitive, and heavy.

Sonographic Diagnosis

Criterion

→ Well-defined, homogeneous, and hypoechoic mass

As synchronous or metachronous tumours are found in 4% of the patients, both testicles should always be scanned.

Sonographic Differential Diagnosis

Differential diagnosis:
◆ Torsion
◆ Infarction
◆ Orchitis
◆ Abscess
◆ Haematoma

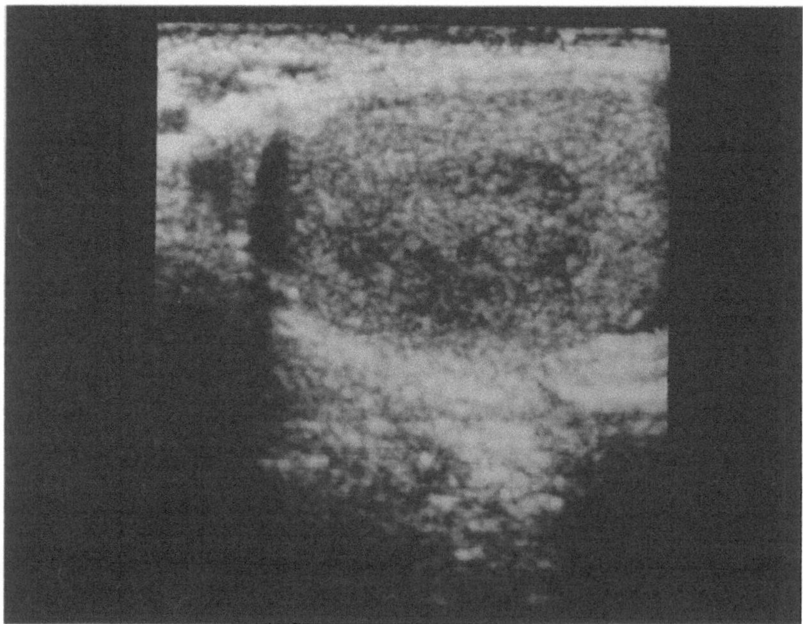

Fig. 14.7. Seminoma. Seminomas account for 50% of primary testicular tumours

14.2.3.6 Teratoma

Clinical Data

Teratoma is the commonest testicular tumour in children whilst seminoma is the commonest in adults.

Sonographic Diagnosis

Criterion

→ Irregular, inhomogeneous, and complex mass
  – Solid areas
  – Cystic areas

Echogenic areas with acoustic shadowing are usually due to cartilaginous or bony elements.

Sonographic Differential Diagnosis

Over the age of 60 years testicular neoplasms are mainly lymphomas or metastases. Intratesticular lesions must be considered malignant until proven otherwise.

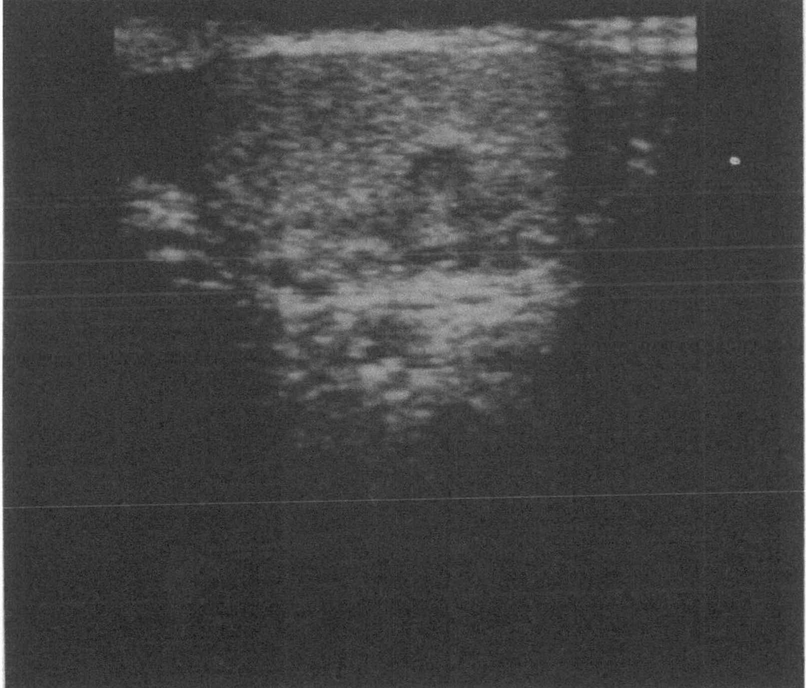

Fig. 14.8. Teratoma. Teratomas account for 10% of primary testicular tumours

14.2.4 Checklist for Reporting

Testicles
- Size
- Contour
- Echopattern

Epididymis
- Size

Spermatic cord

Chapter 15 Uterus

15.1 Imaging Modalities

Sonography is the method of choice to image the uterus. Imaging modalities are:

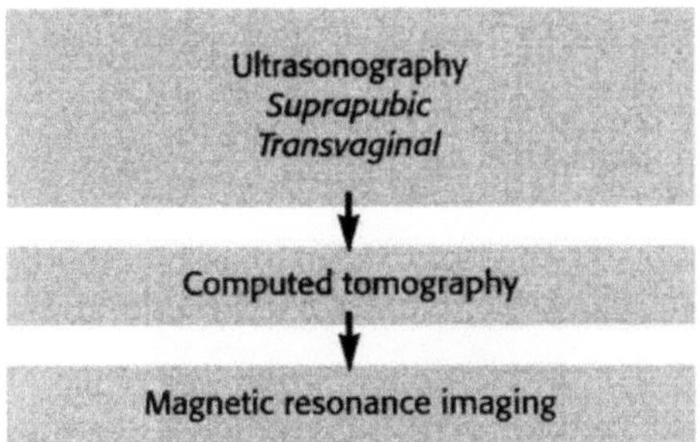

15.2 Ultrasonography

15.2.1 Examination Technique

Gynaecological-obstetrical sonography should be carried out by a specialist. But all sonographers should have a knowledge of the ultrasound anatomy and pathology of the female genital tract to ensure a comprehensive preliminary examination for lower abdominal pain. Similarly, a basic knowledge of the possibilities and limitations of breast sonography is desirable.

It is essential for any patient undergoing pelvic ultrasound to have a full bladder to act as a window through which the pelvic structures can be seen. The patient is examined in supine position with a 3.5- and 5-MHz convex transducer. A sector probe can be used as well. Scans are usually made in the longitudinal and transverse planes.

Transvaginal sonography is far superior to suprapubic.

15.2.2 Sonoanatomy

On a midline longitudinal scan the vagina can be recognized as a tubular structure, with a central linear echo arising from the opposing vaginal surfaces. The uterus lies immediately behind the bladder, and the body of the uterus can be seen to be in conti-

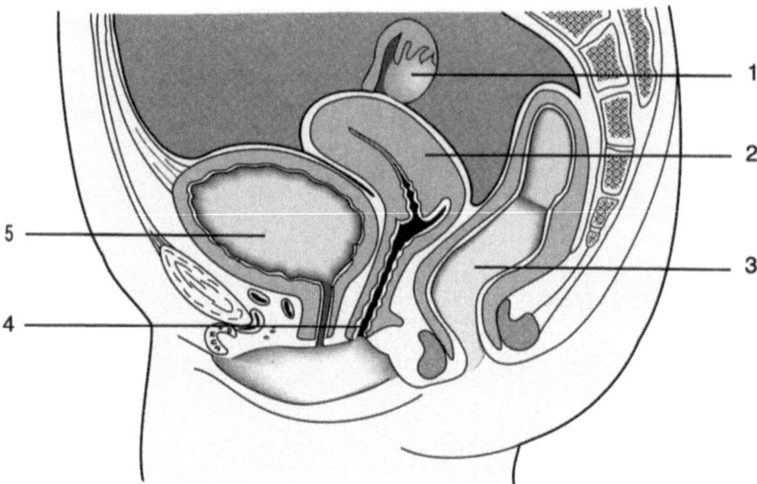

Fig. 15.1. Female pelvis. *1*, Ovary; *2*, uterus; *3*, rectum; *4*, vagina; *5*, bladder

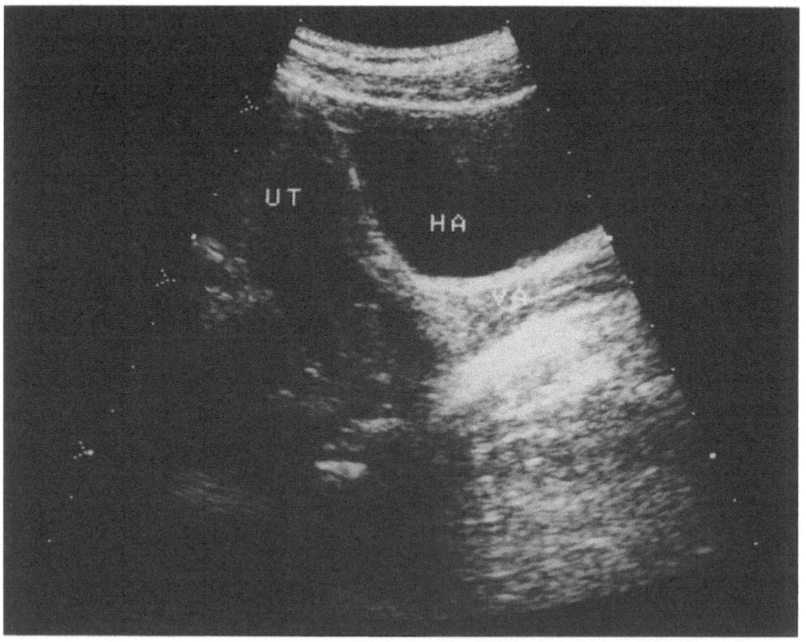

Fig. 15.2. Uterus. Longitudinal scan. *UT*, Uterus; *VA*, vagina; *HA*, bladder

nuity with the cervix and vagina. The myometrium is rather hypoechoic, whereas the endometrial cavity is echogenic.

The precise appearances of the uterus depend upon the age and parity of the patient and also the lie of the uterus. The body of uterus is usually anteflexed or angled slightly forwards in relation to the cervix. The whole uterus is normally anteverted.

Uterine malformations:
◆ Uterus didelphys
◆ Uterus bicornis
◆ Septate uterus

The normal Fallopian tubes are too small to be visualized sonographically.

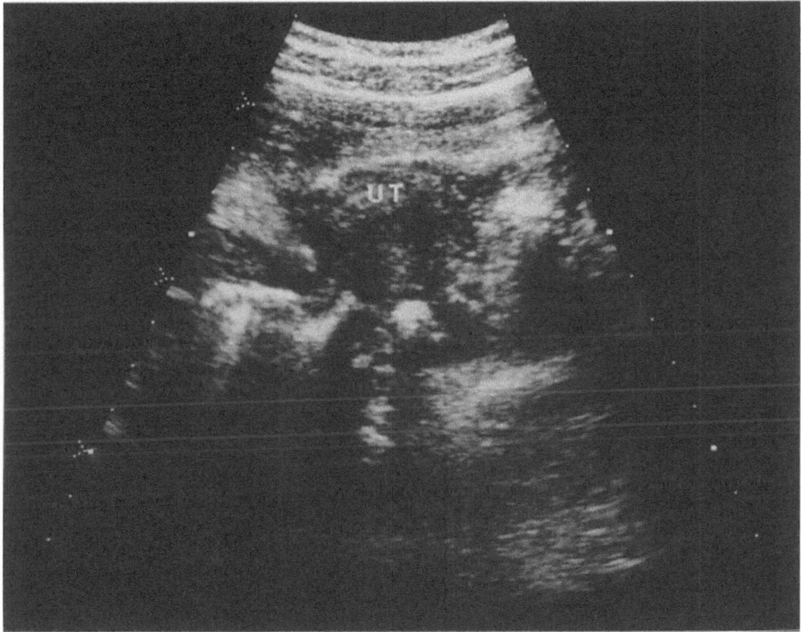

Fig. 15.3. Uterus. Transverse scan. *UT*, Uterus

15.2.2.1 Normal Dimensions

Uterus:
- ◆ Prepuberal
  - Length < 3 cm
  - Width < 1 cm
  - Depth < 1 cm
- ◆ Nullipara
  - Length < 8 cm
  - Width < 4 cm
  - Depth < 4 cm
- ◆ Multipara
  - Length < 9.5 cm
  - Width < 5.5 cm
  - Depth < 5.5 cm
- ◆ Postmenopausal
  - Length < 6 cm
  - Width < 2 cm
  - Depth < 2 cm

15.2.3 Sonopathology

15.2.3.1 Fibroids

Clinical Data

Uterine fibroids are localized proliferations of smooth muscle. Fibroids are often multiple causing lobular uterine enlargement. Patients may present with dysmenorrhoea, painful defecation or dysuria.

Sonographic Diagnosis

Criteria

- → Lobular enlargement
- → Inhomogeneous, hypoechoic masses
- → Anechoic areas due to haemorrhage or necrosis
- → Echogenic foci with acoustic shadowing due to calcification

The endometrial canal may be deviated or even masked.

Sonographic Differential Diagnosis

Pedunculated fibroids may be indistinguishable from ovarian carcinoma.

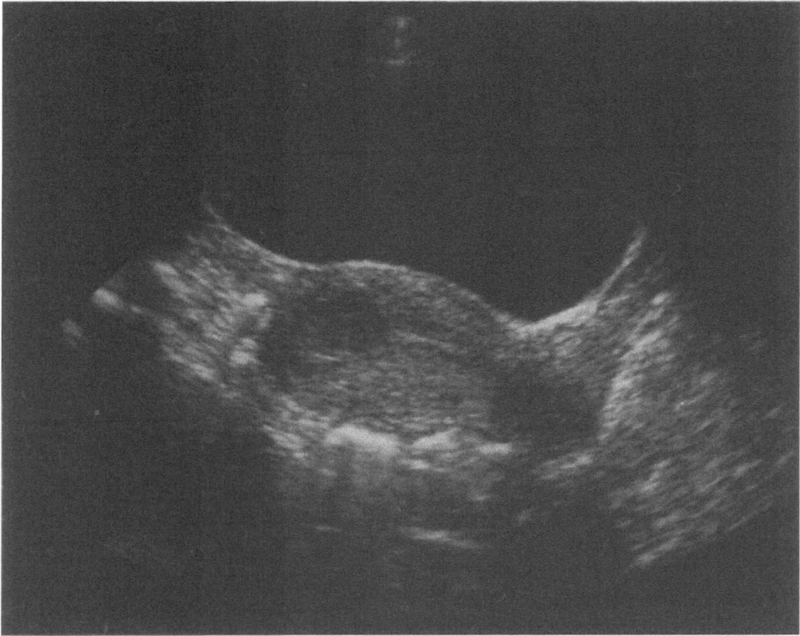

Fig. 15.4. Uterine fibroids. The scan shows two hypoechoic masses in the myometrium

15.2.3.2 Carcinoma

Clinical Data

The cardinal symptom of endometrial carcinoma is inappropriate uterine bleeding, such as any postmenopausal bleeding or recurrent metrorrhagia in the premenopausal patient. The presence of fibroids should not engender complacency regarding abnormal bleeding. A mucoid or watery discharge may precede bleeding by several weeks or months.

Sonographic Diagnosis

Criteria

→ Uterine enlargement
→ Abnormal echotexture
→ Distorted canal

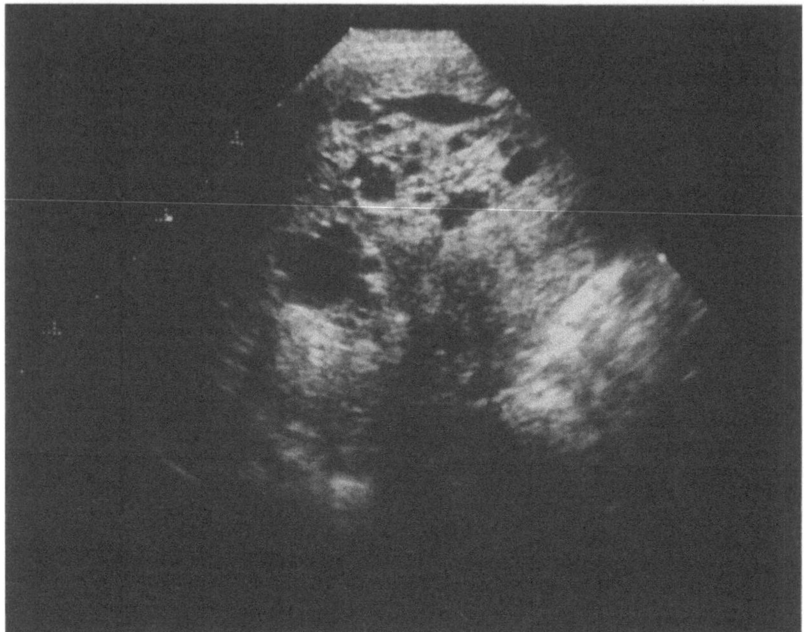

Fig. 15.5. Endometrial carcinoma

Sonographic Differential Diagnosis

The endometrium thickens during the normal menstrual cycle. No endometrium is discernible in the prepuberal or postmenopausal state.

Increased endometrial thickness:
◆ Endometrial carcinoma
◆ Endometrial hyperplasia
◆ Endometrial polyp
◆ Intrauterine pregnancy
◆ Ectopic pregnancy
◆ Oestrogen excess

15.2.4 Checklist for Reporting

Uterus
- Position
- Size
- Contour
- Echopattern

Periuterine space

Chapter 16 Ovaries

16.1 Imaging Modalities

Sonography is the method of choice to image the ovaries. Imaging modalities, are:

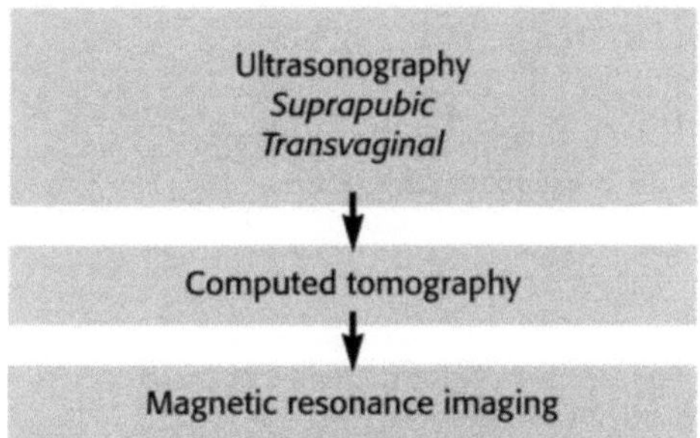

16.2 Ultrasonography

16.2.1 Examination Technique

The ovaries are best imaged when the bladder is full. Also, the intestine should be empty because the left ovary is often hidden behind the filled sigmoid colon. The examination takes place in a supine position with 3.5- and 5-MHz convex or sector transducers. In the transverse section the uterus and the ovaries can mostly be displayed jointly; otherwise the left and right ovaries can be found by moving the transducer cranially and caudally. The ovarian vessels, entering cranio-laterally, are the guiding structures to the ovaries which may have various positions.

16.2.2 Sonoanatomy

The ovaries are suspended from the broad ligament and usually lie lateral to the uterus near the side walls of the pelvis.

The endocrine changes during the menstrual cycle have a great effect on the appearance of the ovaries. During the early phase, several cystic structures are seen representing developing follicles. Around the eighth day of the cycle, one follicle becomes dominant and may reach 2–2.5 cm in diameter prior to ovulation. At ovulation, the follicle

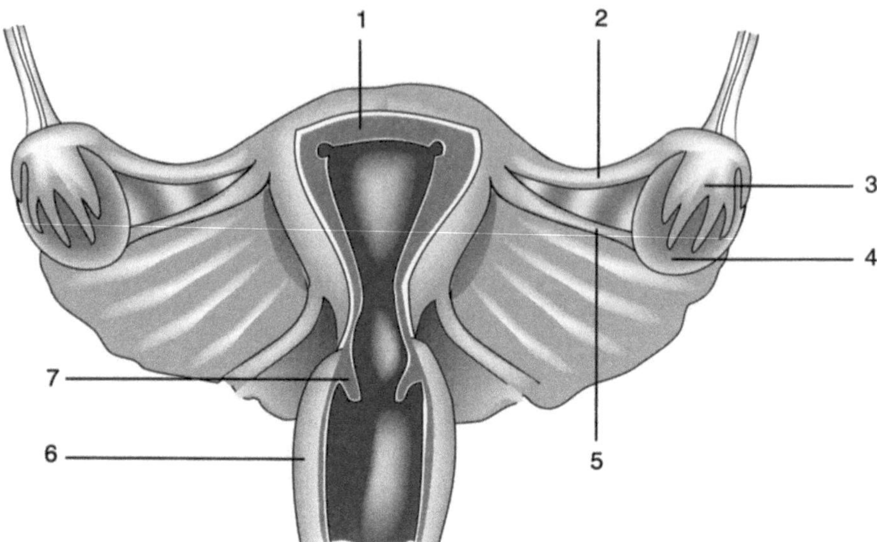

Fig. 16.1. Female genital organs. *1*, Body of uterus; *2*, Fallopian tube; *3*, fimbria; *4*, ovary; *5*, ligament of the ovary; *6*, vagina; *7*, neck of uterus

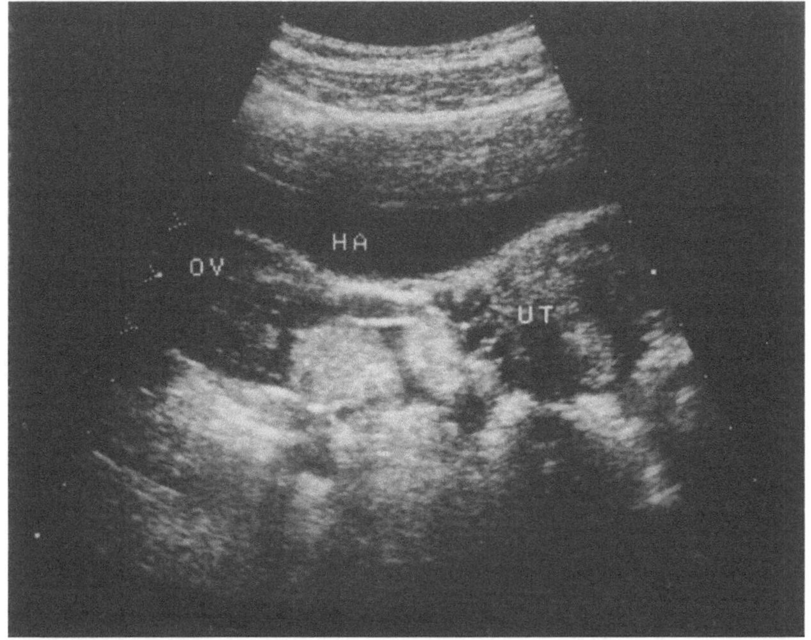

Fig. 16.2. Ovary. *OV*, Ovary; *UT*, uterus; *HA*, bladder

ruptures and immediately decreases in size giving rise to the corpus luteum which degenerates if there is no intervening pregnancy. Immediately after follicle rupture, a small amount of fluid may be visible in the pelvis.

16.2.2.1 Normal Dimensions

Ovaries:
- Prepuberal
  - Length < 2.5 cm
  - Width < 2.5 cm
  - Depth < 2.5 cm
- Puberty
  - Length < 4 cm
  - Width < 2.5 cm
  - Depth < 2.5 cm
- Postmenopausal
  - Length < 3 cm
  - Width < 1.5 cm
  - Depth < 1.5 cm

16.2.3 Sonopathology

16.2.3.1 Cysts

Clinical Data

Ovarian cysts are frequently asymptomatic, but the pressure of an abdominal mass may cause discomfort, aching or heaviness.

Polycystic ovary syndrome:
- Amenorrhoea
- Infertility
- Obesity
- Hirsutism

Sonographic Diagnosis

Criteria

→ Spherical or oval anechoic lesion
→ Sharp and well-defined border
→ Distal acoustic enhancement
→ Prominent posterior border

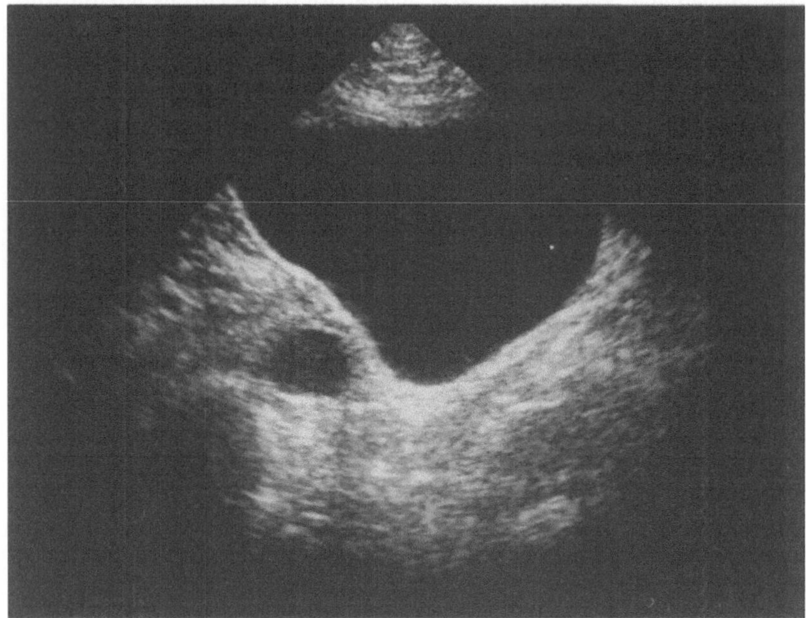

Fig. 16.3. Ovarian cyst

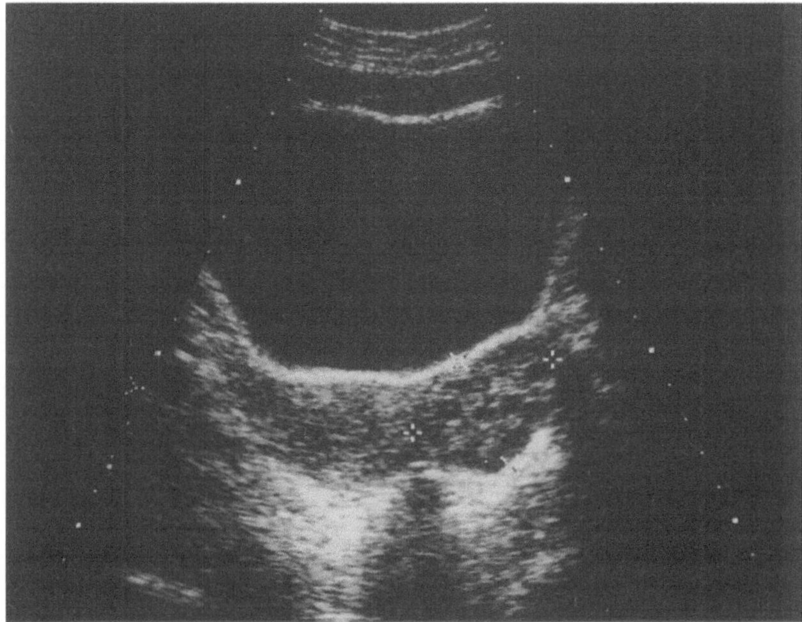

Fig. 16.4. Polycystic ovary syndrome

Physiological cysts show changing dimensions and resolve after ovulation. They may be up to 3 cm in diameter just before ovulation. In polycystic ovary syndrome the ovaries are enlarged and show discrete cysts. An apparently normal ultrasound scan, however, does not exclude the diagnosis. 10% of women with polycystic ovaries develop ovarian tumours.

Sonographic Differential Diagnosis

Cystic ovarian mass:
- Follicular cyst
- Paraovarian cyst
- Corpus luteum cyst
- Theca lutein cyst
- Polycystic ovary syndrome
- Cystic tumour
- Ectopic pregnancy
- Loculated ascites
- Bowel loop

Bilateral ovarian enlargement:
- Polycystic ovary syndrome
- Cystic disease
- Ovarian tumour

16.2.3.2 Endometriosis

Clinical Data

The clinical manifestations of endometriosis are pelvic pain, pelvic mass, dysmenorrhoea, and infertility. Midline pelvic pain pre- or perimenstrually, particularly beginning after several years of pain-free menses, may occur. Such dysmenorrhoea is an important diagnostic clue. Endometriotic implants on the ovary can form an endometrioma, i.e. a cystic mass of endometriosis localized to an ovary, giving rise to a pelvic mass. Occasionally, rupture or leakage from an endometrioma may be associated with acute abdominal pain.

Sonographic Diagnosis

Criterion

→ Hyperechoic, complex, hypoechoic or anechoic lesion

The sonographic appearance depends upon the state of the blood within the cyst. Fresh blood is anechoic but becomes hyperechoic as it clots.

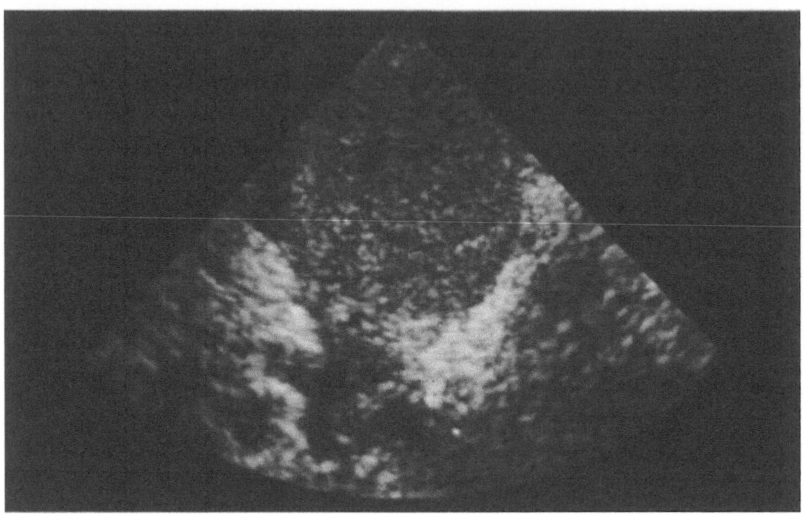

Fig. 16.5. Chocolate cyst of the ovary

Sonographic Differential Diagnosis

Chocolate cysts may be impossible to differentiate from solid masses. The most important differential diagnoses are mucinous cystadenoma and cystadenocarcinoma.

16.2.3.3 Dermoid

Clinical Data

Dermoids are tumours originating from the germ cells which can produce almost all known tissue components of the body, for example, hair, teeth, and fat. They may be bilateral.

Sonographic Diagnosis

Criteria

→ Usually hyperechoic lesion
→ Frequently acoustic shadowing
→ Variable appearance due to tissue components
   - Hair
   - Teeth
   - Fat

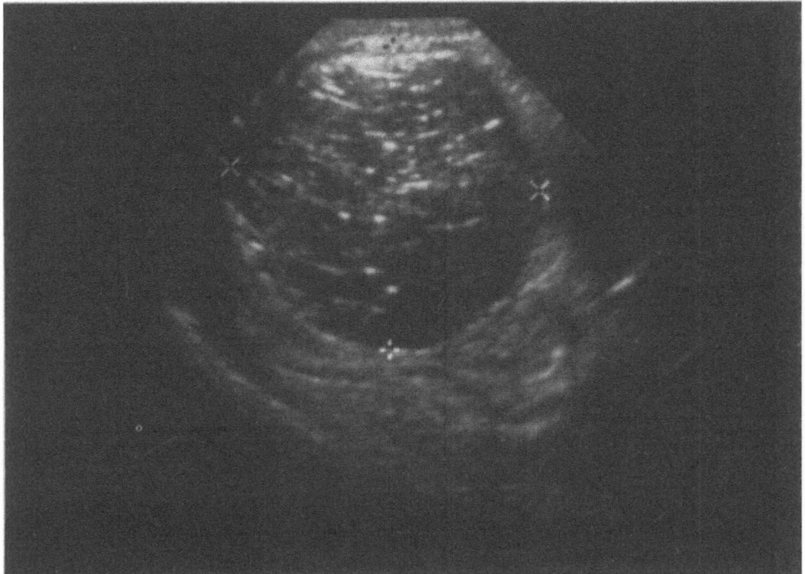

Fig. 16.6. Ovarian dermoid

Sonographic Differential Diagnosis

Differential diagnosis:
◆ Calcified uterine fibroid
◆ Bowel loop

16.2.3.4 Carcinoma

Clinical Data

An ovary may grow to considerable size before clinical signs appear. The earliest symptoms are lower abdominal discomfort and mild digestive complaints. Abdominal swelling due to ovarian enlargement or ascitic fluid, pain, anaemia, and cachexia occur very late in the course.

Meig's syndrome:
◆ Ovarian tumour
◆ Hydrothorax
◆ Ascites

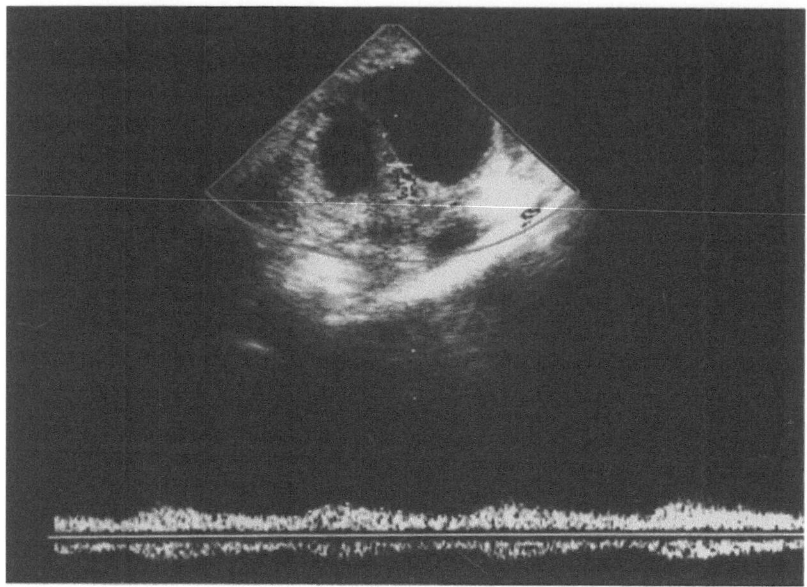

Fig. 16.7. Ovarian carcinoma

Sonographic Diagnosis

Criteria

→ Multiloculated cyst
  – Cyst with solid component
  – Cyst with thick septa
→ Ascites

Sonography is a sensitive means of detecting ovarian masses. Benign and malignant tumours, however, cannot be reliably differentiated by ultrasonography. A unilocular cyst with a diameter of less than 5 cm is nearly always benign.

Sonographic Differential Diagnosis

Pelvic and adnexal masses:
◆ Uterine mass
◆ Tubal mass
◆ Ovarian mass
◆ Bladder mass
◆ Bowel mass
◆ Pelvic mass
◆ Ectopic pregnancy

◆ Vascular anomalies
◆ Endometriosis
◆ Abscess
◆ Haematoma
◆ Lymphocele

16.2.4 Checklist for Reporting

Ovaries
• **Position**
• **Size**
• **Contour**
• **Echopattern**

Chapter 17 Breast

17.1 Imaging Modalities

Imaging modalities are:

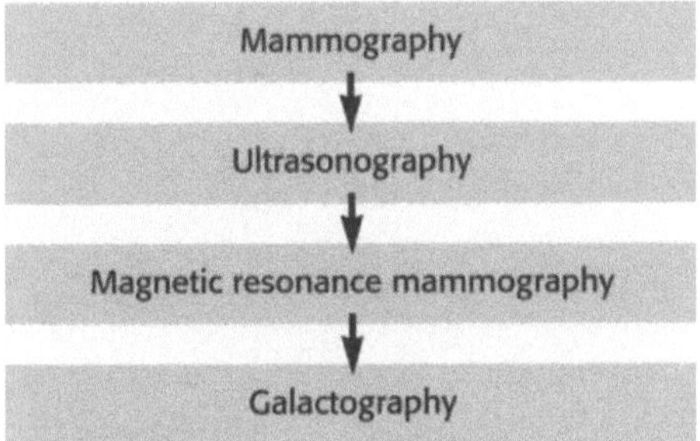

17.2 Ultrasonography

17.2.1 Examination Technique

Sonography is a valuable adjunct to clinical examination and mammography for determining the size and location of a lesion, especially in young women with dense breasts and women who have undergone augmentation mammoplasty. It is excellent for the guidance of cytologic aspirations. Sonography of the breast is mainly used in the differential diagnosis of masses already detected by palpation or mammography. Cystic and solid structures can be differentiated from a size of 3 mm. The accuracy of breast ultrasound in differentiating benign from malignant masses depends upon the presence of typical sonographic criteria.

The patient is examined lying slightly on the left or right side. The arm of the side to be examined is positioned behind the head. The examination is carried out with a 7.5-MHz transducer and with gentle compression of the breast. Every quadrant must be examined thoroughly. The region immediately posterior to the nipple is difficult to assess.

With ultrasound of the breast no clearly defined or exactly reproducible section levels can be recommended. For documentation purposes the following information is therefore needed:

◆ Side
◆ Quadrant
◆ Landmarks
  - Distance from the nipple
  - Distance from the sternum
  - Distance from the clavicle
  - Distance from the ribs

17.2.2 Sonoanatomy

The parenchymal tissue of the breast is embedded between the hyperechoic skin and the hypoechoic subcutaneous tissue anteriorly, and the pectoral fascia and the pectoralis muscle posteriorly.

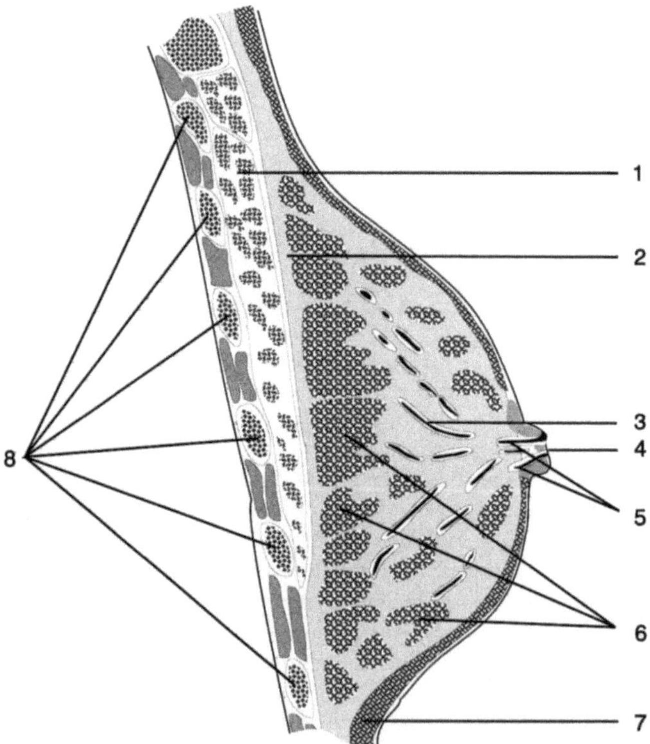

Fig. 17.1. Breast. *1*, Pectoralis major muscle; *2*, pectoral fascia; *3*, lactiferous duct; *4*, nipple; *5*, lactiferous sinuses; *6*, parenchymal tissue; *7*, subcutaneous fat; *8*, ribs

◆ Breast in young women
- High content of connective tissue
- Homogeneous, hyperechoic parenchymal tissue
◆ Breast in older women
- High content of fatty tissue
- Inhomogeneous, hypoechoic parenchymal tissue

17.2.2.1 Normal Dimensions

Breast:
◆ Lactiferous ducts < 2 mm

17.2.3 Sonopathology

17.2.3.1 Cysts

Clinical Data

Cysts are usually asymptomatic.

Sonographic Diagnosis

Criteria

→ Spherical or oval anechoic lesion
→ Sharp and well-defined border
→ Distal acoustic enhancement
→ Prominent posterior border

Breast cysts can also be multiloculated and septic.

Sonographic Differential Diagnosis

Cystic structures with internal echoes:
◆ Reverberation
◆ After aspiration
◆ After biopsy
◆ Haemorrhage
◆ Abscess
◆ Breast carcinoma
◆ Tumour necrosis

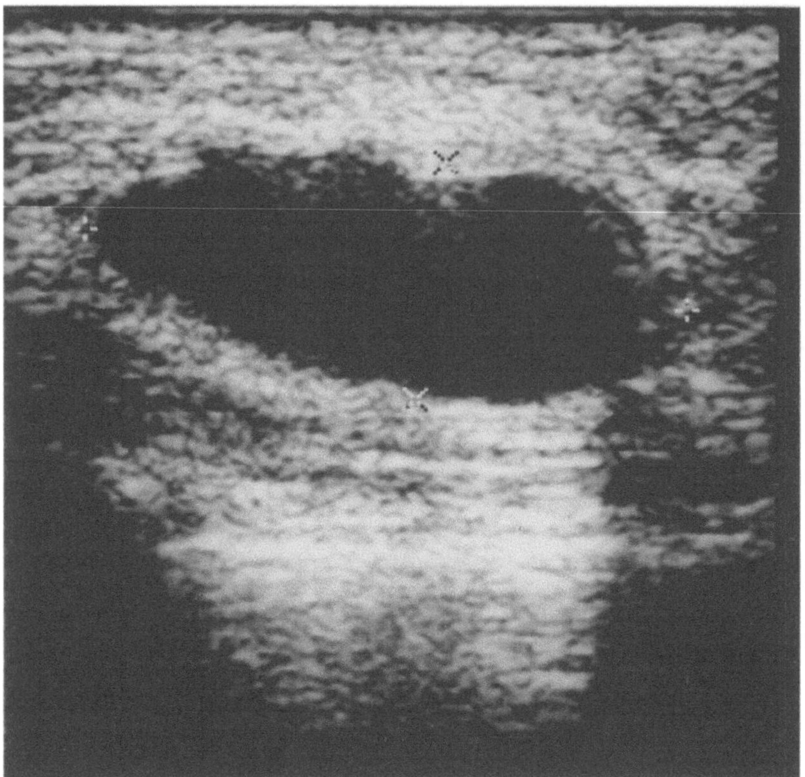

Fig. 17.2. Breast cyst

17.2.3.2 Fibroadenoma

Clinical Data

Fibroadenomas are the most common benign breast tumours. As a pathologic entity they rank third behind fibrocystic disease and carcinoma, respectively. These tumours, seen most frequently in young women, have a firm, rubbery consistency and are well circumscribed.

Sonographic Diagnosis

Criteria
→ Oval hypoechoic mass
→ Smooth, hyperechoic border
→ Slight acoustic enhancement

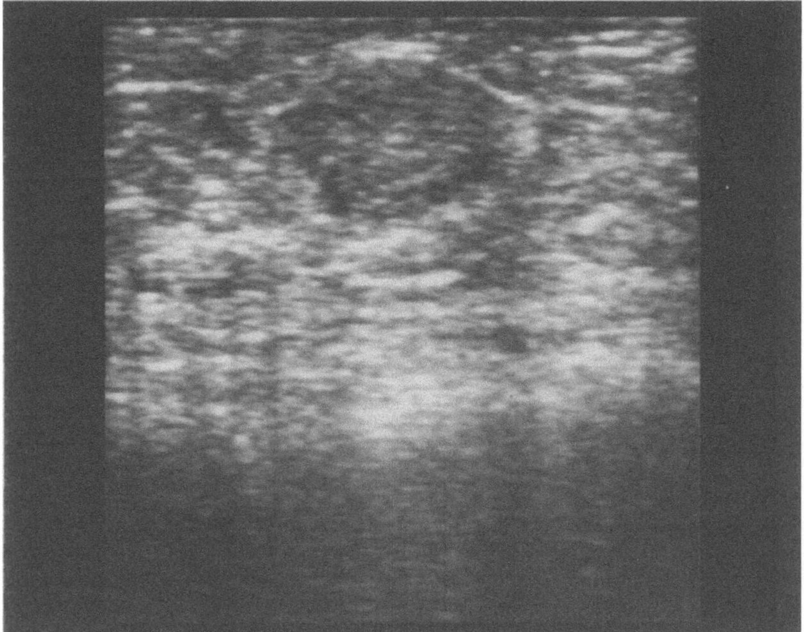

Fig. 17.3. Breast fibroadenoma

Calcifications may occur in fibroadenomas; they are seen as echogenic foci with distal acoustic shadowing.

Sonographic Differential Diagnosis

Breast carcinoma.

17.2.3.3 Carcinoma

Clinical Data

Most breast cancers appear as a slow-growing, painless mass, though a vague discomfort may be present. Retracted nipple, bleeding from the nipple, distorted areola. Attachment of the mass to surrounding tissues, including the underlying fascia and the overlying skin. Axillary and supraclavicular lymph nodes may be present.

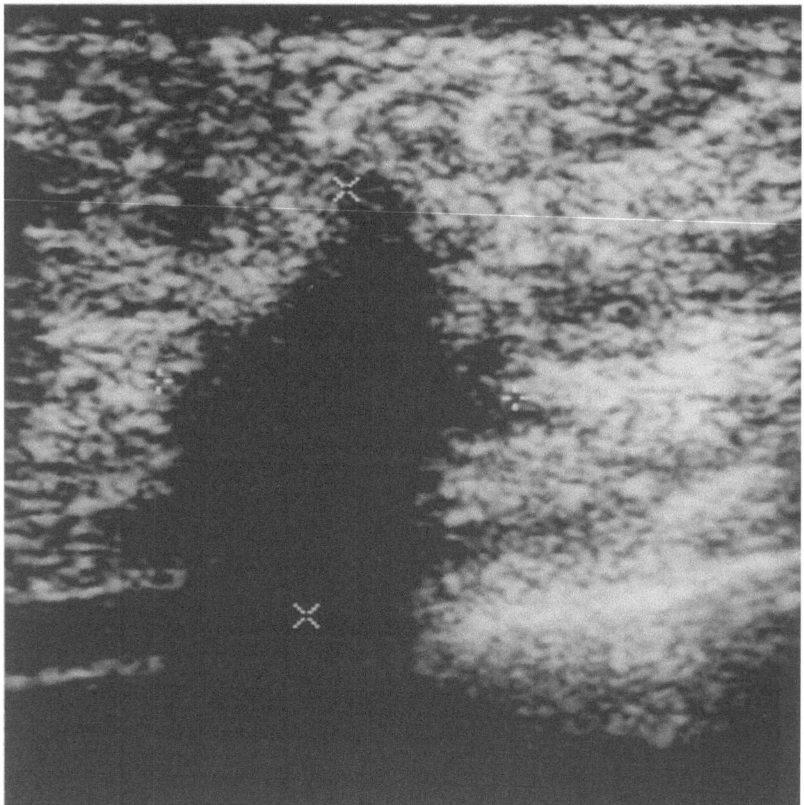

Fig. 17.4. Breast carcinoma

Sonographic Diagnosis

Criteria

→ Spherical hypoechoic mass
→ Irregular border
→ Distal shadowing

Other findings may include:
◆ Lymph node metastases
◆ Liver metastases

Sonographic Differential Diagnosis

Solid lesions should be considered malignant until proven otherwise.

17.2.4 Checklist for Reporting

Breast
- **Shape**
- **Echopattern**
- **Acoustic enhancement**
- **Acoustic shadowing**
- **Compressibility**
- **Skin**
- **Pectoral fascia**

Axilla

Supraclavicular fossa

Liver

Chapter 18 Thyroid

18.1 Imaging Modalities

Sonography is the method of choice to image the thyroid. Imaging modalities are:

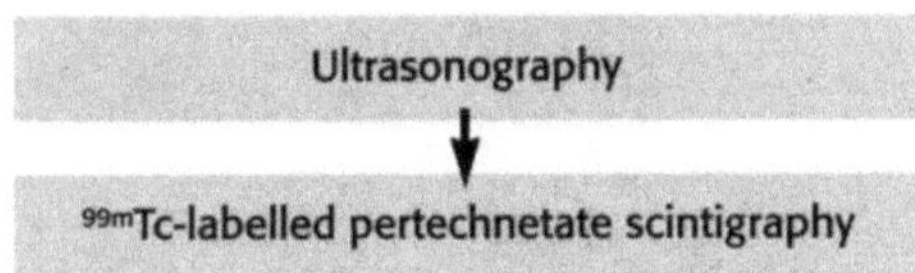

18.2 Ultrasonography

18.2.1 Examination Technique

The thyroid gland is examined with the head in a reclining position with a 7.5-MHz linear probe. To display the lobes and isthmus, longitudinal and transverse sections are made. Retrosternal parts of the thyroid can only be seen to a limited extent.

18.2.2 Sonoanatomy

The thyroid gland is normally situated in the lower neck and consists of two lobes joined by an isthmus that crosses the anterior tract of the second and third tracheal rings. The lobes have an ellipsoid configuration with a pointed superior pole and poorly defined inferior pole merging medially toward the isthmus. A pyramidal lobe is frequently present and in most instances is attached to the left lobe. The thyroid gland is closely fixed to the anterior and lateral aspects of the trachea by loose connective tissue. A fibrous capsule, which invests the gland, is connected to the pretracheal fascia, causing the thyroid to move upward with deglutition.

Lying lateral to each lobe are the carotid artery, the internal jugular vein, and the sternocleidomastoid muscle.

The thyroid gland has a very characteristic finely homogeneous echotexture.

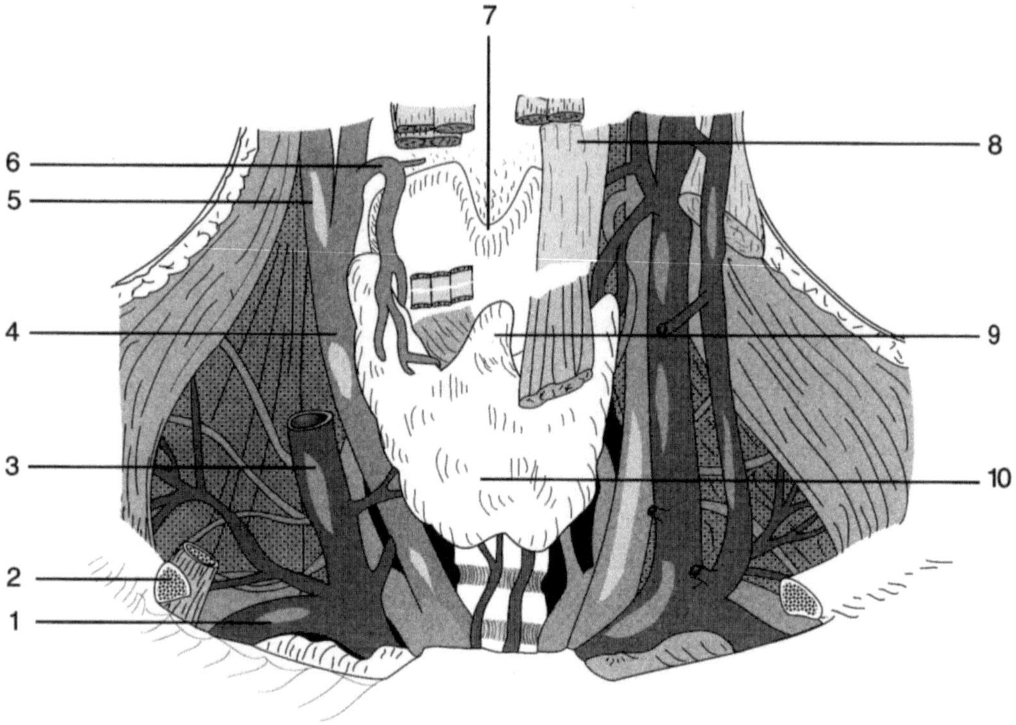

Fig. 18.1. Cervical region. *1*, Subclavian vein; *2*, clavicle; *3*, internal jugular vein; *4*, common carotid artery; *5*, carotid bifurcation; *6*, superior thyroid artery; *7*, thyroid cartilage; *8*, hyoid muscles; *9*, pyramidal lobe; *10*, thyroid gland

18.2.2.1 Normal Dimensions

Thyroid:
◆ Length < 5 cm
◆ Width < 2 cm
◆ Depth < 1.5 cm
◆ Isthmus < 1.5 cm

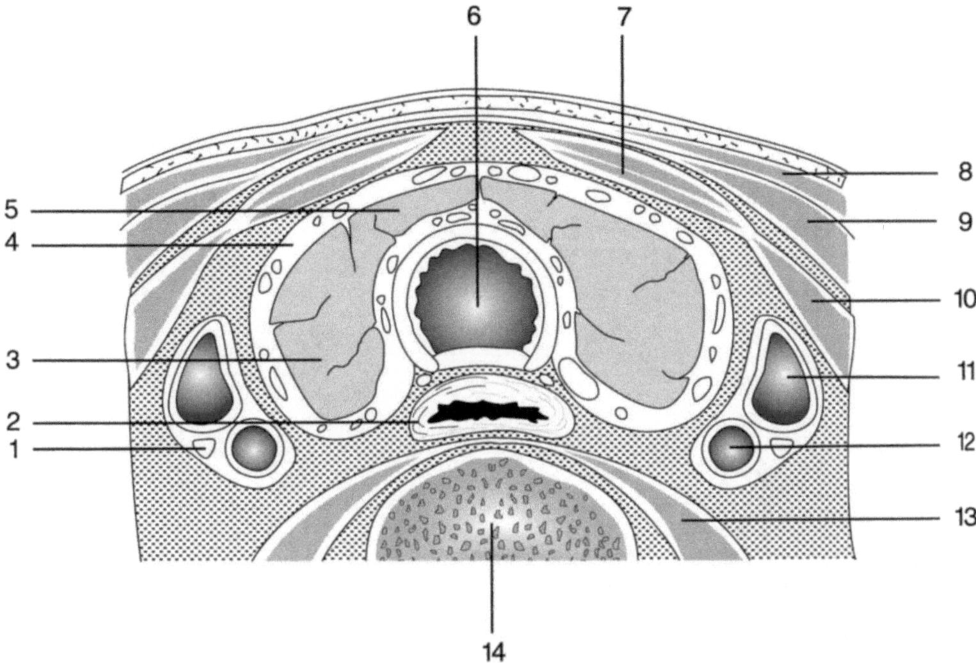

Fig. 18.2. Thyroid region. *1*, Vagus nerve; *2*, oesophagus; *3*, thyroid lobe; *4*, thyroid capsule; *5*, isthmus; *6*, trachea; *7*, sternohyoid muscle and sternothyroid muscle; *8*, platysma; *9*, sternocleidomastoid muscle; *10*, omohyoid muscle; *11*, internal jugular vein; *12*, common carotid artery; *13*, scalenus anterior muscle and scalenus medius muscle; *14*, vertebral body

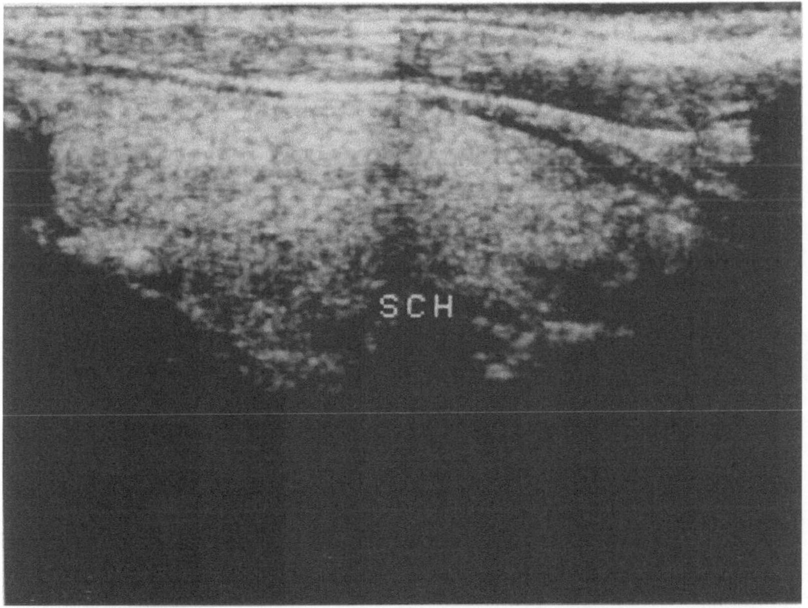

Fig. 18.3. Thyroid gland. Longitudinal scan. *SCH,* Thyroid gland

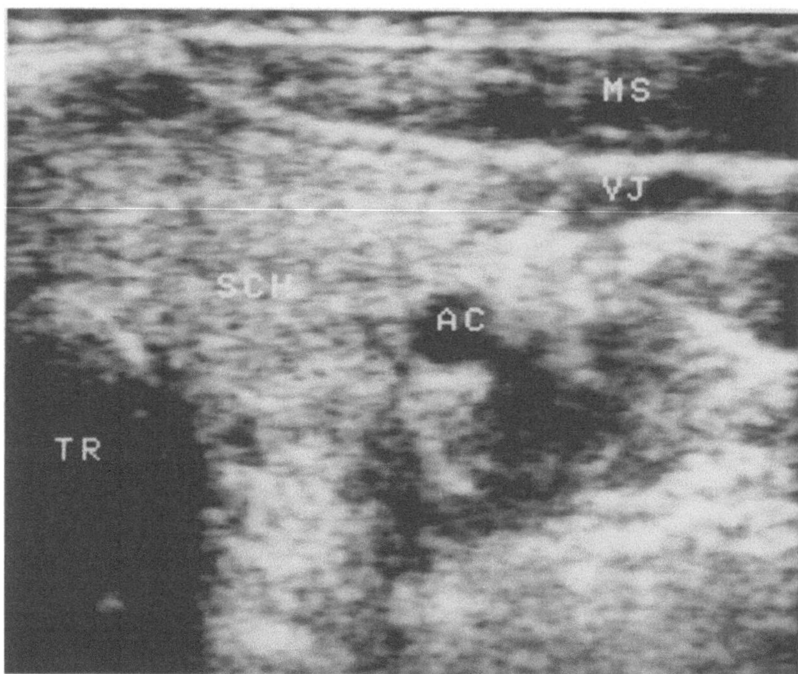

Fig. 18.4. Thyroid gland. Transverse scan. *SCH*, Thyroid gland; *AC*, carotid artery; *VJ*, internal jugular vein; *MS*, sternocleidomastoid muscle; *TR*, trachea

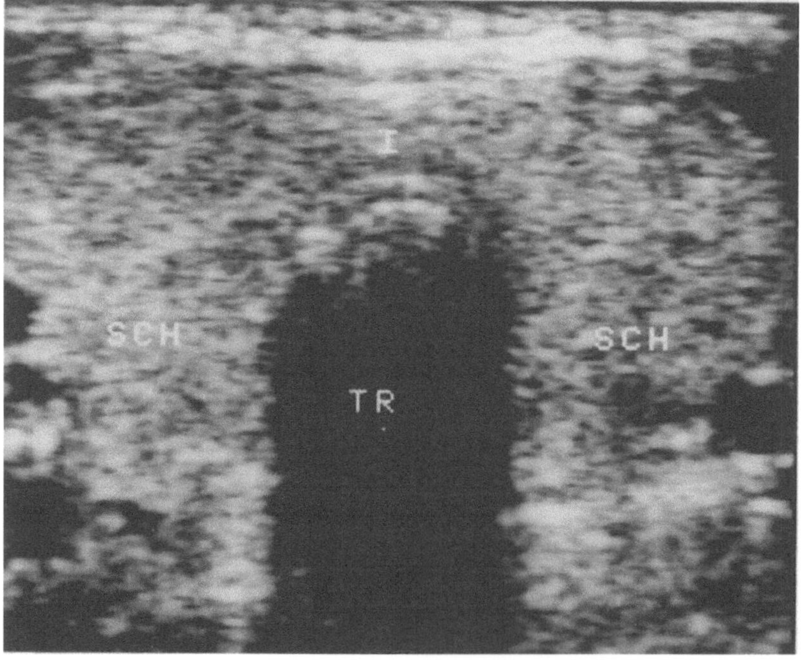

Fig. 18.5. Thyroid gland. Transverse scan. *SCH*, Thyroid gland; *I*, isthmus; *TR*, trachea

18.2.3 Sonopathology

18.2.3.1 Thyroiditis

Clinical Data

Thyroiditis:
◆ Autoimmune thyroiditis (Hashimoto's disease)
◆ Subacute thyroiditis (De Quervain's disease)
◆ Woody thyroiditis (Riedel's disease)

In subacute thyroiditis, the thyroid usually becomes acutely enlarged, firm, tender, and painful, in a patient who is unwell and feverish.

Sonographic Diagnosis

Criteria
→ Enlarged thyroid gland
→ Focal hypoechoic areas
→ Tenderness

Nodular structures may be present within the thyroid gland, in which case differentiation from carcinoma is difficult.

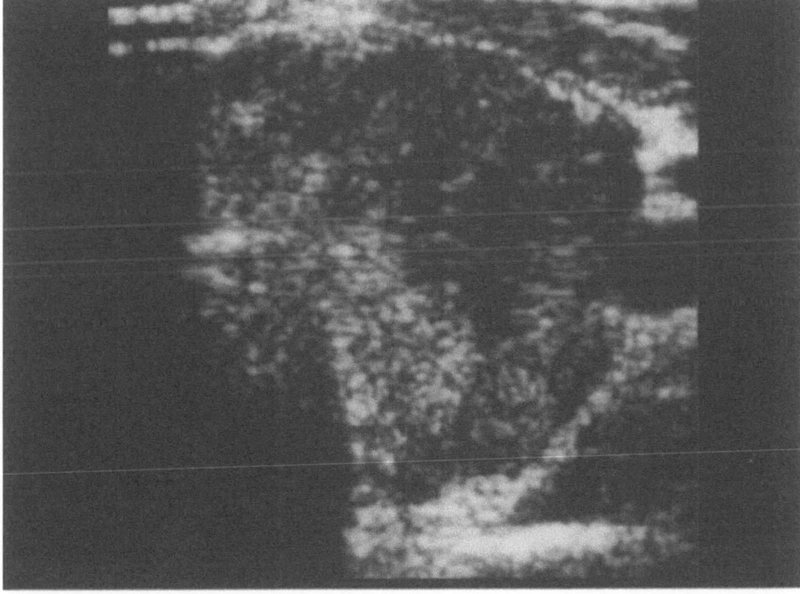

Fig. 18.6. Subacute thyroiditis (De Quervain's disease)

Sonographic Differential Diagnosis

Diffusely hypoechoic thyroid gland:
- Acute thyroiditis
- Autoimmune thyroiditis (Hashimoto's disease)
- Graves' disease

Graves' disease is characterized by pulsatile hypervascularization. High flow velocities are present in systole, with much lower or even absent flow in diastole. This pulsatile pattern differentiates Graves' disease from the more continuous flow pattern throughout the cardiac cycle seen in thyroiditis. With treatment the vascularization pattern returns to normal.

18.2.3.2 Cysts

Clinical Data

Cysts are usually incidental findings.

Sonographic Diagnosis

Criteria
→ Spherical or oval anechoic lesion
→ Sharp and well-defined border
→ Distal acoustic enhancement
→ Prominent posterior border

Sonographic Differential Diagnosis

Lymph nodes.

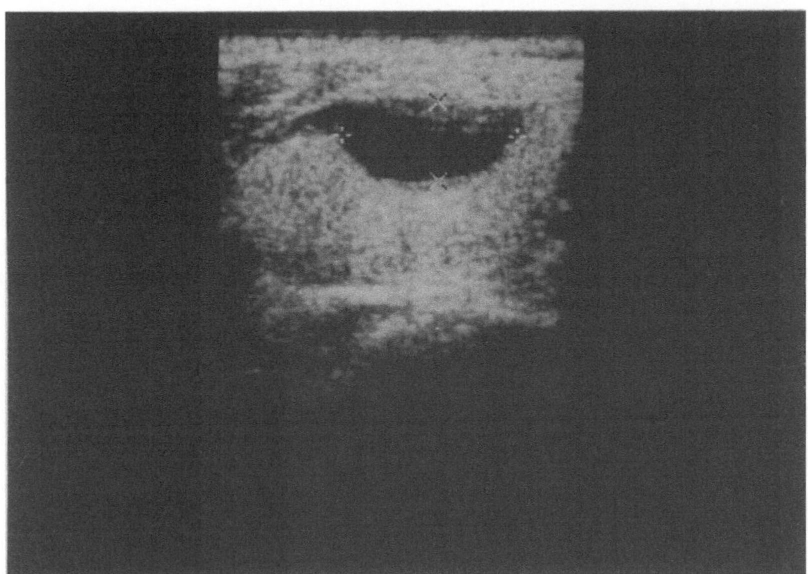

Fig. 18.7. Thyroid cyst

18.2.3.3 Goitre

Clinical Data

A goitre is an enlarged thyroid gland. The term simple goitre is used for the diffuse non-toxic goitre.

Sonographic Diagnosis

Criteria

→ Enlarged thyroid gland
→ Nodules
→ Degenerative changes
  – Cysts
  – Calcifications

Sonographic Differential Diagnosis

Differential diagnosis:
◆ Adenoma
◆ Carcinoma

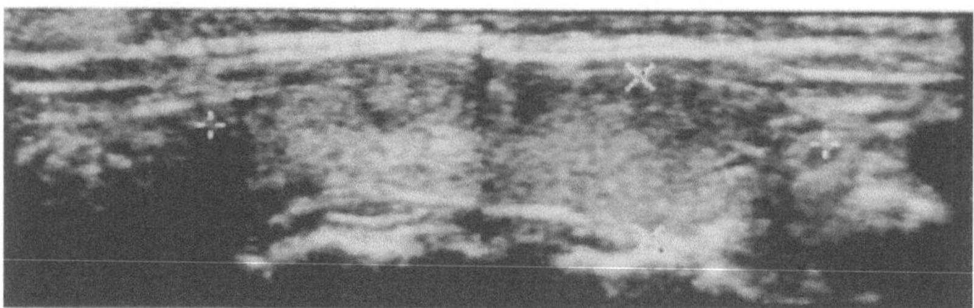

Fig. 18.8. Goitre. Longitudinal scan showing diffuse enlargement of the thyroid gland. A nodule can be visualized in the cranial pole of the lobe

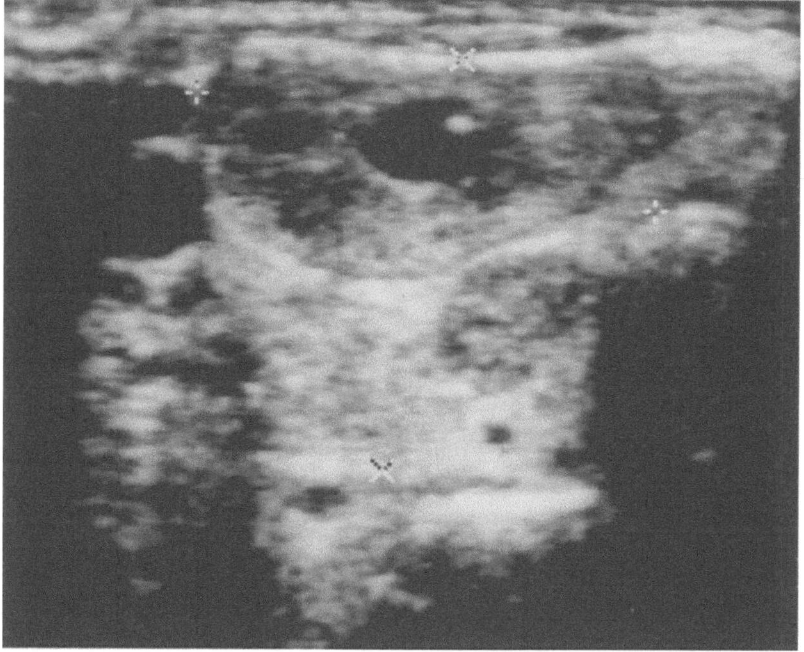

Fig. 18.9. Goitre. Transverse scan showing several nodules with cystic areas

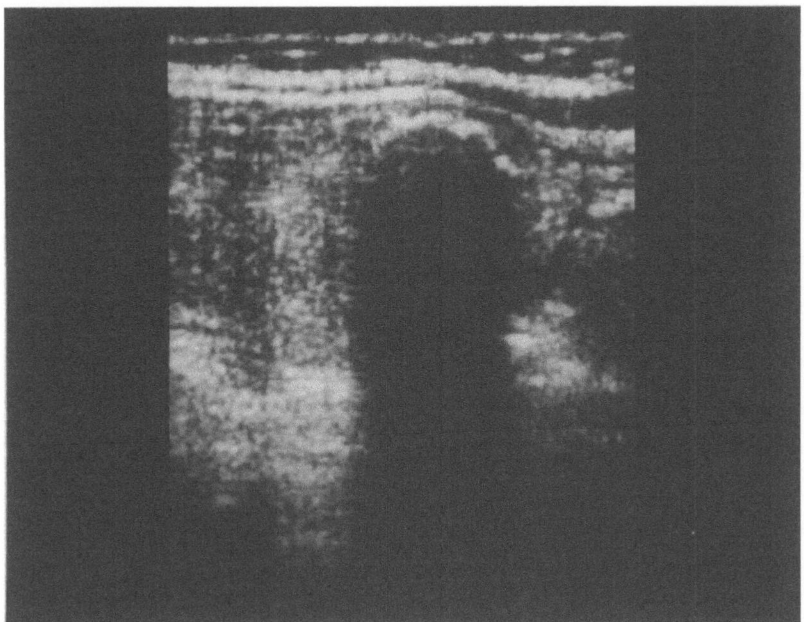

Fig. 18.10. Goitre. The curvilinear echogenic line with distal acoustic shadowing is due to calcification

18.2.3.4 Adenoma

Clinical Data

Clinical features of thyrotoxicosis include diminished tolerance of warm temperatures, palpitations, dyspnoea, weakness, fatigue, nervousness, irritability, tremor, weight loss with increased appetite.

Sonographic Diagnosis

Criterion

→ Nodule
  - Solitary or multiple
  - Well-demarcated from adjacent tissue
  - Hypo-, iso- or hyperechoic
  - Halo sign

The halo sign is a thin hypoechoic margin completely encircling the nodule. Colour Doppler often demonstrates hypervascularity within this region.

Simple thyroid adenomas show no evidence of central hypervascularization, whereas autonomous adenomas have both central and peripheral hypervascularization.

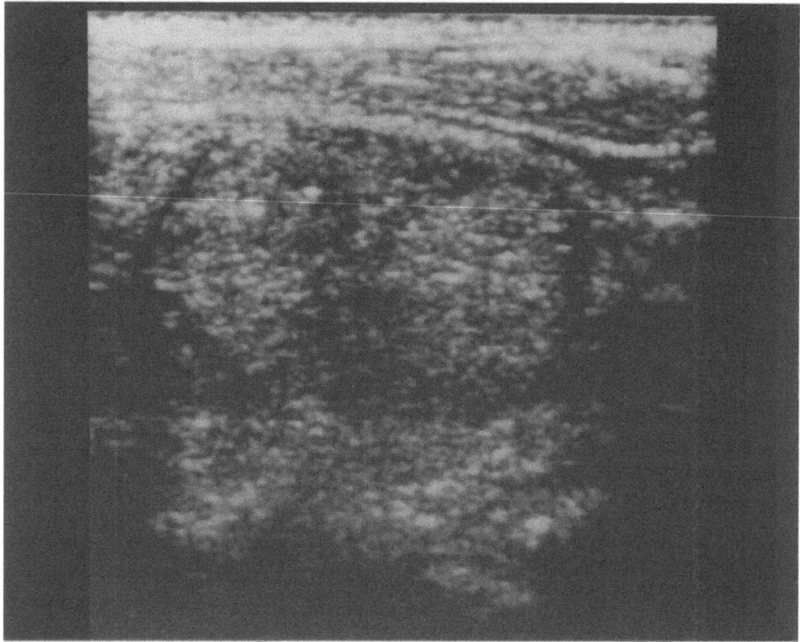

Fig. 18.11. Thyroid adenoma. The nodules are encircled by a thin hypoechoic margin, the so-called halo

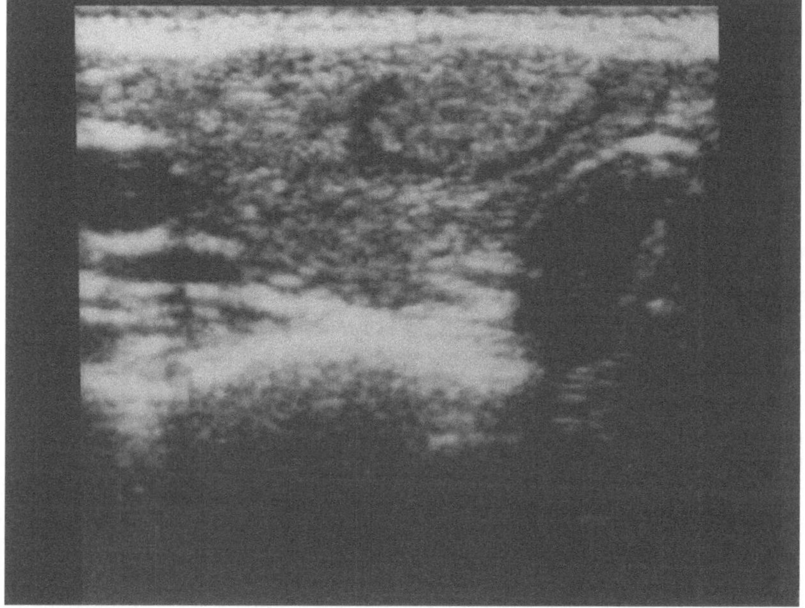

Fig. 18.12. Thyroid adenoma. Note the halo sign

Sonographic Differential Diagnosis

Hyperechoic nodules without evidence of local invasion or adjacent lymphadenopathy are usually low-risk lesions.

18.2.3.5 Carcinoma

Clinical Data

A solitary hard nodule in the thyroid gland should raise suspicion of carcinoma. When enlarged lymph nodes can also be palpated the diagnosis is almost certain.

Histologically, thyroid carcinomas can be divided into four types:
◆ Follicular
◆ Papillary
◆ Anaplastic
◆ Medullary

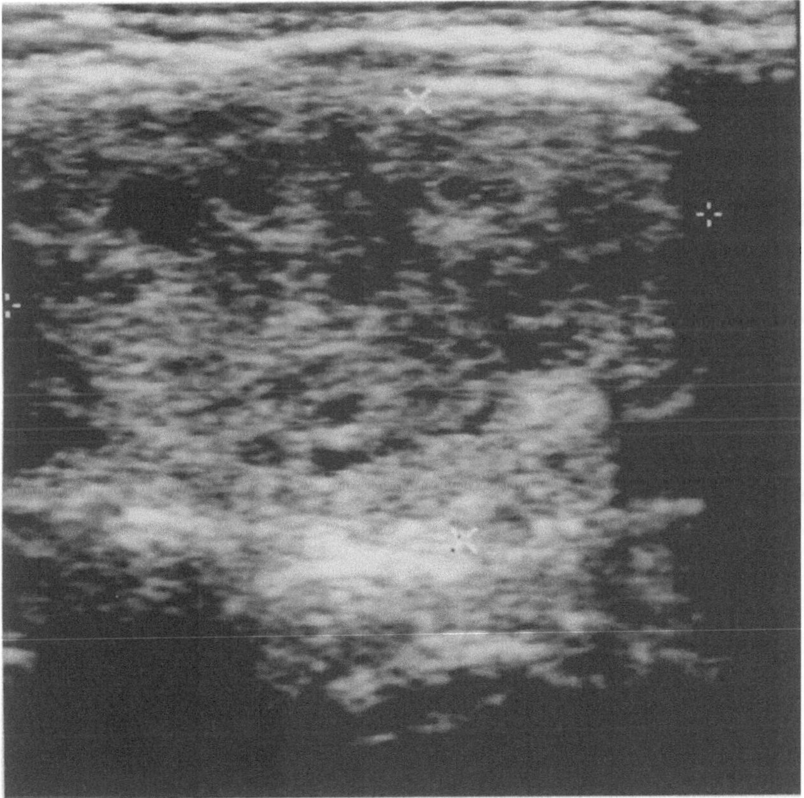

Fig. 18.13. Thyroid carcinoma

Sonographic Diagnosis

Criterion

→ Ill-defined, usually hypoechoic mass

Thyroid carcinomas can present with a wide variety of sonomorphological and vascular patterns.

Sonographic Differential Diagnosis

The tendency to invasion of surrounding structures is one of the few reliable signs of malignancy. Cervical lymphadenopathy may also be associated with thyroid malignancy.

18.2.3.6 Lymphadenopathy

Clinical Data

Aetiology:
- Inflammation
- Tumour

Sonographic Diagnosis

Criterion

→ Well-defined, usually hypoechoic mass

Tenderness usually indicates inflammation.

Sonographic Differential Diagnosis

Differential diagnosis:
- Vessel
- Muscle

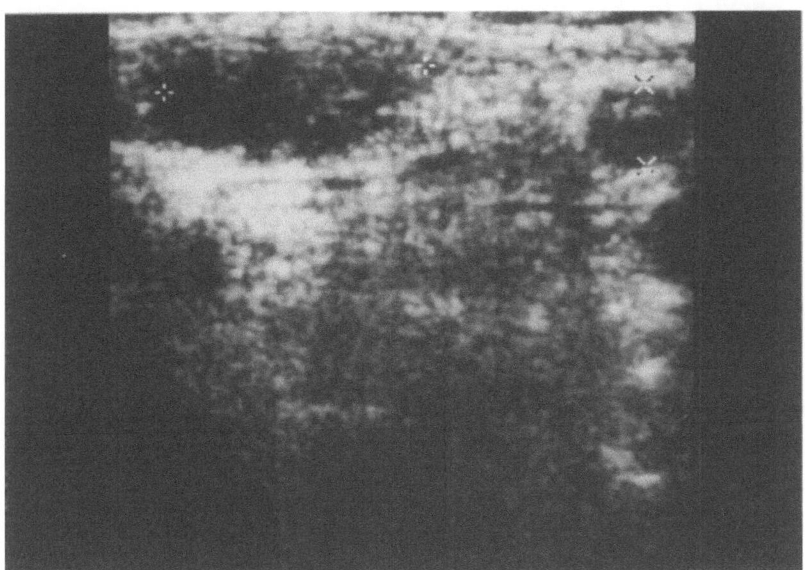

Fig. 18.14. Cervical lymphadenopathy. Longitudinal scan

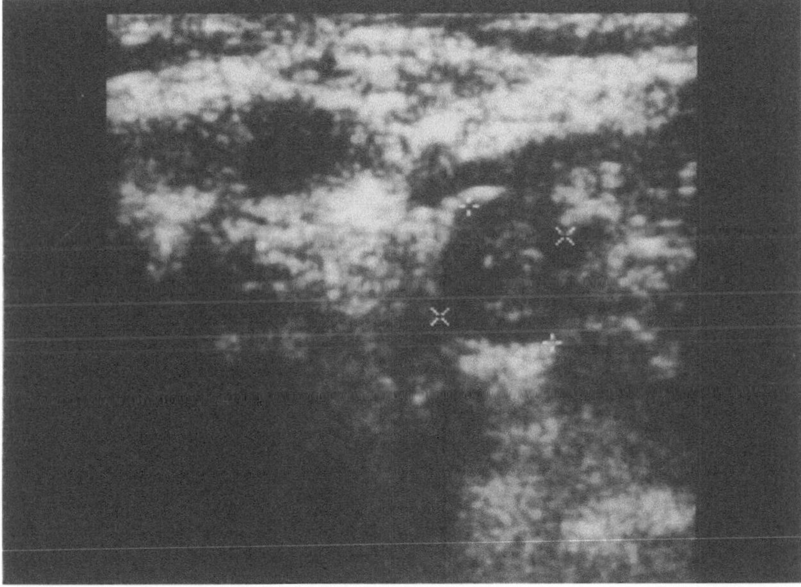

Fig. 18.15. Cervical lymphadenopathy. Transverse scan

18.2.4 Checklist for Reporting

Thyroid
- **Position**
- **Size**
- **Contour**
- **Echopattern**
- **Mobility on swallowing**

Parathyroid

Vessels
- **Common carotid artery**
- **Internal jugular vein**

Lymph nodes

Trachea
- **Narrowing**
- **Displacement**

Chapter 19 Parathyroid

19.1 Imaging Modalities

Sonography is the method of choice to image the parathyroid. Imaging modalities are:

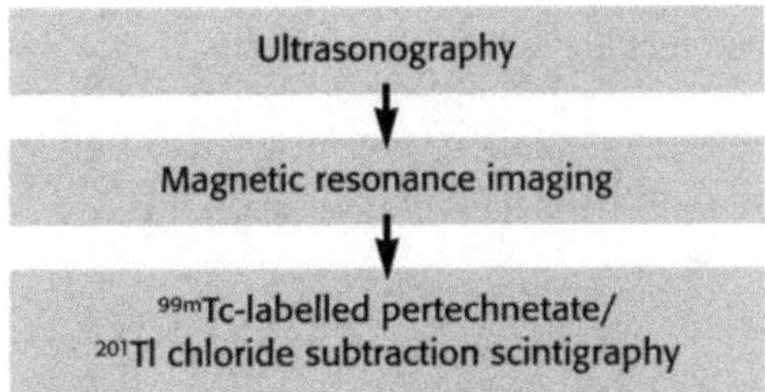

19.2 Ultrasonography

19.2.1 Examination Technique

The examination of the parathyroid gland is performed – as with the thyroid gland – with a 7.5-MHz linear probe. The neck is tilted backwards. Normal parathyroid glands are not generally identified by sonography.

19.2.2 Sonoanatomy

The parathyroid glands have a variable location. There are usually four: two upper and two lower. The superior pair are often significantly larger and therefore easier to find. The parathyroid glands are most commonly located along the dorsal surface of the thyroid gland.

Atypically positioned parathyroid tissue:
◆ In the thymus
◆ In the mediastinum
◆ In the thyroid gland
◆ Behind the oesophagus
◆ In the parapharyngeal region

19.2.2.1 Normal Dimensions

Parathyroid:
- Length < 7 mm
- Width < 5 mm
- Depth < 2 mm

19.2.3 Sonopathology

19.2.3.1 Adenoma

Clinical Data

The clinical features of hyperparathyroidism include renal stones, osteitis fibrosa cystica (von Recklinghausen's disease), and peptic ulcer. About 80% of patients with primary hyperparathyroidism have a parathyroid adenoma, 15% hyperplasia of all the parathyroid glands, and a small percentage underlying parathyroid carcinoma.

Sonographic Diagnosis

Criterion

→ Homogeneous, hypoechoic nodule

Parathyroid adenomas are mainly:
- Posterior to the thyroid
- Anterior to the longus colli muscle
- Lateral to the trachea
- Medial to the common carotid artery

Colour Doppler readily demonstrates the hypervascular pattern in parathyroid adenomas.

Sonographic Differential Diagnosis

Differential diagnosis:
- Thyroid cyst
- Thyroid adenoma
- Thyroid carcinoma
- Longus colli muscle
- Common carotid artery
- Internal jugular vein
- Oesophagus

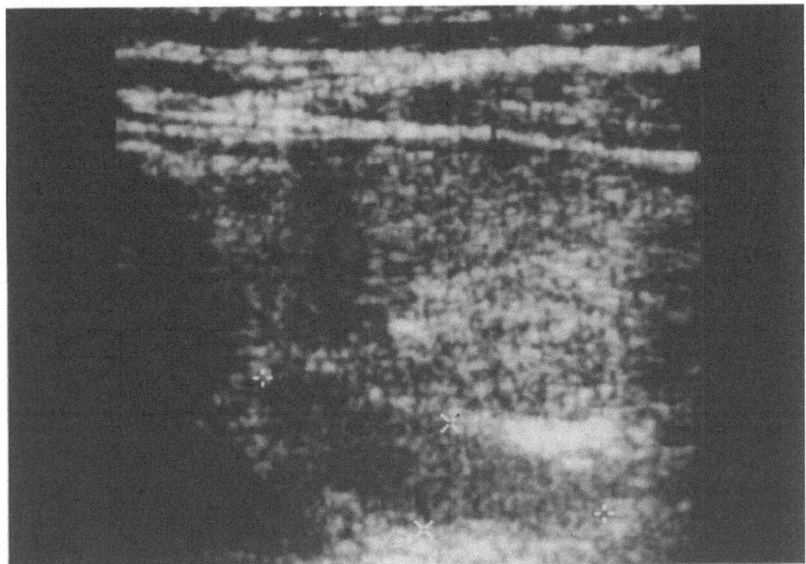

Fig. 19.1. Parathyroid adenoma. Longitudinal scan

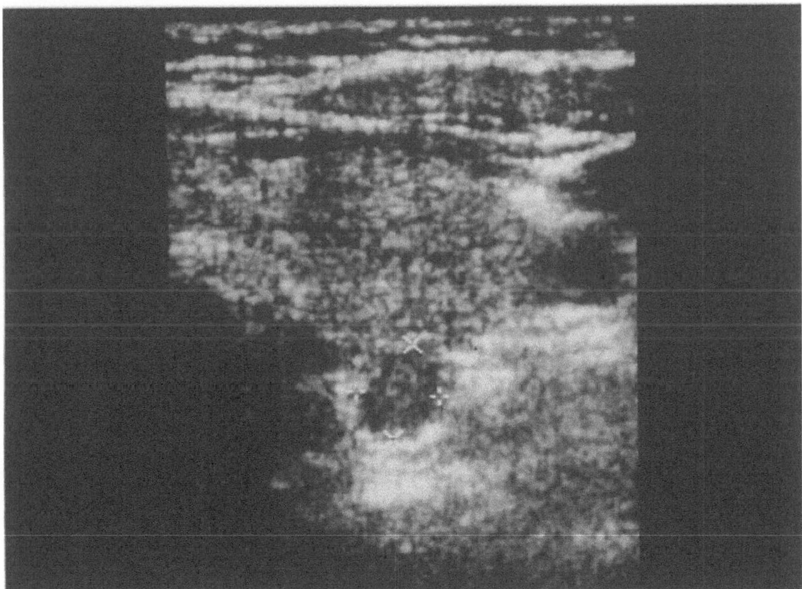

Fig. 19.2. Parathyroid adenoma. Transverse scan

19.2.4 Checklist for Reporting

Parathyroid
- Size

Chapter **20** Vessels

20.1 Imaging Modalities

Imaging modalities are:

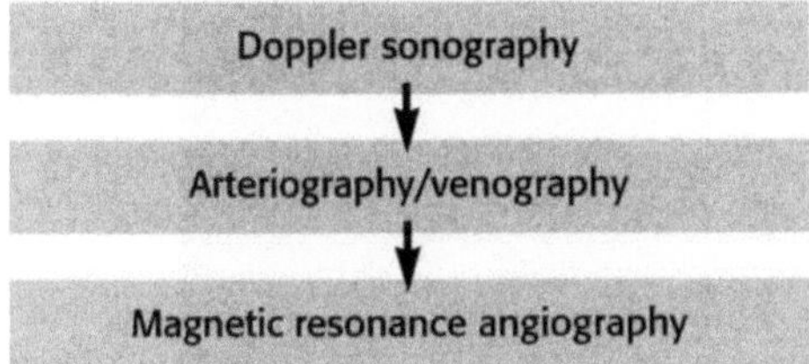

20.2 Ultrasonography

20.2.1 Examination Technique

The sonoanatomy and sonopathology of the abdominal vessels – particularly the aorta and the inferior vena cava – were explained in the chapter on retroperitoneum. Here is discussed briefly the diagnosis of some clinically relevant vein thromboses.

The superficial veins are examined in longitudinal and transverse sections with 7.5-MHz transducers.

20.2.2 Sonoanatomy

In the longitudinal plane, vessels are seen as anechoic tubes. They are circular structures in the transverse plane.

20.2.2.1 Normal Dimensions

Veins:
◆ Portal vein < 1.5 cm
◆ Splenic vein < 1 cm

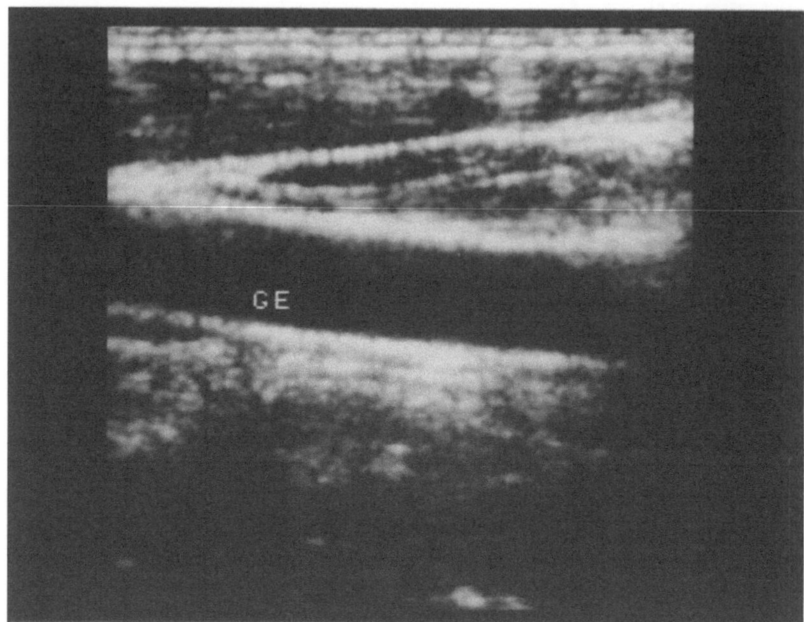

Fig. 20.1. Vessel. Longitudinal scan. *GE*, Vessel

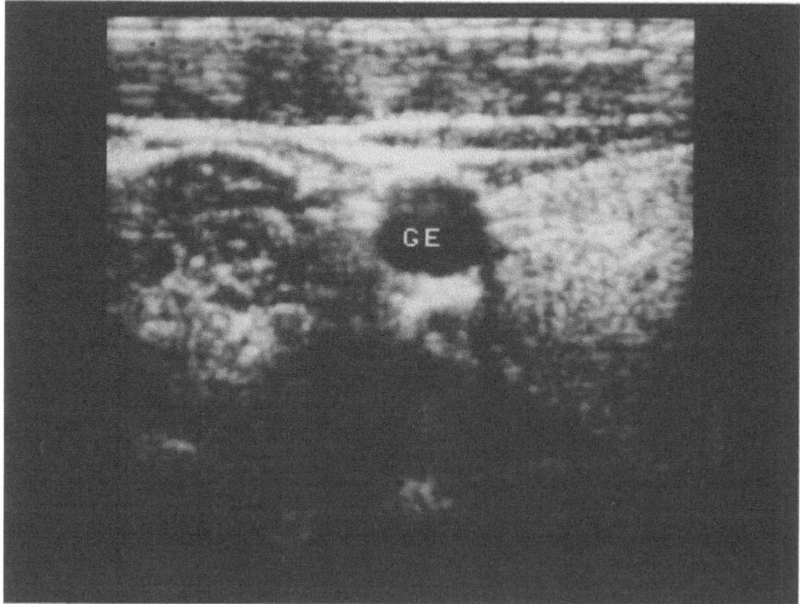

Fig. 20.2. Vessel. Transverse scan. *GE*, Vessel

20.2.3 Sonopathology

20.2.3.1 Jugular Vein Thrombosis

Clinical Data

Aetiology:
- Prolonged venous compression
- Inflammatory conditions
- Tumour
- Surgery
- Catheter
- Heart disease
- Intravenous drug abuse

Thrombosis of the internal jugular vein can affect the subclavian vein.

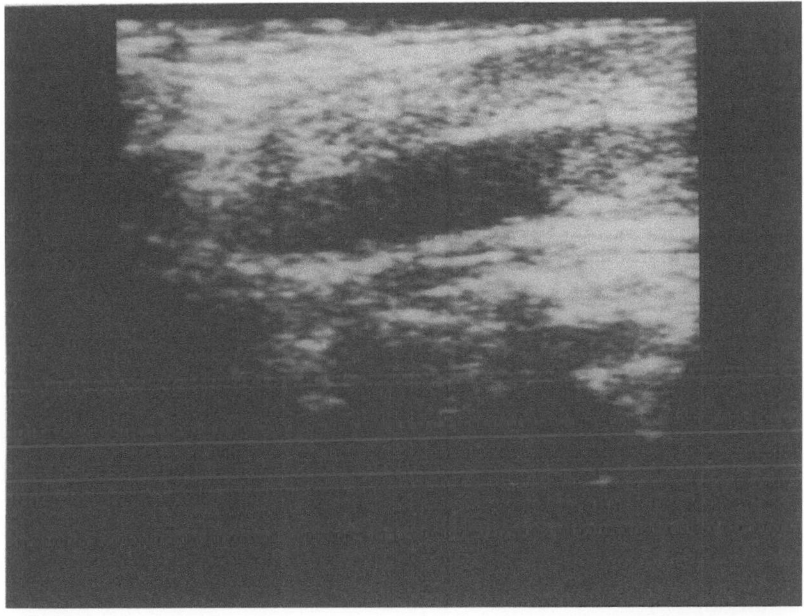

Fig. 20.3. Jugular vein thrombosis. The echogenic thrombus appears slightly inhomogeneous; the vein is incompressible

Sonographic Diagnosis

Criteria

→ Intraluminal hypoechoic material in recent thrombus
→ Intraluminal hyperechoic material in old thrombus
→ Loss of compressibility
→ No augmentation during Valsalva's manoeuvre

Sonographic Differential Diagnosis

In recent thrombosis of the internal jugular vein, the lumen is nearly anechoic, but no flow signals can be recorded within the vessel.

20.2.3.2 Portal Vein Thrombosis

Clinical Data

Aetiology:
◆ Liver disease
◆ Pancreatitis
◆ Cholecystitis
◆ Tumour
◆ Coagulation disorders

In many patients, no aetiologic factor can be identified. The clinical effect of portal vein thrombosis depends upon the location and extent of the thrombosis, and the rapidity with which it develops. Portal hypertension is the end result.

Sonographic Diagnosis

Criteria

→ Intraluminal hypoechoic material in recent thrombus
→ Intraluminal hyperechoic material in old thrombus
→ Evidence of portal hypertension
    - Collateral circulation
    - Splenomegaly
    - Ascites

Sonographic Differential Diagnosis

Non-visualization of the portal vein is strongly suspicious of occlusion.

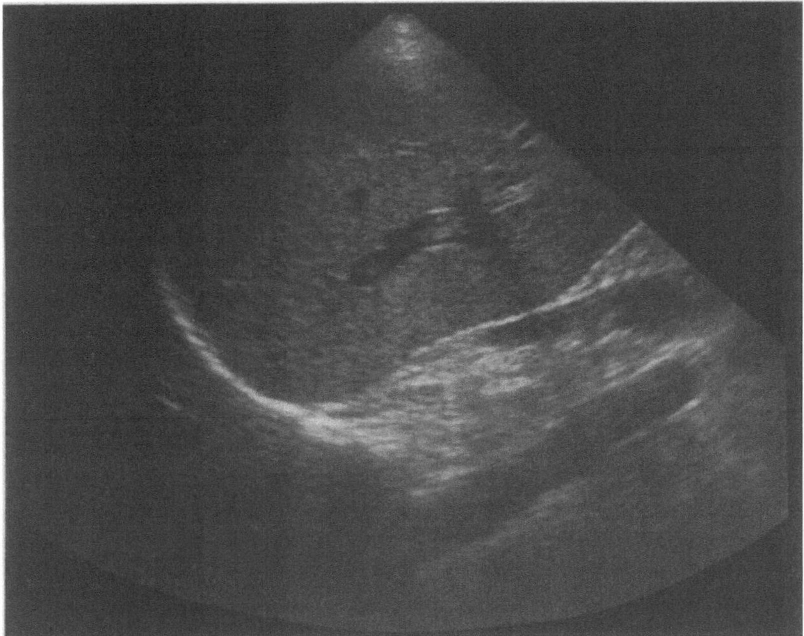

Fig. 20.4. Portal vein thrombosis

20.2.3.3 Femoral Vein Thrombosis

Clinical Data

Clinical features of thrombosis.

Sonographic Diagnosis

Criteria

→ Intraluminal hypoechoic material in recent thrombus
→ Intraluminal hyperechoic material in old thrombus
→ Loss of compressibility

Sonographic Differential Diagnosis

Colour Doppler is a suitable alternative to venography. In malignant disease, for example, compression or displacement of the veins by enlarged lymph nodes is better assessed by sonography than by venography.

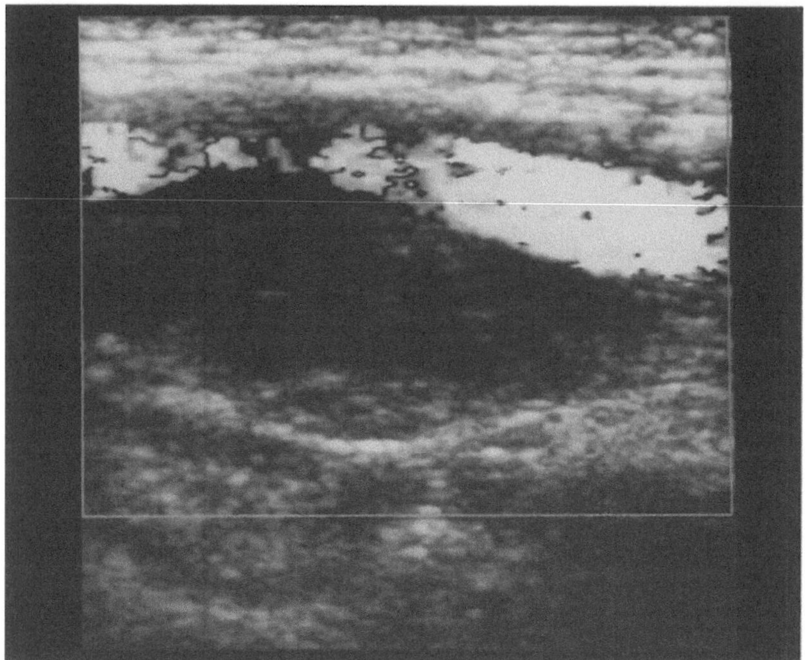

Fig. 20.5. Femoral vein thrombosis

20.2.4 Checklist for Reporting

Vessels
- **Position**
- **Course**
- **Diameter**
- **Wall**
- **Echopattern**
- **Pulsatility**
- **Compressibility**

Chapter ㉑ Musculoskeletal System

21.1 Imaging Modalities

Imaging modalities are:

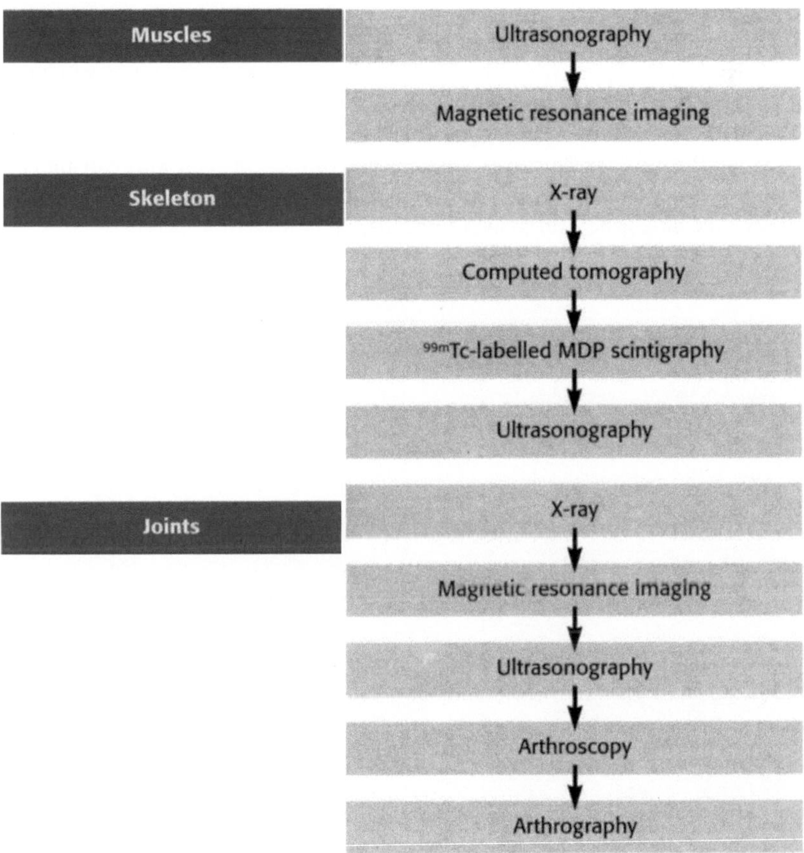

21.2 Ultrasonography

21.2.1 Examination Technique

No patient preparation is needed. Both longitudinal and transverse sections must be performed. In order to assess better the extent of post-traumatic injuries, a dynamic study is required. A comparative study of the normal contralateral muscle avoids errors. The ideal probe is a linear 7.5-MHz; a 5-MHz transducer is required to study large muscle groups as well as hip joints in older babies. Tendons and ligaments are better studied with a 10-MHz small parts probe and with the adjunct of a stand-off pad to compensate for the limited contact surface during active and passive movements.

21.2.2 Sonoanatomy

The muscles have a striped pattern with thin oblique bright connective septa on a hypoechoic background. On dynamic study the striations become more prominent and the echogenicity of the muscle decreases temporarily. Each muscle is surrounded by an echogenic fascia. Within large muscles vessels are commonly seen and can be confirmed by colour Doppler. The veins obliterate during contraction. Scanning of the opposite unaffected side is helpful to avoid pitfalls.

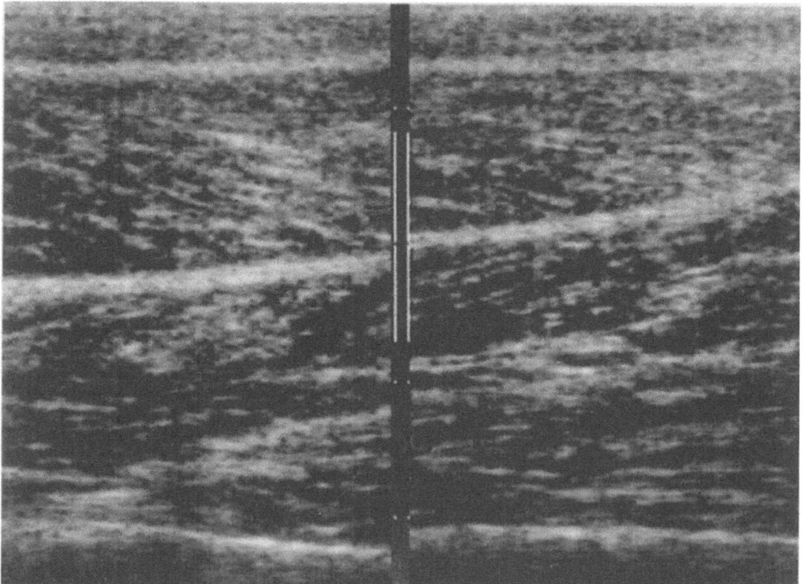

Fig. 21.1. Muscle. Longitudinal scan of the calf, showing the gastrocnemius and soleus muscles with the typical echogenic perimysium, above the hypoechoic muscle fibres, divided by parallel connective striae. The intermuscular fascia is bright. In the soleus muscle a large anechoic vein is seen

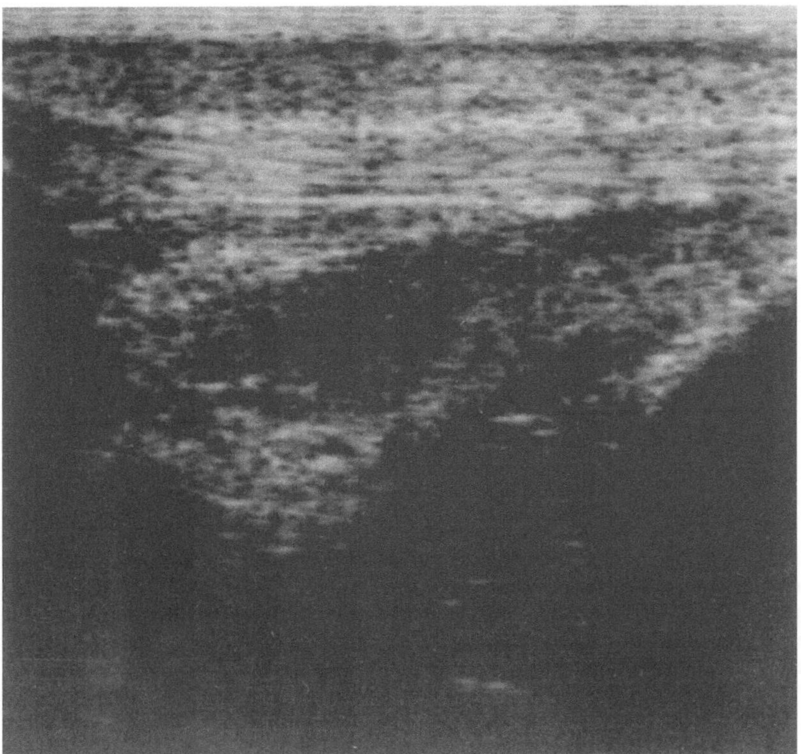

Fig. 21.2. Patellar tendon. Longitudinal scan of the normal patellar tendon extending from the patella to the tibial tuberosity. It shows the hyperechoic fibrillar structure of the tendon, anterior to the hypoechoic infrapatellar bursa and the fat pad of the knee (Hoffa's body)

The tendons and ligaments have a homogeneous, hyperechoic fibrillar structure which does not change on dynamic study. Most of them are surrounded by a synovial sheath and the synovial bursa can be seen in close relation to them. A narrow band of hypoechoic fibrocartilage joins the tendon to its bone insertion. The synovial bursae are seen as flat hyperechoic lines; they can be distended by a small physiological amount of fluid, therefore appearing anechoic.

The neonatal hip is a poorly ossified, therefore hypoechoic structure. The bony hyperechoic landmarks are the ileal margin and the acetabular promontory. The cartilage structures are the acetabular roof, the femoral epiphysis, and the triradiate cartilage.

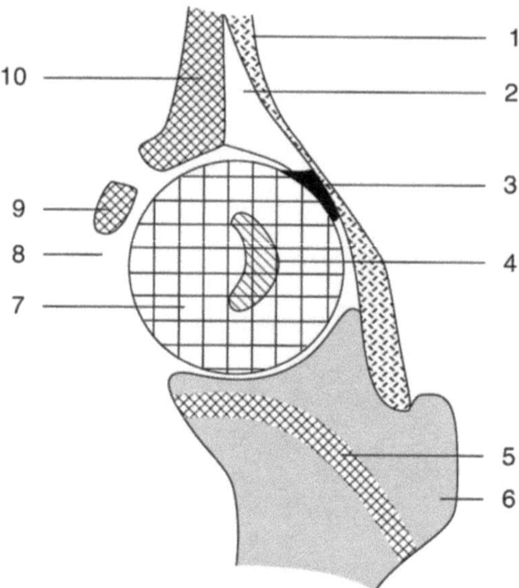

Fig. 21.3. Neonatal hip. *1*, Superior extent of the joint capsule; *2*, hyaline cartilage of the acetabular roof; *3*, fibrocartilaginous labrum of the acetabulum; *4*, small ossific proximal epiphyseal femoral nucleus; *5*, fibro-osseous boundary of the femoral shaft; *6*, greater trochanter; *7*, unossified femoral head; *8*, triradiate cartilage of the acetabulum; *9*, deep portion of the ileum; *10*, lateral bony margin of the ileum

21.2.2.1 Normal Dimensions

Tendons:
◆ Achilles tendon 6 mm
◆ Quadriceps tendon 5 mm
◆ Patellar tendon 3 mm
◆ Long biceps tendon 2 mm
Ligaments 2–3 mm
Synovia in physiologically distended bursae 2 mm

Neonatal hip:
◆ α Angle > 60°
◆ β Angle < 55°

Shoulder:
◆ Rotator cuff
  – Anteriorly 6 mm
  – Posteriorly 4 mm

No definite normal dimensions are given for muscles as they depend upon the patient's age and activity and, in the same patient, on the dominant side.

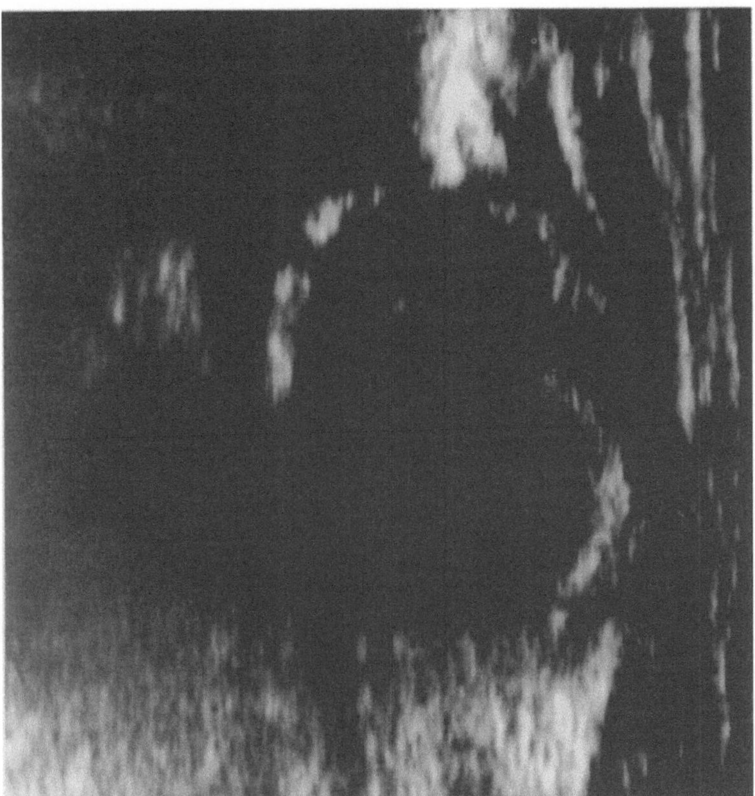

Fig. 21.4. Neonatal hip. Coronal scan parallel to the midline of the femoral head. The hip is imaged vertically with the baby in lateral decubitus position and with the hips slightly flexed. The head of the baby is towards the superior part of the image, the acetabular fossa towards the left of the image, and the probe over the region of the greater trochanter; to the right, gluteus minimus and medius muscles with the gluteal intermuscular septum. The lateral bony margin of the ileum is straight and the bony acetabular promontory is well formed, the hyaline cartilage of the acetabular roof is thin and the acetabular labrum is in a good position

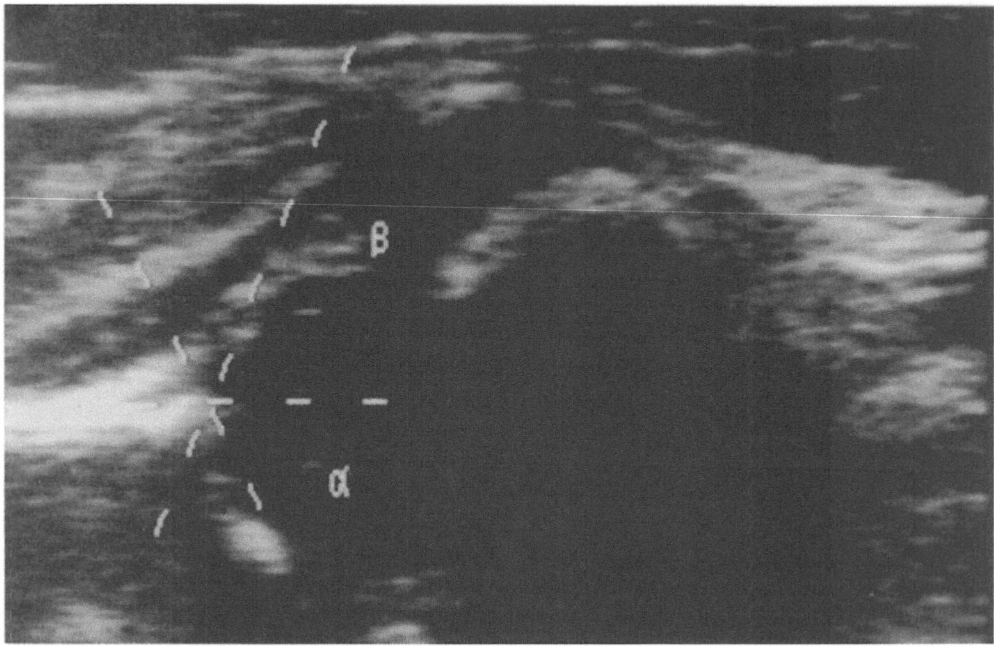

Fig. 21.5. Neonatal hip. The Graf's method lines have been drawn over the image. The baseline lateral to the ileum margin, and the roof line which goes from the triradiate cartilage to the bony contour of the acetabular roof, measure the α angle or bony angle. The β angle is measured between a line drawn from the labrum of the bony contour of the acetabular roof and the baseline

21.2.3 Sonopathology

21.2.3.1 Muscle Trauma

Clinical Data

In the acute stage the pain is associated with dysfunction and haematoma.

Sonographic Diagnosis

Criteria

→ Hyperechoic acute haemorrhage
→ Blurred edges
→ Bulging of the muscle profile
→ Hypoechoic resolving haematoma

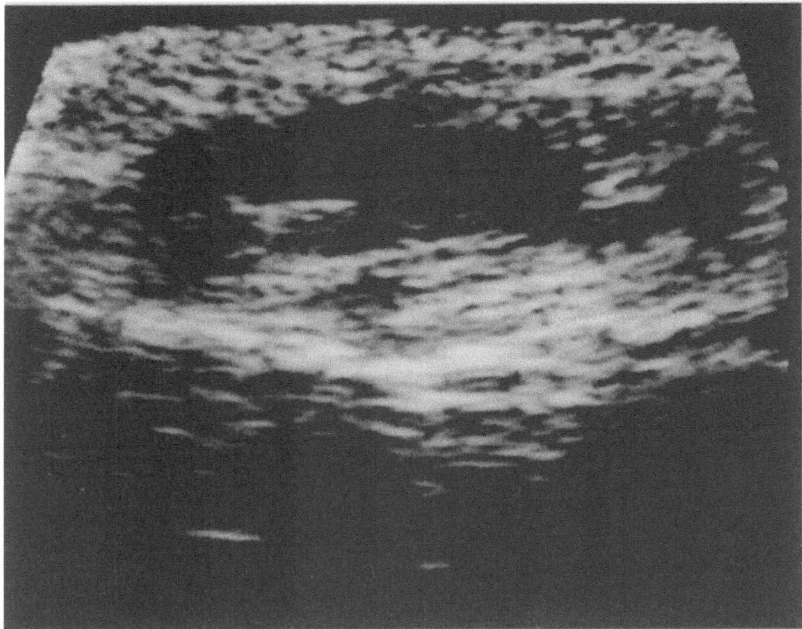

Fig. 21.6. Muscle rupture of the long head of the biceps femoris muscle (longitudinal scan), characterized by an anechoic collection due to discontinuity in muscle fibres and an associated liquefying haematoma with thin internal fibrinous strands

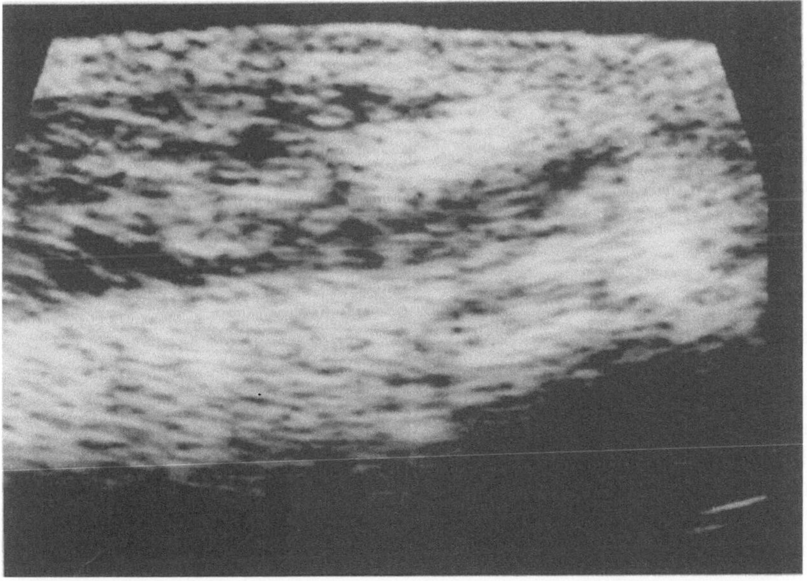

Fig. 21.7. Fibrous scar in the rectus femoris muscle. Longitudinal scan. The echogenic area abuts the epimysium of the muscle

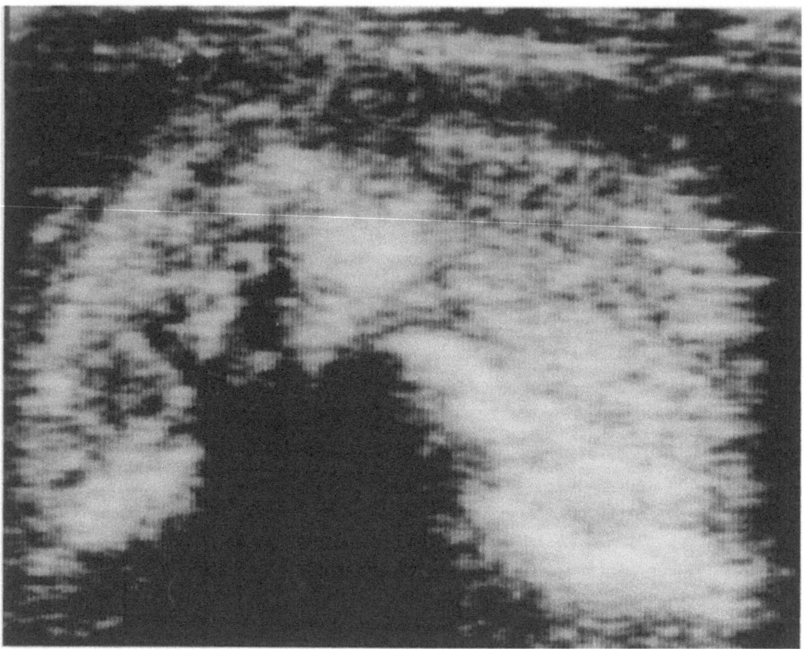

Fig. 21.8. Ossification of muscle haematoma of the vastus intermedius muscle: post-traumatic myositis ossificans. Transverse scan. Typical bright foci from the calcific nucleus with acoustic shadowing

With time the sonographic appearance of muscle trauma changes. Findings may then include:
- Complete restitutio ad integrum
- Permanent serous cyst
- Fibrous hyperechoic scar
- Calcified foci with acoustic shadowing
- Muscular hernia

Sonographic Differential Diagnosis

Differential diagnosis:
- Soft tissue mass
- Prominent veins
- Capillary haemangioma

Prominent veins (varices) can mimick partial muscle rupture.

21.2.3.2 Tendons Injury

Clinical Data

Incomplete tears cause local tenderness with associated swelling. Complete tears give rise to dysfunction and well-localized pain with skin depression at the site of retraction of the ruptured tendon.

Sonographic Diagnosis

Criteria

→ Partial tear
  - Focal hypoechoic lesion
  - Hypoechoic collection at the tendon insertion
→ Complete tear
  - Hypoechoic gap between hyperechoic fragments
  - Strong echo with acoustic shadowing in bone avulsion

Tiny hypoechoic defects next to the site of tear are signs of associated degenerative changes.

Sonographic Differential Diagnosis

Differential diagnosis:
◆ Insertion tendinitis
◆ Focal tendinitis
◆ Intratendinous xanthomas

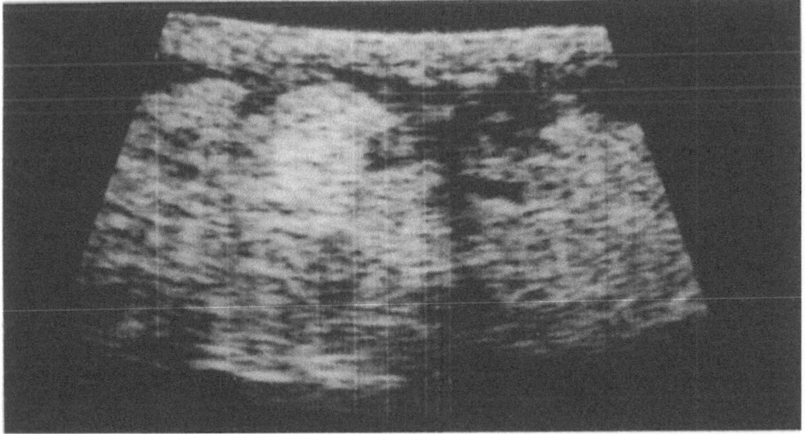

Fig. 21.9. Achilles tendon rupture. The longitudinal scan shows the full thickness gap of the tendon which is swollen. The cleft between the torn fragments is filled with hypoechoic haemorrhagic fluid and clots. The epitendineum also is interrupted

21.2.3.3 Ligament Injury

Clinical Data

Joint laxity under stress manoeuvre. Pain, swelling, haematoma.

Sonographic Diagnosis

Criteria

→ Complete tear
  - Hypoechoic or anechoic haematoma separating the free ends of the ligament
  - Anechoic collection surrounding the ligament
→ Partial tear
  - Focal thickening
  - Focal hypoechoic area
→ Resolution
  - Restitutio ad integrum
  - Hyperechoic tissue to fill the gap
  - Total or partial reabsorption of the effusion
→ Non-union
  - Focal thinning of the ligament
  - Hypertrophic granulation tissue with hypoechoic mass
  - Bright calcium deposits

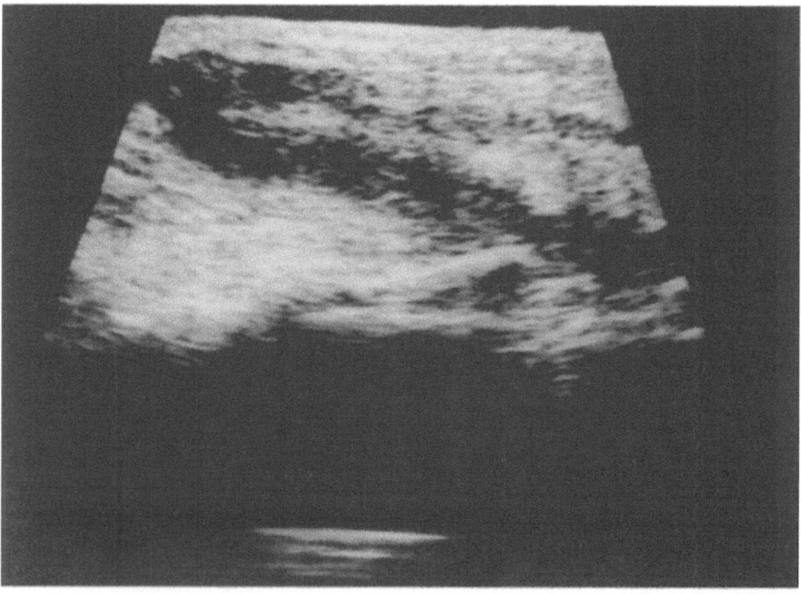

Fig. 21.10. Rupture of the anterior fibulotalar ligament. Detachment of the cranial part of the ligament, with surrounding hypoechoic haematoma. The soft tissues are diffusely swollen

Sonographic Differential Diagnosis

The clinical history is typical.

21.2.3.4 Baker's Cyst

Clinical Data

This acquired growth pathology never presents before the age of 10 years. There is a swollen localized area next to the joint. Spontaneous pain, exacerbated by compression. Patients with longstanding rheumatoid arthritis.

Sonographic Diagnosis

Criteria

→ Anechoic fluid
→ Clear margins
→ Debris due to haemarthros or inflammatory arthropathy
→ Angular margins and extension down to the calf when ruptured

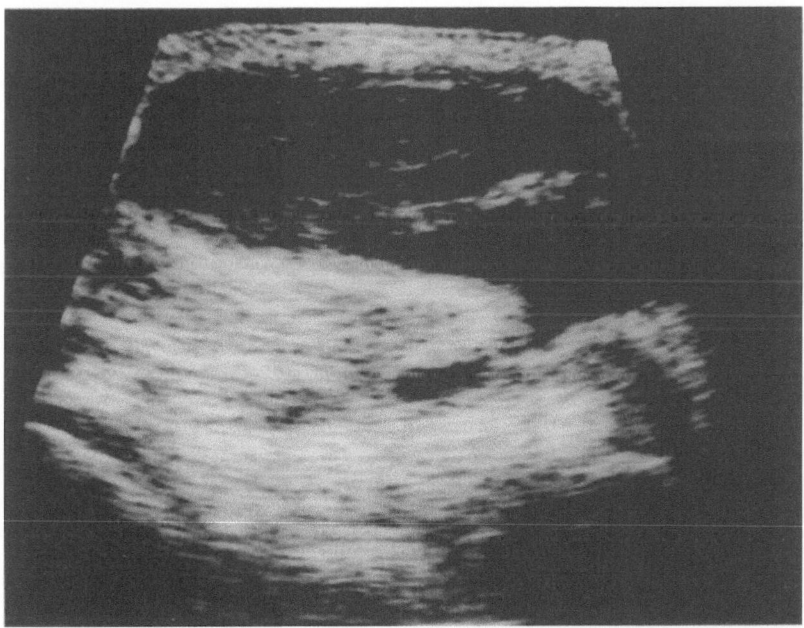

Fig. 21.11. Baker's cyst. Transverse scan of the popliteal fossa. The large anechoic cavity contains internal strands. In this case it is possible to trace the origin of the gastrocnemius-semimembranosus bursa back to the joint space

Sonographic Differential Diagnosis

Differential diagnosis:
◆ Popliteal aneurysm
◆ Adventitious cystic degeneration of the popliteal artery
◆ Synovioma

21.2.3.5 Rotator Cuff Injury

Clinical Data

Pain. Limited shoulder movements, especially abduction.

Sonographic Diagnosis

Criteria

→ Absence of tendon
→ Hypoechoic focal defect within the hyperechoic tendon
→ Focal atrophy of the tendon
→ Distended subacromio-subdeltoid bursa
→ Increased amount of fluid in the biceps tendon sheath

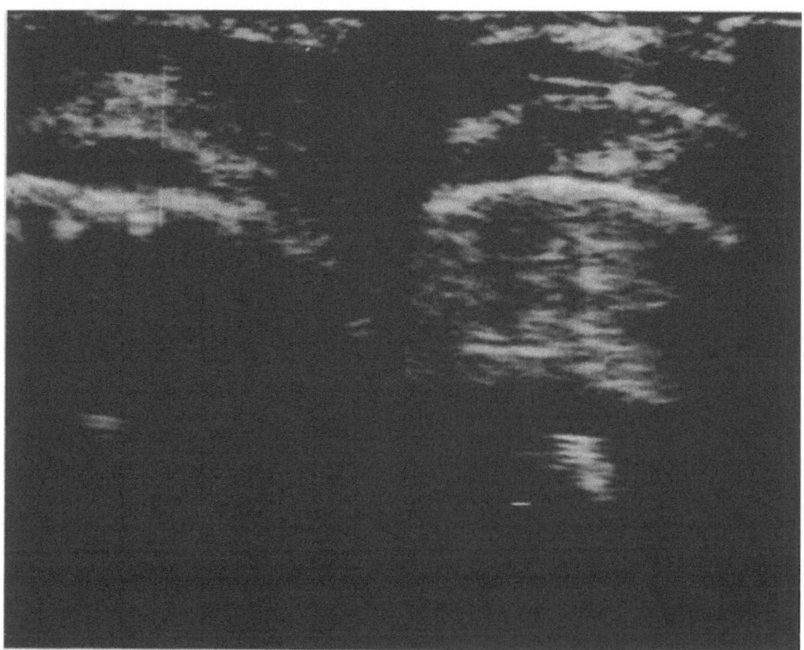

Fig. 21.12. Shoulder. Split screen image. *Right*, normal round, hyperechoic biceps tendon; *left*, absence of the biceps tendon, replaced by a fluid-filled sheath. Fluid is seen within the subacromial-subdeltoid bursa between the tendon sheath and the deltoid muscle anteriorly

Sonographic Differential Diagnosis

Differential diagnosis:
◆ Septic arthritis with distended bursa
◆ Rheumatoid arthritis pannus

21.2.3.6 Tumours

Clinical Data

Patients tend to present late; therefore the lesion is usually large.

Sonographic Diagnosis

Criteria

→ Complex, predominantly hypoechoic mass
→ Usually well-defined margins

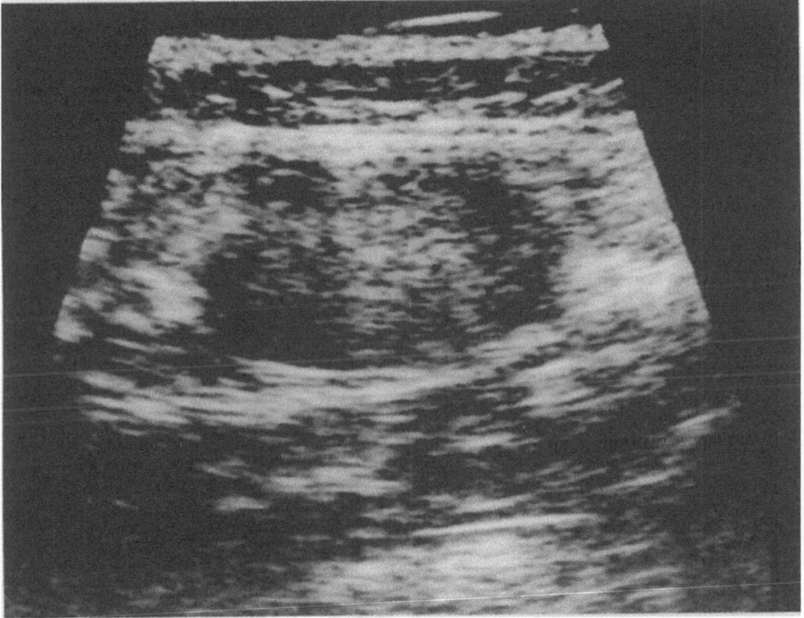

Fig. 21.13. Sarcoma of the thigh. Mixed echopattern; solid mass with lobulated margins, located in the vastus intermedius muscle; in the antero-superior aspect the edge is irregular, probably from infiltration of the muscle fascia, with an echotexture suggestive of necrosis

Sonographic Differential Diagnosis

It is unusual for ultrasound to miss a soft tissue tumour, while the histological diagnosis is rather difficult.

21.2.3.7 Hip Dislocation

Clinical Data

In severe cases the diagnosis at birth is straightforward.

Sonographic Diagnosis

Criteria

→ Shallow acetabulum
→ Steep acetabular roof
→ Wide hyperechoic acetabulum cartilage
→ Lateral and cranial displacement of the labrum
→ Femoral epiphysis outside the acetabulum

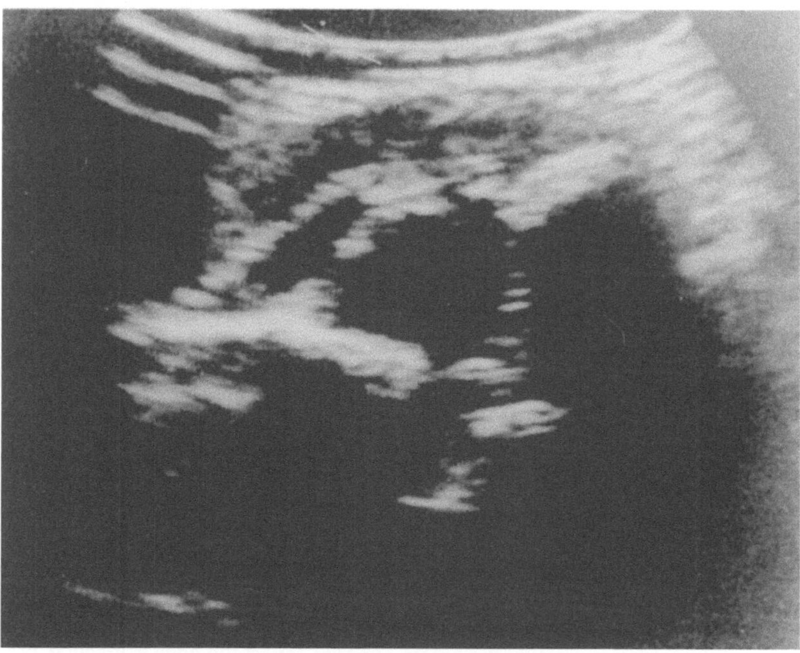

Fig. 21.14. Subluxated hip. The unossified femoral epiphysis is markedly dislocated supero-laterally. The bony acetabular roof is flat, with a shallow acetabulum

Sonographic Differential Diagnosis

The accuracy of ultrasonography in the diagnosis of hip dislocation is very high, even in borderline hips the dynamic manoeuvre displaces the femoral head.

21.2.4 Checklist for Reporting

Musculoskeletal system
- **Change in thickness**
- **Change in echopattern**
- **Diastasis of fragments**
- **Bulging of fascia or sheath**
- **Accompanying fluid collection**
- **Dynamic study**
- **Opposite side**

Chapter 22 Skin

22.1 Imaging Modalities

Imaging modalities are:

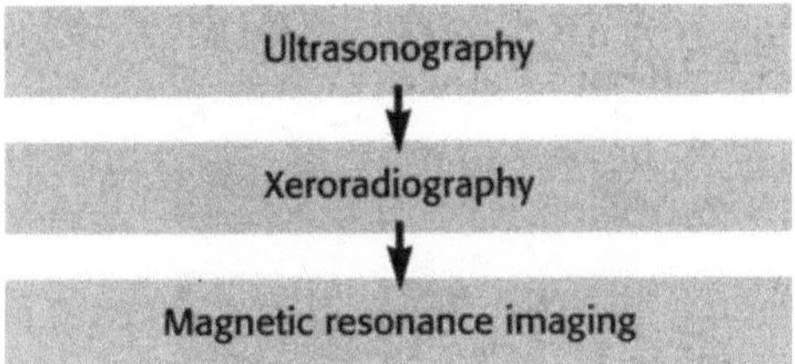

22.2 Ultrasonography

22.2.1 Examination Technique

No patient preparation is needed; it is seldom necessary to cut the hair overlying the lesion. The probe must be perpendicular to the skin surface. A comparative scan of normal skin on the contralateral side of the body should precede the study of the palpable nodule.

The ideal probe to study this very superficial structure is a 10-MHz transducer. Nowadays there are commercially available 13- to 15- and even 20-MHz probes which give very detailed images, but provide poor information on the surrounding extension of the lesion. If only a 7.5-MHz transducer is available it is necessary to use a 2 mm thick stand-off pad.

22.2.2 Sonoanatomy

It is possible to image the skin layers down to the superficial fascia which separates the underlying muscle. The epidermis is a thin, linear, hyperechoic structure. The dermis is barely distinguishable from the epidermis as it is also hyperechoic, but it contains tiny hypoechoic cavities due to the bulbus piliferus. The subcutaneous tissue is a hypoechoic layer which contains thin bright strands due to connective fibres interposed among the fat lobules. Its deep margin is sharply delineated as the superficial fascia is a hyperechoic well-defined structure, parallel to the skin surface and in close contact to the muscle.

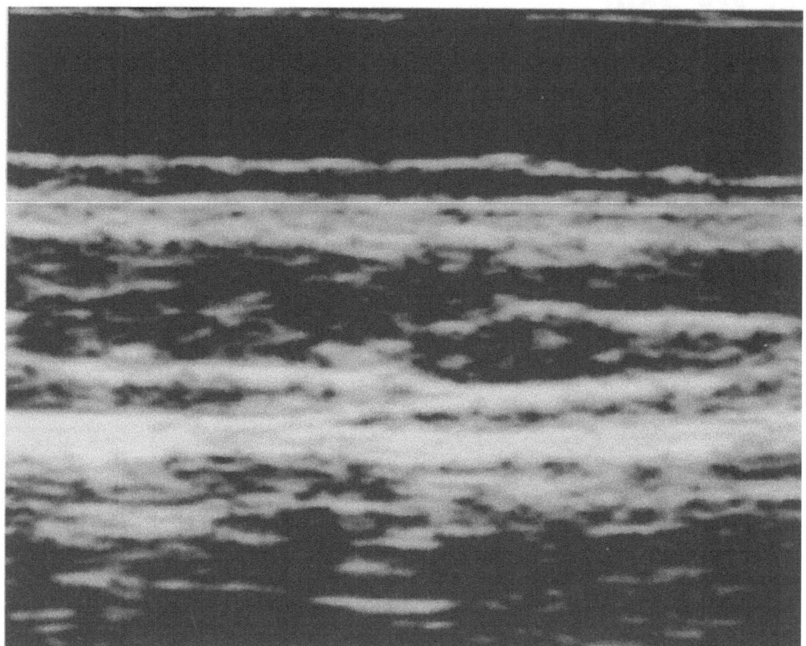

Fig. 22.1. Skin. A stand-off pad was used. The epidermis appears as an echogenic line. The dermis is homogeneous and bright, due to its high content of collagen. The subcutaneous tissue is hypoechoic and contains thin bright strands, due to connective fibres of separation between the fat lobules. The deep limit is clear cut by the hyperechoic superficial fascia

22.2.2.1 Normal Dimensions

Skin:
- Epidermis 1–2 mm
- Dermis 2–3.5 mm
- Subcutis 5–20 mm

The thickness of the subcutaneous layer varies depending upon the body habit, the site and the amount of fat in the region to be examined.

22.2.3 Sonopathology

22.2.3.1 Cyst

Clinical Data

Palpable, elevated nodule, mobile and slightly compressible; congenital or post-traumatic.

Sonographic Diagnosis

Criteria

→ In the subcutaneous layer
→ Spherical or oval anechoic lesion
→ Sharp and well-defined border
→ Distal acoustic enhancement
→ Prominent posterior border

The sebaceous and mucinous cysts tend to be hypoechoic, fairly homogeneous, with smooth edges and often with posterior enhancement.

The value of ultrasound in the diagnosis of cysts is to assess the real size of the lesion.

Sonographic Differential Diagnosis

The differential diagnosis of cysts includes haemangiomas and small cavity lymphangiomas which show change of shape and displacement of fluid under probe compression.

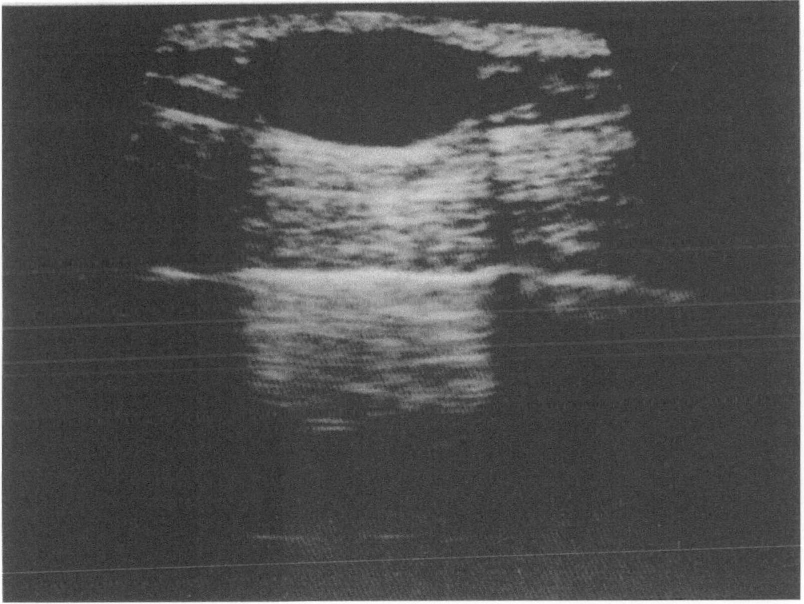

Fig. 22.2. Subcutaneous cyst

22.2.3.2 Lipoma

Clinical Data

Palpable, elevated nodule, highly mobile, soft, pliable; when large its border can be difficult to appreciate. Typically located in the neck, forearm, and dorsum.

Sonographic Diagnosis

Criteria

→ In the subcutaneous layer
→ Hypoechoic mass
→ Clear cut, bright contour
→ Thin internal bright strands

Large lipomas are not well encapsulated; this ultrasound finding is important for surgical planning. In the skin fat tends to be hypoechoic, while fat accumulation in the muscle, liver, and kidney is hyperechoic.

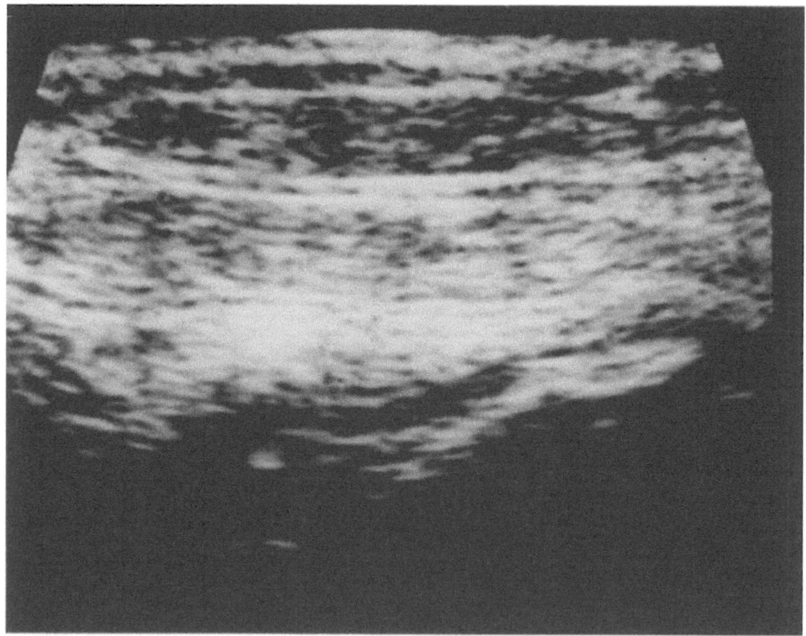

Fig. 22.3. Lipoma

Sonographic Differential Diagnosis

Differential diagnosis:
◆ Fibroma
◆ Dermatofibroma

Dermatofibromas tend to be small and are less compressible.

22.2.3.3 Haemangioma

Clinical Data

Soft swelling, highly compressible. Under compression its colour can disappear as the blood lake empties.

Sonographic Diagnosis

Criteria
→ In the dermis
→ Can reach the epidermis
→ Completely anechoic
→ Thin or thick septa
→ Debris due to thrombosis
→ Bright echoes with acoustic shadowing due to calcification

Colour Doppler may be valuable in identifying the feeding and draining vessels. Sometimes the flow within the lesion can be too slow to be detected on Doppler.

Sonographic Differential Diagnosis

Differential diagnosis:
◆ Cyst
◆ Lymphangioma
◆ Mucinous cyst

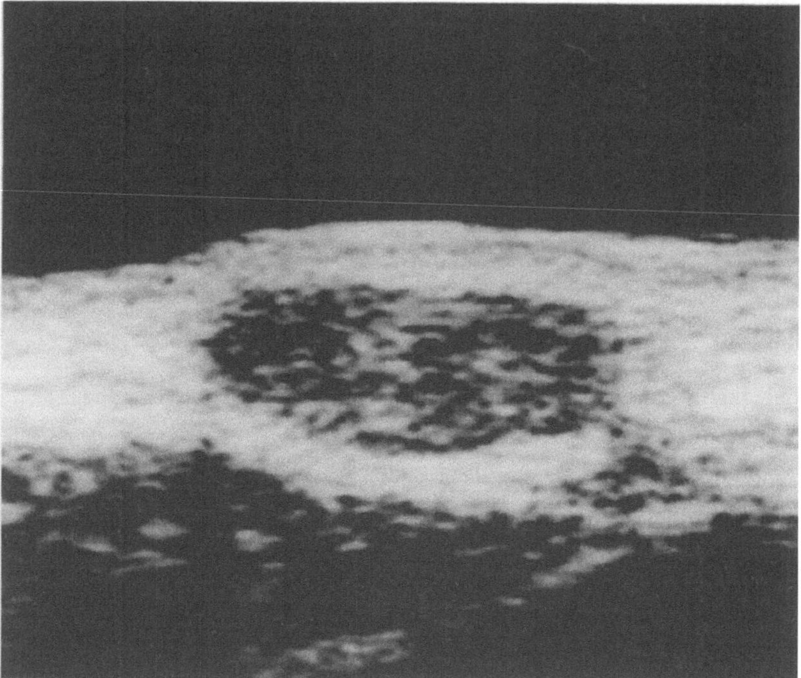

Fig. 22.4. Haemangioma. The lesion shows a well-defined margin with a fairly homogeneous echopattern depending upon the lack of internal blood lakes

22.2.3.4 Basal Cell Epithelioma

Clinical Data

Superficial brown lesion, typically in skin areas exposed to the sun.

Sonographic Diagnosis

Criteria

→ In the epidermis
→ Hypoechoic lesion
→ Slightly inhomogeneous depending upon the orientation of the cells
→ Fuzzy edges, especially posteriorly
→ Acoustic enhancement when stroma is thick

The surrounding epidermis is slightly hypoechoic due to sun exposure degeneration, therefore the lateral edges of the nodule are not clear cut. During the examination it is

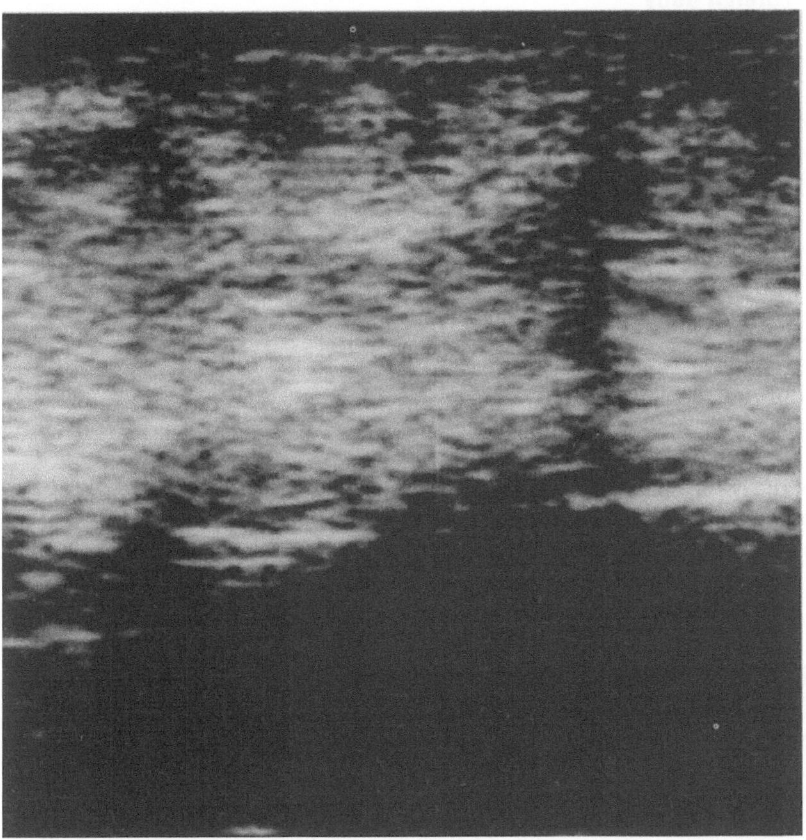

Fig. 22.5. Basal cell epithelioma. A very flat, superficial nodular lesion with an extension into the subcutaneous layer. The deep margin is not clear cut

possible to apply traction on the surrounding skin which appears hyperechoic due to the process of elastosis while the tumour remains hypoechoic.

Sonographic Differential Diagnosis

Differential diagnosis:
◆ Spinal cell epithelioma
◆ Large melanoma

Melanomas are superficial, fairly anechoic lesions with clear cut edges; however in case of accompanying proliferative reaction the contours of the lesion become fuzzy.

22.2.3.5 Foreign Body

Clinical Data

History of an accident, wound or recent surgical treatment with persistence of pain. In the acute stage the site of entrance of the foreign body is still present; later it can be masked by a scar.

Sonographic Diagnosis

Criteria

→ Small or large bright echo
→ Posterior reverberations
→ Hypoechoic halo

In case of really tiny foreign bodies the surrounding subcutaneous inflammatory reaction helps in detecting the included material. The ultrasound aspect is non-specific, but the patient's history is diagnostic. Once the foreign body is identified its relationship to adjacent structures should be carefully documented. In difficult cases a needle can be inserted under ultrasound guidance.

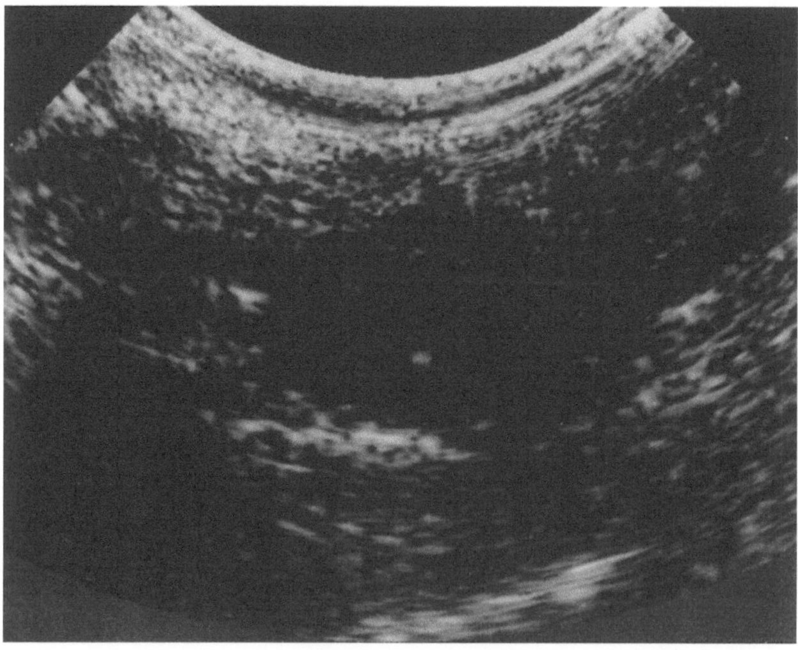

Fig. 22.6. Foreign body. The foreign material is hyperechoic (a piece of glass from a windscreen). The surrounding hypoechoic halo is due to granulation tissue. By ultrasound the size of a foreign body can be easily determined

Sonographic Differential Diagnosis

The patient's history is pathognomonic.

22.2.4 Checklist for Reporting

Skin
- Layer of origin
- Shape
- Edge
- Echopattern
- Posterior echogenicity
- Compressibility

Chapter 23 Neonatal Brain

23.1 Imaging Modalities

Imaging modalities are:

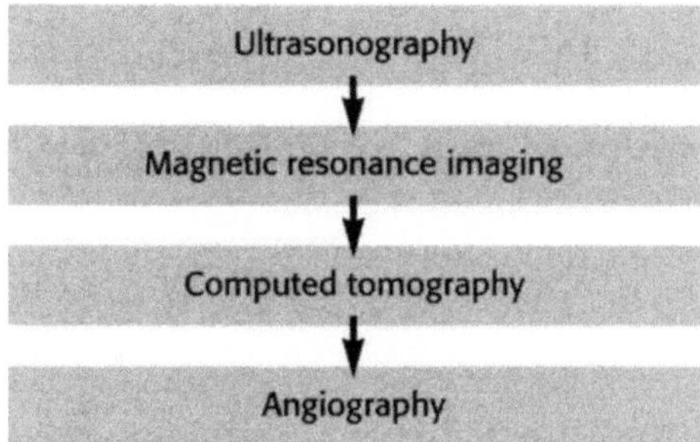

23.2 Ultrasonography

23.2.1 Examination Technique

The examination requires a 7.5- or 5-MHz sector transducer. No preparation or sedation is needed. Premature infants can be scanned within the incubator. In older children feeding during the examination can reduce movement. The anterior fontanelle is the window used to obtain sagittal and coronal views. A dense growth of scalp hair does not obscure the view if a large amount of coupling gel is used.

23.2.2 Sonoanatomy

The middle portion of the brain is occupied from top to bottom by the 3rd ventricle, the 4th ventricle, and the Sylvian aqueduct. In premature infants these structures can be mildly dilated, while in the full term newborn they are barely seen. Slightly lateral to these structures there are the frontal, temporal, and occipital horns, the body and the atrium of the lateral ventricle. In the floor of the body and atrium the highly vascular hyperechoic choroid plexus can be seen. Around the ventricular complex there are the gyri, the caudate nucleus, and the thalamus; between the latter structures lies the germinal matrix in the ependymal layer. At the periphery the Sylvian fissure appears as a hyperechoic, pulsatile, inverted Y-shaped structure.

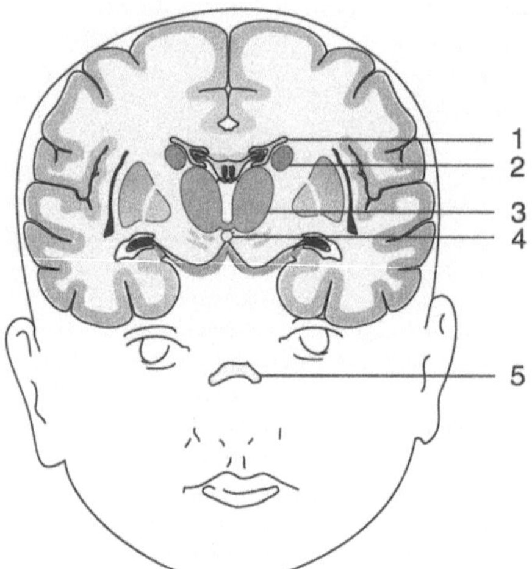

Fig. 23.1. Coronal section of the brain. *1*, Anterior horn of lateral ventricle; *2*, head of caudate nucleus; *3*, thalamus; *4*, 3rd ventricle; *5*, 4th ventricle

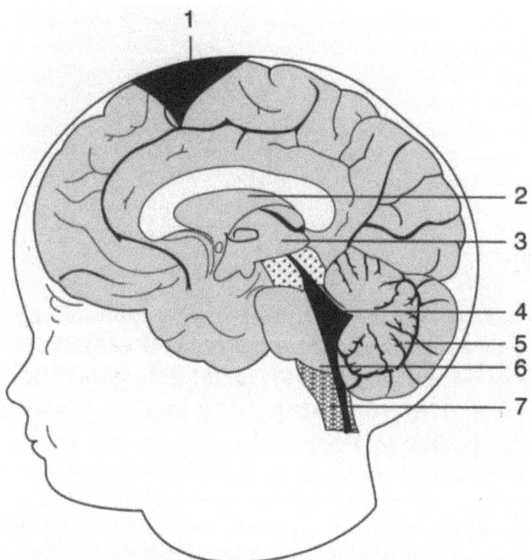

Fig. 23.2. Sagittal section of the brain. *1*, Anterior fontanelle; *2*, lateral ventricle; *3*, 3rd ventricle; *4*, 4th ventricle; *5*, cerebellum; *6*, pons; *7*, medulla oblongata

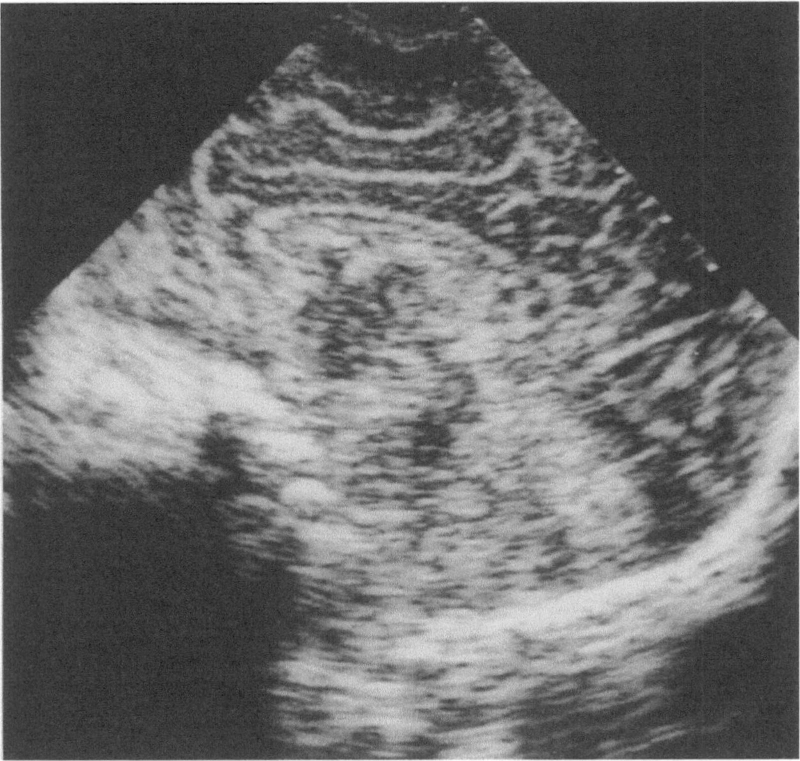

Fig. 23.3. Brain. Sagittal scan. The inferior echoes delineate the anterior, middle, and posterior fossa. The curvilinear hypoechoic structure in the midline is the corpus callosum. The 3rd and 4th ventricles are physiologically obliterated. In the posterior fossa the main structure is the cerebellum

23.2.2.1 Normal Dimensions

Brain:
- Hemispherical width 33 mm
- Biventricular width at caudate nucleus 25 mm
- Frontal horn at foramen of Monro 10 mm

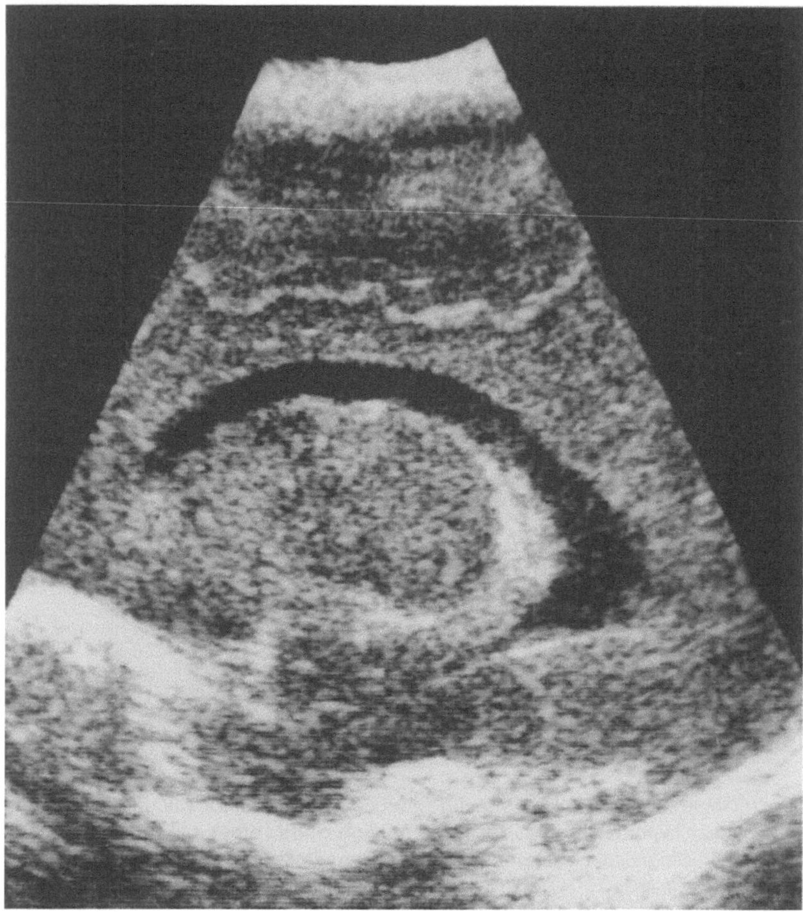

Fig. 23.4. Brain. Parasagittal scan. Mild dilatation of the lateral ventricle. The hyperechoic structure posterior to the head of the caudate nucleus and the thalamus is the choroid plexus

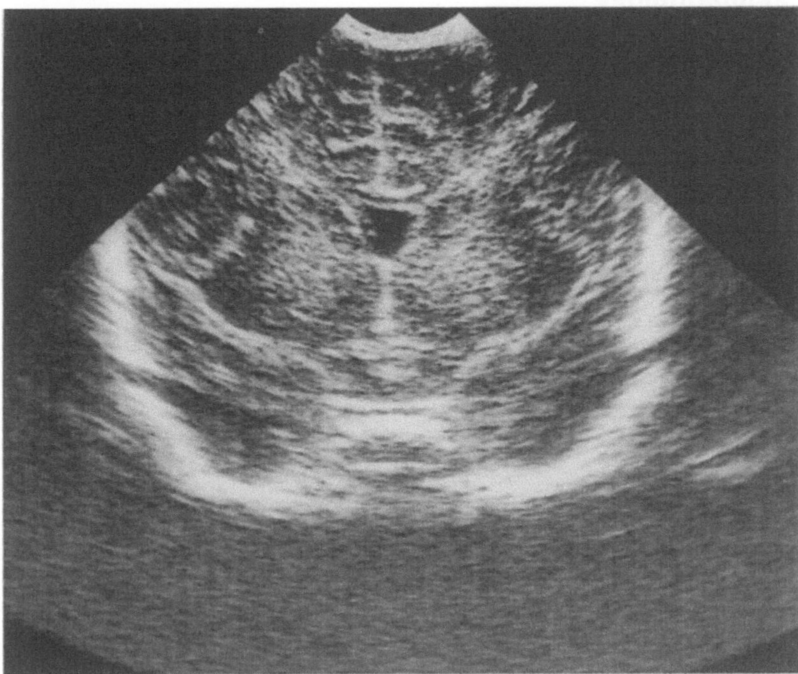

Fig. 23.5. Brain. Middle coronal scan. The superior midline linear echogenic structure is the interhemispheric fissure. The thin perpendicular hypoechoic line is the corpus callosum with the anechoic cavum septi pellucidi, physiologically seen up to two months. In the normal infant the frontal horns are barely seen. Inferolateral to them the head of the caudate nucleus and the thalamus are seen. The Y-shaped structure next to the parietal bone is the Sylvian fissure with the middle cerebral artery

23.2.3 Sonopathology

23.2.3.1 Haemorrhage

Clinical Data

The infant presents with seizures, hypotonia, and cyanosis.

Sonographic Diagnosis

Criteria

→ Acute
  - Hyperechoic
  - Homogeneous
→ Chronic
  - Complex
  - Inhomogeneous

With time the sonographic appearance of haemorrhage changes. Findings may then include:
◆ Complete resolution
◆ Residual linear echoes
◆ Porencephalic cyst
◆ Obstructive hydrocephalus

Subependymal haemorrhage:
◆ Premature infant
◆ At caudothalamic groove
◆ Hyperechoic, round
◆ Often bilateral

Intraventricular haemorrhage:
◆ Full term infants
◆ Echogenic filling of the ventricle, complete as with a cast or focal with clots
◆ Cerebrospinal fluid-clot level in the occipital horn
◆ Ventricular dilatation
◆ Hyperechoic ventricular wall

Sonographic Differential Diagnosis

Differential diagnosis of subependymal haemorrhage:
◆ Leukomalacia
◆ Anterior attachment of the choroid plexus
◆ Artefact from the frontal horn wall
◆ Basal ganglia haemorrhage

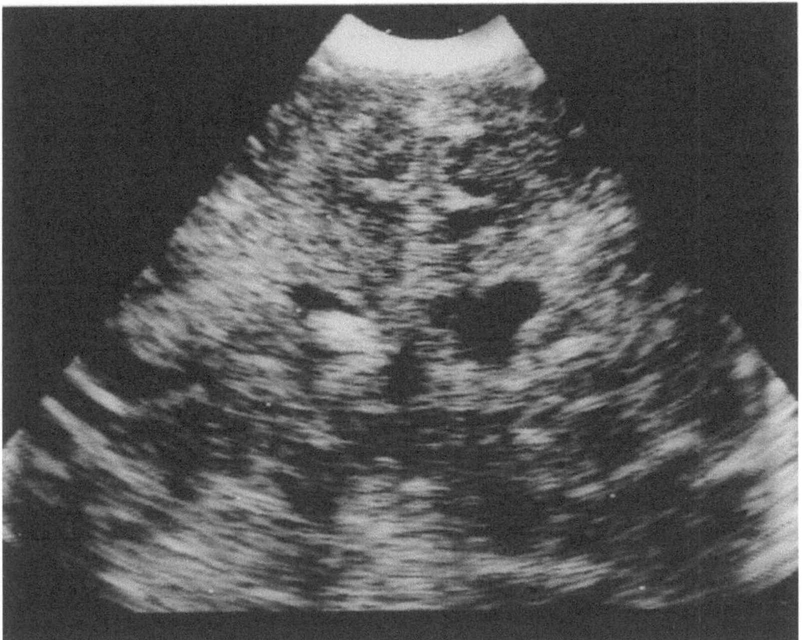

Fig. 23.6. Subependymal haemorrhage at the level of the floor of the right frontal horn. Anterior coronal scan. The lesion is hyperechoic and occupies part of the lumen of the horn

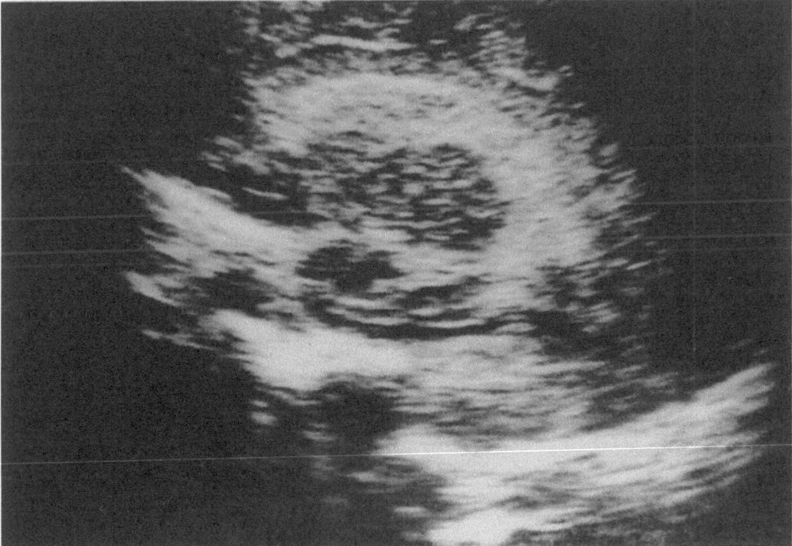

Fig. 23.7. Intraventricular haemorrhage. Parasagittal scan. The homogeneously hyperechoic acute bleeding occupies the lateral ventricle entirely

Differential diagnosis of intraventricular haemorrhage:
◆ Choroid plexus bleeding
◆ Ventriculitis

23.2.3.2 Congenital Anomalies

Clinical Data

Facial deformities, head circumference large for age, bulging anterior fontanelles. Delay in neurological development, psychomotor abnormalities.

Sonographic Diagnosis

Criteria

→ Posterior fossa cyst
→ Dysgenesis of the vermis
→ Hypoplasia of the cerebellar hemispheres
→ Superior elevation of the tentorium
→ Hydrocephalus

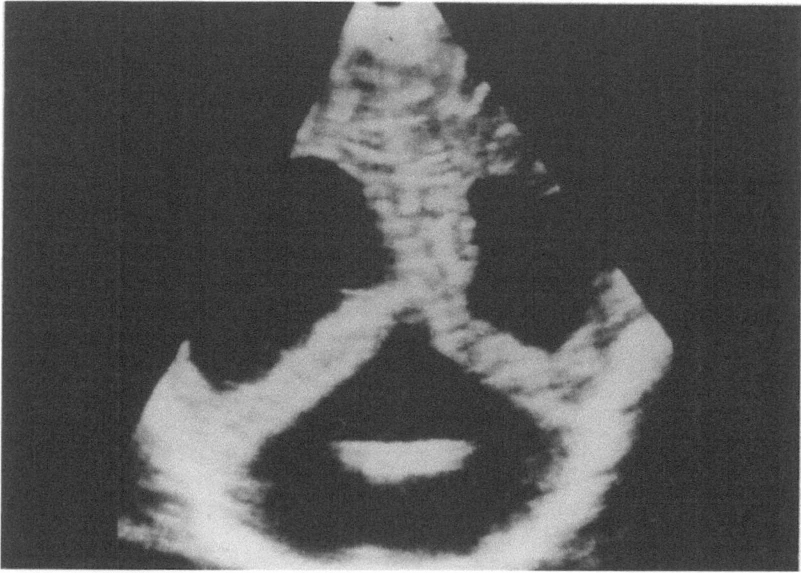

Fig. 23.8. Dandy-Walker syndrome. Posterior coronal scan. The anechoic anterolateral cavities are the dilated occipital horns of the lateral ventricles. The posterior midline fluid-filled cavity is the very distended 4th ventricle in which the tip of the drainage catheter is seen as a linear bright echo

Sonographic Differential Diagnosis

Differential diagnosis:
- Posterior fossa arachnoid cyst
- Enlarged cisterna magna

23.2.3.3 Infection

Clinical Data

In congenital disease the head can be enlarged. In early stage of post-natal infection there are only a few clinical signs. Later the patients present with neurological disorders and generalized sepsis symptoms. Bulging anterior fontanelle.

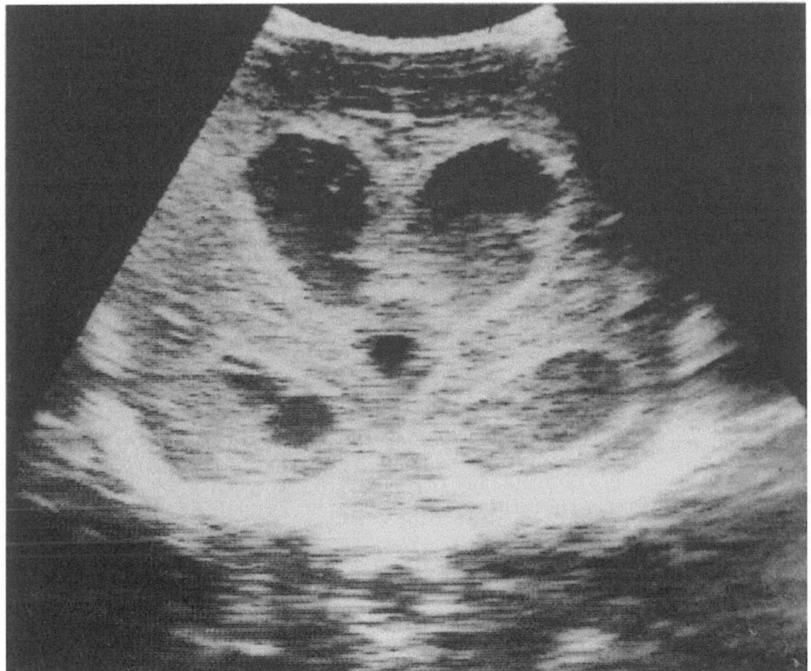

Fig. 23.9. Meningoencephalitis due to *Escherichia coli*. Anterior coronal scan. The infected brain parenchyma is hyperechoic; the ventricular walls are very thick and bright due to ventriculitis. The lateral ventricular system and the 3rd ventricle are dilated and contain hyperechoic fibrinous strands and debris

Sonographic Diagnosis

Criteria

→ Increased echogenicity of brain
→ Ventricular dilatation
→ Thick ventricular walls
→ Strands within the ventricles
→ Abscess formation
→ Extra-axial fluid collection
→ Porencephalic cyst

Sonographic Differential Diagnosis

Differential diagnosis:
◆ Encephalomalacia
◆ Hydrocephalus
◆ Subdural, subarachnoid haemorrhage

23.2.3.4 Tumours

Clinical Data

Rapidly enlarging head, cerebral hypertension. Seizures. Palsy.

Sonographic Diagnosis

Criteria

→ Supratentorial complex mass
→ Ventricular obstruction
→ Hydrocephalus
→ Displacement of midline structures

Sonographic Differential Diagnosis

The mass, usually very large, does not pose any diagnostic problem. Even in a case of severe hydrocephalus the obstructive mass is readily seen.

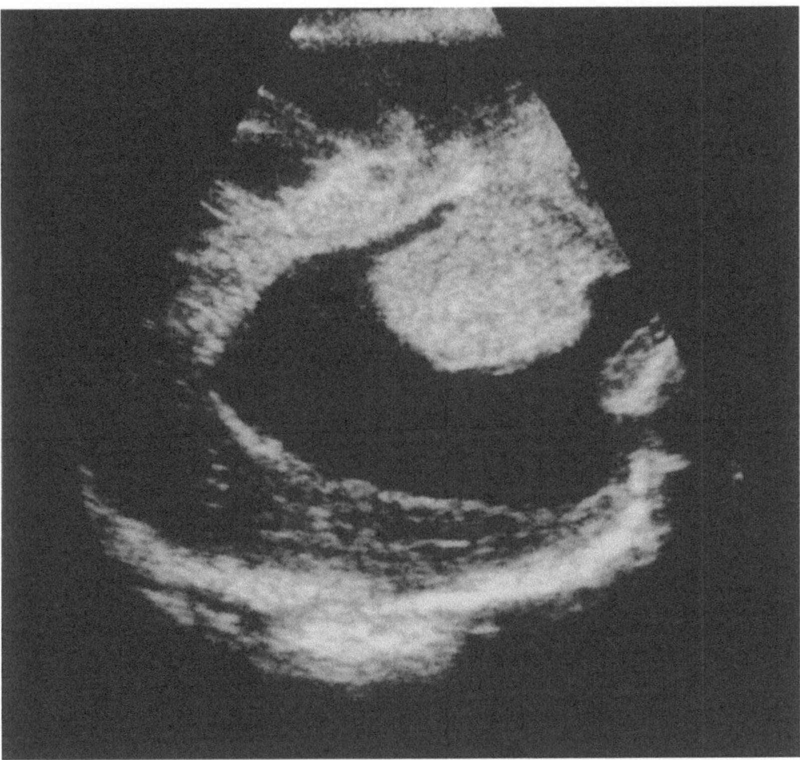

Fig. 23.10. Choroid plexus papilloma. Parasagittal scan. The anechoic cystic cavity is the very dilated atrium of the lateral ventricle with a hyperechoic soft tissue mass, arising from its wall

23.2.4 Checklist for Reporting

Brain
- **Symmetry of the anatomical landmarks in the two hemispheres**
- **Size of the ventricles**
- **Echogenic material within the ventricles**
- **Focal lesions next to the ventricular system or embedded in the parenchyma**

24.1 Introduction

The first clinical applications of the Doppler principle in ultrasound date back to 1954, but this technique became widely available for the detection of foetal heart only in the middle 1960s. The determination of vessel patency, blood flow, and organ perfusion has been a goal of diagnostic imaging with varying success by angiography, computed tomography, and magnetic resonance imaging as well as Doppler sonography. However, Doppler ultrasound has evolved slowly compared to other applications of diagnostic ultrasound. Recent advances in colour Doppler technology have resulted in an explosion of new clinical applications. It is one of the fastest growing yet possibly least understood modality in ultrasound today.

24.2 What Is Doppler?

The Doppler technique measures the changes in the frequency of reflected ultrasound when the target is moving. The frequency increases if the target moves towards the transducer and vice versa. The Doppler shift frequency is described by the formula: $f_D = 2 f_0 \, v \cos \theta / c$, where f_D is the Doppler frequency shift, f_0 is the incident frequency, v is the flow velocity, θ is the angle between the path of the central ultrasound beam and the direction of flow, and c is the speed of sound in human tissue.

Simple Doppler devices (continuous-wave Doppler) offer velocity information without depth resolution and are therefore used only in the examination of superficial vessels. However, due to very poor image resolution and long acquisition time (typically 5–10 min) these systems are no longer used except for foetal heart monitoring.

24.3 Duplex Doppler

Duplex Doppler or pulsed Doppler implies simultaneous real-time B-mode ultrasound imaging and acquisition of Doppler information from a single point within the imaged area (Figs. 24.1, 24.2).

Conventional B-mode scanning is performed in the normal manner and the target vessel is identified. The ultrasound beam must be directed to obtain as small an angle as possible with the long axis of the vessel. A sample gate can be placed over the area of interest. The scanner converts the Doppler frequency information into graphical wave form: the Doppler spectrum (Figs. 24.1, 24.2). Flow towards the transducer appears above the base line of the spectral Doppler graph whereas flow away from the transducer appears below the base line. This display shows the instantaneous velocity and direction of blood flow within the vessel during the examination. The most commonly used information from the Doppler spectrum are:

- Peak velocity
- Mean velocity
- Spectrum broadening
- Pulsatility index (PI)
- Resistance index (RI)

Indices of pulsatility are ratios of Doppler shift frequencies and hence are independent of the Doppler angle (between beam and vessel). The PI measures the difference between the maximum (peak systolic) and minimum (end diastolic) value divided by the mean value of the waveform over the cardiac cycle. The PI conveys the pulsatility of the Doppler shift frequency of the signal from an artery. The RI, also known as Pourcelot Index, is an index of pulsatility defined as the difference between the maximum and minimum Doppler shifts divided by the maximum.

With a high peripheral resistance, i.e. no, low or reversal of diastolic flow, the PI increases (Fig. 24.1), whereas low resistance flow, i.e. flow continuing during diastole, reduces the PI (Fig. 24.2). The PI is used to assess the flow in arteries. As a general rule the PI is reduced if the peripheral bed supplied by the artery has reduced resistance to blood flow and vice versa, for example, arteries supplying brain (internal carotid artery), kidney (renal artery), liver (hepatic artery) have a low PI, while arteries supplying limbs (subclavian artery, femoral artery) have a high PI. Increase in the PI indicates increased stiffness of the organ and can be used as an indication of the severity of disease, for example, cirrhosis, renal transplant rejection, and intra-uterine growth retardation. Spectral broadening is associated with stenosis of the vessel which can be quantified by the degree of broadening.

However, the resolution of B-mode ultrasound is not good enough to identify small parenchymal vessels, which are especially important in neovascularization and in the normal vascularization of organs such as the breast, ovary, kidney, and liver. Thus the value of a simultaneous display of the real-time image and Doppler, the main advantage of Duplex, is limited. Another major limitation is that the flow information is obtained only from a small region. Hence it is important to perform careful sampling of the sites within the vessel lumen where flow disturbances are most likely to be found. Like continuous wave Doppler, this technique is too time-consuming for routine application on its own.

24.4 Colour Doppler

Colour Doppler allows the evaluation of flow characteristics throughout an entire image combined with a high resolution B-mode display of the vessel wall and surrounding tissue features. Signals from red blood cells are displayed in colour as a function of their motion towards or away from the transducer. Conventionally, colours are set to display blood flow towards the transducer in red and flow away in blue. Various shades of red and blue are used to indicate the relative velocity of the moving red blood cells. Usually lighter shades indicate higher velocity, however this depends upon the choice of settings. The equipment allows the user to select the optimum range/window of velocities depending upon the requirement, for example, for subclavian artery, femoral artery, aorta, heart, and all other major vessels where blood flow has a higher velocity, a higher velocity scale is used, whereas for veins, intraparenchymal vessels, and tumour vasculature, a lower velocity scale is required. By displaying all colour Doppler data in real-time and in two dimensions, normal as well as abnormal vessels can be located relatively quickly and their anatomical positions and patterns can be elucidated. The colour Doppler image serves as a map to guide the placement of the pulse Doppler gate. Thus colour Doppler not only opens the way for precisely directed velocity measurements, but offers unique anatomical information that may be of value in its own right. Usually colour Doppler is performed first and then, depending upon the need, pulsed Doppler is used to obtain various flow measurements from the Doppler spectrum.

24.5 Clinical Applications

24.5.1 General Applications

General clinical applications are:
- Presence of blood flow (Figs. 24.3–24.6)
  - Arterial stenosis
  - Venous thrombosis
- Direction of blood flow (Figs. 24.7, 24.8)
  - Portal hypertension
  - Varicose veins
  - Shunts
- Characterization of altered flow (Figs. 24.9, 24.10)
  - Renal transplant rejection
  - Renal/carotid artery stenosis
  - Intra-uterine growth retardation
  - Arteriovenous fistula
- Tumour vascularization (Fig. 24.11)
- Tissue characterization (Figs. 24.12–24.14)
- Tissue perfusion
  - Placenta
  - Neonatal brain

- Intraoperative imaging
- Follow-up examinations
  - After liver/kidney transplantation
  - After embolization
  - After angioplasty

24.5.2 Specific Applications

24.5.2.1 Vessels

Duplex Doppler of peripheral vessels with B-mode imaging and colour Doppler provides both anatomical imaging of the vessel and flow velocity information.

Carotid Arteries

Atherosclerosis of the cerebral arteries accounts for two thirds of cerebrovascular accidents with a predilection for the extracerebral arteries. Their role in cerebrovascular disease and easy accessibility to ultrasound has made carotid Doppler one of the most common indications.

Clinical indications:
- Neurological deficit
- Carotid bruit
- Degree of stenosis
- Before vascular surgery
- Follow-up after endarterectomy
- Screening in elderly

Findings (Figs. 24.3, 24.4):
- Increased velocities at the point of stenosis
- Spectral broadening distal to stenosis due to flow disturbance

On colour Doppler narrowing of the vessel can be more easily identified; this is especially true for differentiating between a complete thrombosis and a very high grade stenosis (> 90%), which can be difficult by spectral Doppler alone.

The degree of stenosis can be assessed from velocity measurements and flow pattern, especially if the diameter reduction is greater than 50%. This has influenced clinical decisions in selecting patients for surgery and follow-up.

Peripheral Arteries

Clinical indications:
- Suspected occlusive disease (from aorta to popliteal trifurcation)
- Screening procedure prior to angiography or angioplasty
- Follow-up after arterial surgery and dilatation

Leg Veins

Clinical indications:
◆ Suspected deep venous thrombosis
◆ Follow-up in deep venous thrombosis
◆ Varicose veins

Colour Doppler has been proved to be an accurate and suitable replacement for venography in the diagnosis of venous thrombosis (Figs. 24.5, 24.6), and venography is reserved for those cases in whom there is a diagnostic dilemma. Colour Doppler, however, is not very sensitive in detecting thrombosis of calf veins because of wide variation of the normal anatomy.

24.5.2.2 Liver

Doppler ultrasound of the hepatic circulation permits the acquisition of useful physiological and functional information from the liver. The hepatic vein waveform is a sensitive but non-specific indicator of the presence of liver disease, and the degree of deviation from the normal pattern may allow an estimation of the severity of the disease. The examination of the portal vein signal permits the detection and grading of more severe cases of liver disease and allows the assessment of the adequacy of shunting procedures. The examination of the hepatic artery waveform is seldom of direct value but does allow the estimation of the degree of vascularity of hepatic tumours and the success of therapeutic embolization. It is also helpful in liver transplant patients.

Hepatic Circulation

Clinical indications:
◆ Chronic liver disease (cirrhosis)
◆ Budd-Chiari syndrome
◆ Portal vein thrombosis
◆ Liver tumours
◆ Monitoring of secondary biliary cirrhosis in childhood

Chronic liver disease (cirrhosis) (Fig. 24.8):
◆ Portal vein
  – Usually normal
  – Loss of respiratory variation
  – Absent postprandial increase in flow
  – Decrease in velocity flow
◆ Hepatic vein
  – Flattening of the hepatic vein waveform (degree of flattening proportional to the severity of liver disease)
◆ Hepatic artery
  – Normal or increased diastolic flow

Budd-Chiari syndrome:
- Failure to detect flow from hepatic veins (segmental occlusion not uncommon)
- Reversal of flow (if all hepatic veins are thrombosed, blood can only leave via portal vein)

Liver tumours:
- Haemangiomas usually show no signals
- Primary and secondary tumours show flow on colour Doppler
- Hepatoma and large haemangiomas may show reversal of flow in portal vein
- Hepatic veins may show high flow if draining a tumour

24.5.2.3 Kidney

Clinical indications:
- Renal artery stenosis
- Tumours such as Wilms' tumour and renal cell carcinoma to detect involvement of the renal vein and the inferior vena cava (Fig. 24.15)

Renal artery stenosis:
- High systolic flow (increased velocity)
- Reduced diastolic flow
- Spectral broadening due to turbulence of flow in the post-stenotic segment
- Limitations
  - Difficulties in visualizing the renal arteries, especially the left
  - 25% of kidneys may have multiple renal arteries
  - Time consuming

Renal Transplants

The superficial position and high perfusion of renal transplants makes them particularly suitable for ultrasound and Doppler scanning (Fig. 24.9).

Clinical indications:
- Renal artery stenosis (not as in the native kidney, it can be diagnosed confidently, as the anatomy of the renal artery and the site of anastomosis are already known)
- Renal vein stenosis
- Renal vein thrombosis
- Arteriovenous fistula following surgery or biopsy (use of colour Doppler in subsequent biopsies is essential to avoid the possibility of bleeding) (Fig. 24.10)
- Perfusion of parenchyma
- Quality of flow as increase in resistance may indicate rejection/acute tubular necrosis

◆ Limitations
  – Mild rejection may not show any changes
  – Cannot differentiate between rejection and acute tubular necrosis

24.5.2.4 Oncology

Malignant tumours larger than a few millimetres in diameter stimulate the growth of new blood vessels by secreting angiogenesis factor. The neovascularization:

◆ penetrates the lesion from its periphery
◆ consists of thin-walled blood vessels that lack a muscular layer
◆ often shows chaotic anastomoses and shunts

The multiplicity of vessels, their disordered pattern, and the arteriovenous shunts of these tumour vessels give rise to flow that can be detected as:

◆ High velocity signals
◆ Low resistance flow (Fig. 24.2)

In oncology, colour Doppler provides an immediate and reasonable representation of the vascular anatomy that allows tissues to be characterized. In many applications this is helpful in discriminating between benign and malignant masses. These tumour flow signals have been detected in carcinomas of the breast, thyroid, kidney, liver, pancreas, ovaries, and uterus (Fig. 24.11). B-mode ultrasound with colour Doppler has been found to be the most reliable screening method for early detection of ovarian and endometrial cancers.

Currently colour Doppler is also used for indicating:
◆ Prognosis
◆ Response to chemotherapy
◆ Success of tumour embolization
◆ Differentiation between scarring and tumour recurrence on the basis of negative colour Doppler findings

24.5.2.5 Neurology

High resolution ultrasonography of the infant brain in the investigation and management of various abnormalities, especially in the assessment of hydrocephalus and periventricular haemorrhage, is now well established. Colour Doppler angiography with the help of spectral Doppler allows detailed studies of intracranial vascular abnormalities such as:

◆ Arteriovenous malformations
◆ Arterial and venous occlusive processes

Colour Doppler, by improving the anatomical as well as the physiological information on ultrasound images, has changed the way in which examinations are conducted. Colour Doppler is the most significant advance since the transition from static to real-time imaging. Colour Doppler has become an integral part of most ultrasound examinations.

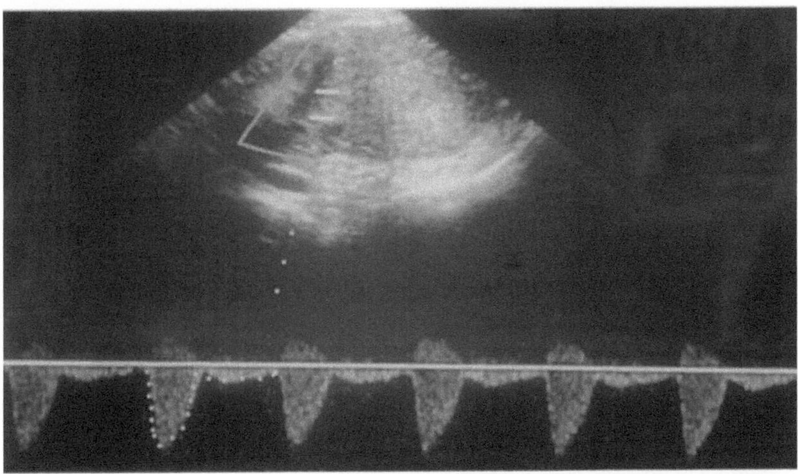

Fig. 24.1. Duplex Doppler of the uterine artery – high resistance flow. High systolic and minimal diastolic flow indicates high resistance flow (blood is flowing away from the transducer, hence Doppler spectrum is below the zero line)

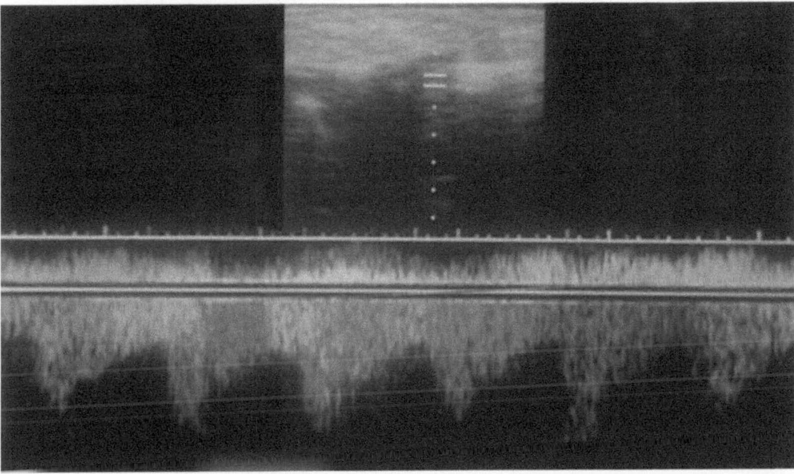

Fig. 24.2. Duplex Doppler of breast carcinoma – low resistance flow. High and continuous flow through diastole indicates relatively low resistance flow

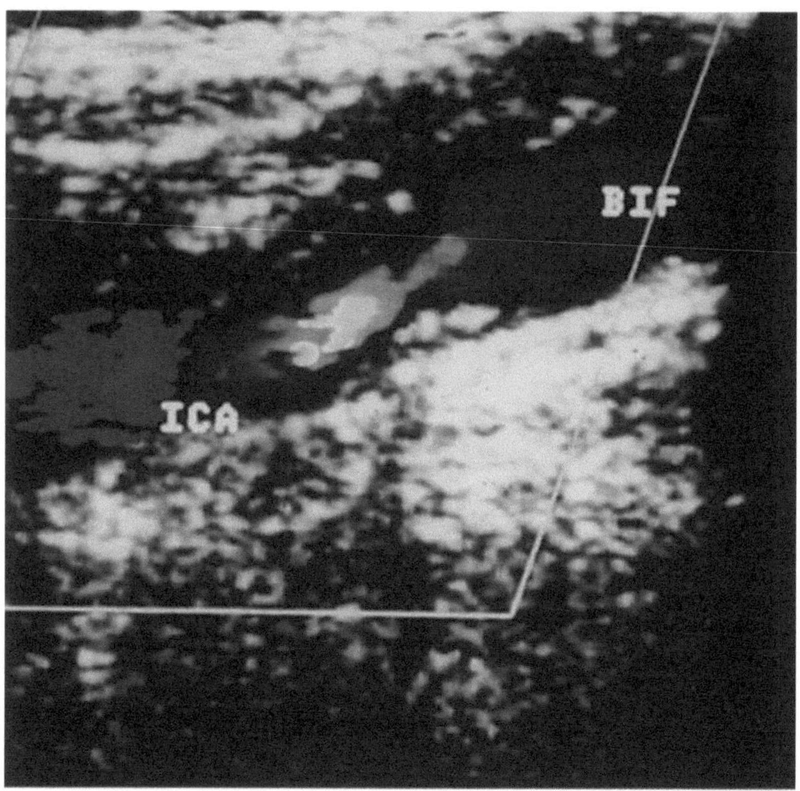

Fig. 24.3. Internal carotid artery stenosis. Longitudinal view of the internal carotid artery (*ICA*) shows a tight stenosis just at its origin. A part of the carotid bifurcation (*BIF*) is also seen

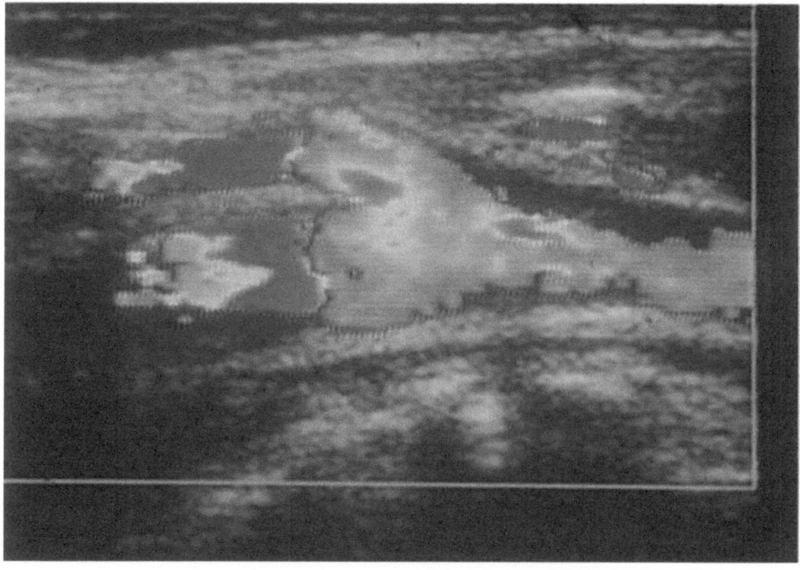

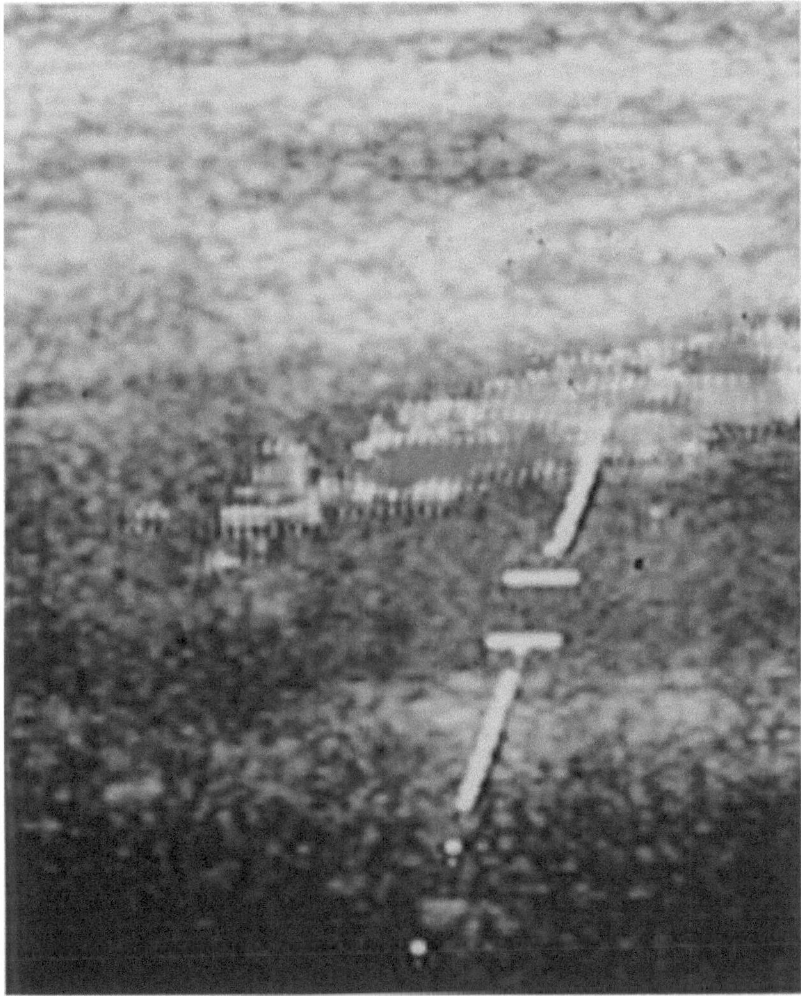

Fig. 24.5. Complete thrombotic occlusion of the femoral vein. Longitudinal view of the femoral vein in the mid thigh showing a good flow in the femoral artery and none in the femoral vein, which is confirmed on Duplex Doppler

◀ **Fig. 24.4.** Common carotid artery and its bifurcation showing partial thrombosis of the common carotid artery just below its bifurcation

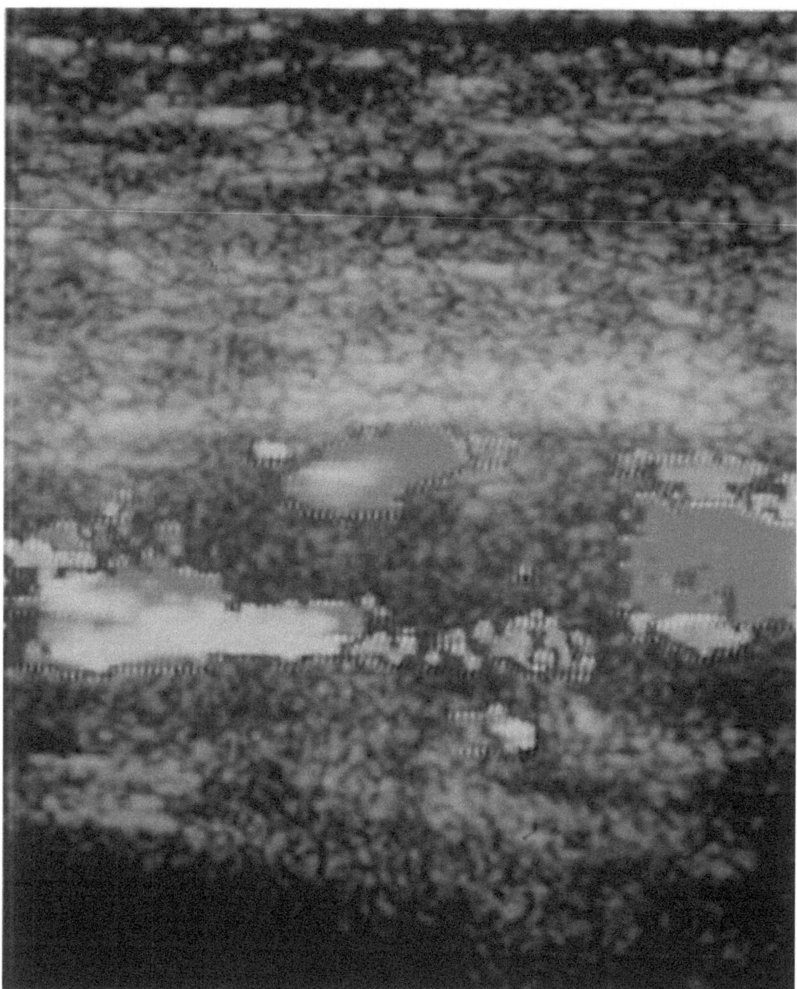

Fig. 24.6. Deep venous thrombosis with partial recanalization

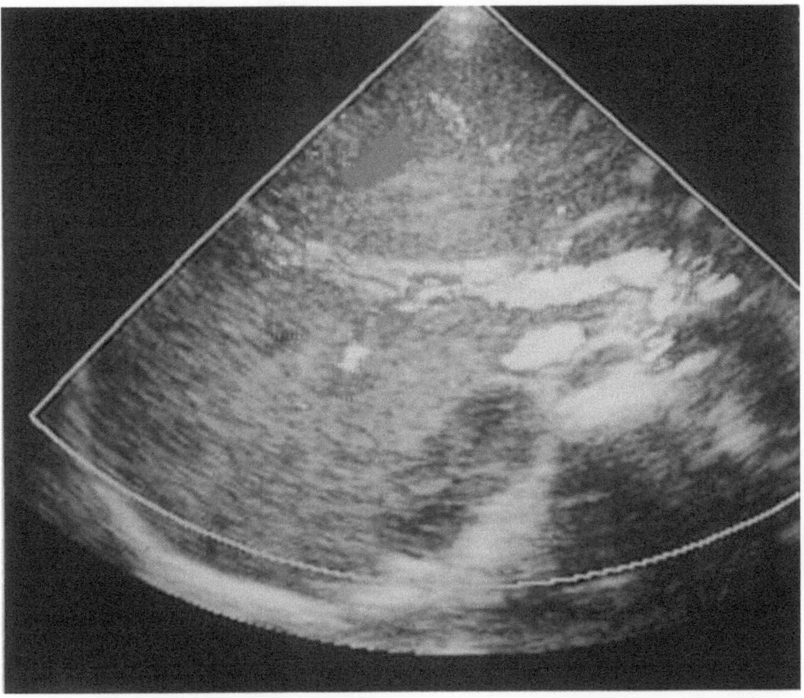

Fig. 24.7. Normal portal vein and its branches on colour Doppler

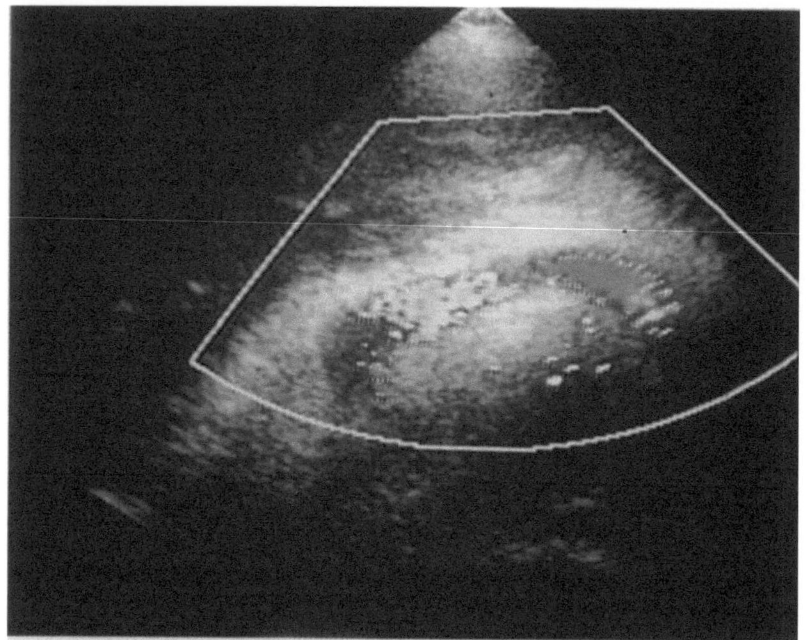

a

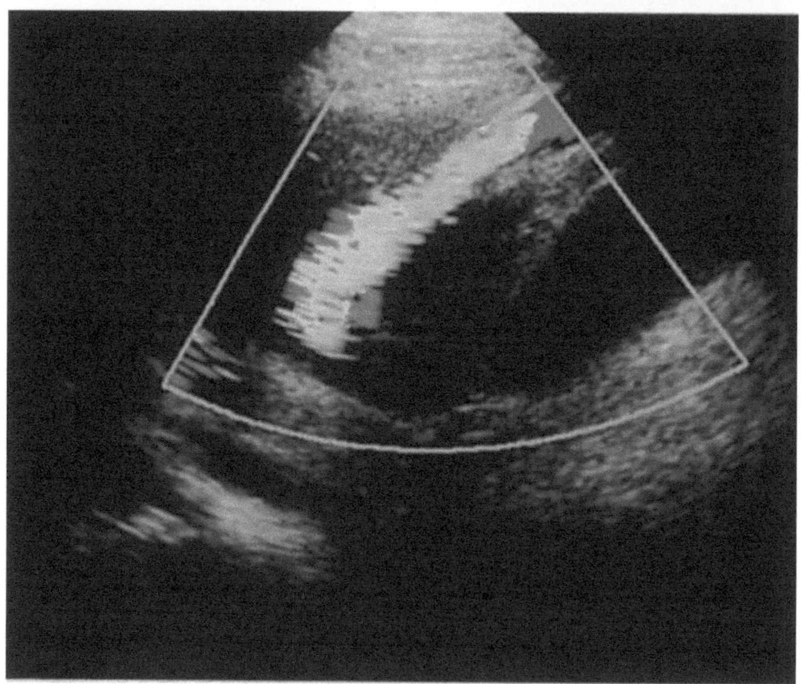

b

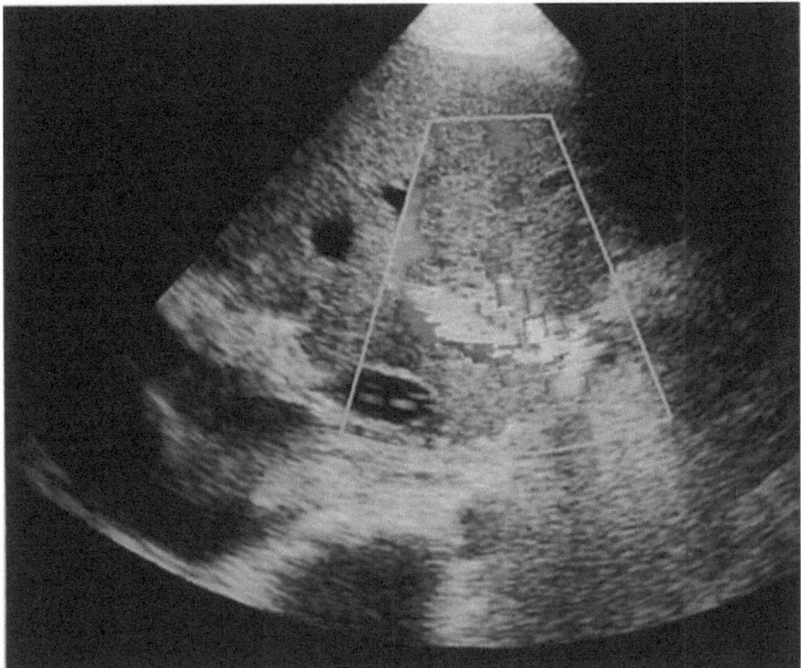

c

Fig. 24.8 a–c. Colour Doppler in portal hypertension. Reversed flow in the splenic vein. **a** Transverse view of the upper abdomen showing reversal of flow in the splenic vein (according to the chosen colour settings, flow towards the transducer should be *red* and flow away from the transducer *blue* – which is reversed). **b** Recanalization of the umbilical vein. **c** Portal cavernoma

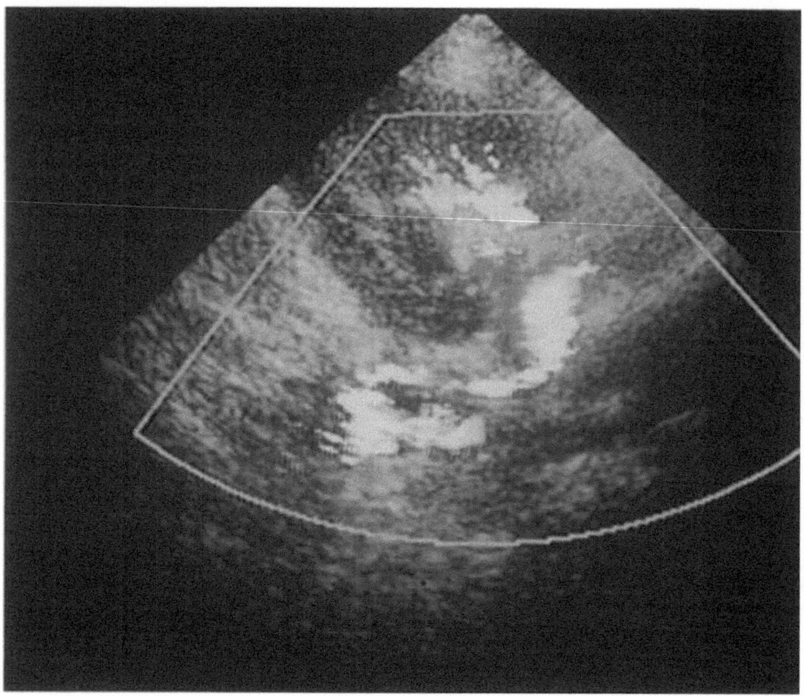

Fig. 24.9. Transverse section of a transplant kidney showing vascular anatomy of renal vessels

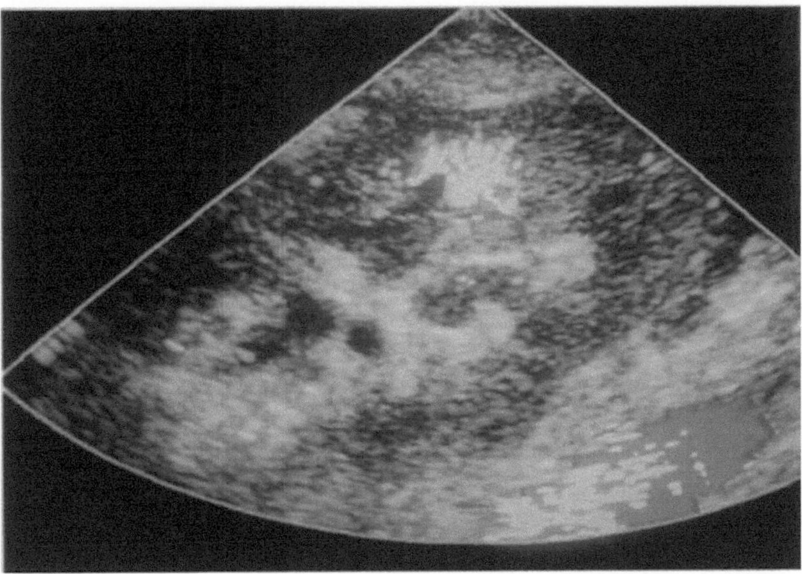

Fig. 24.10. Post-biopsy arteriovenous fistula in a transplant kidney

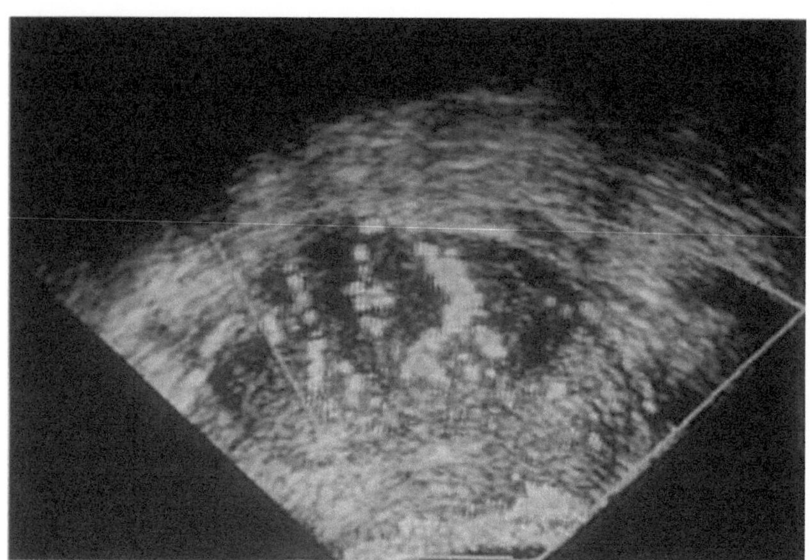

a

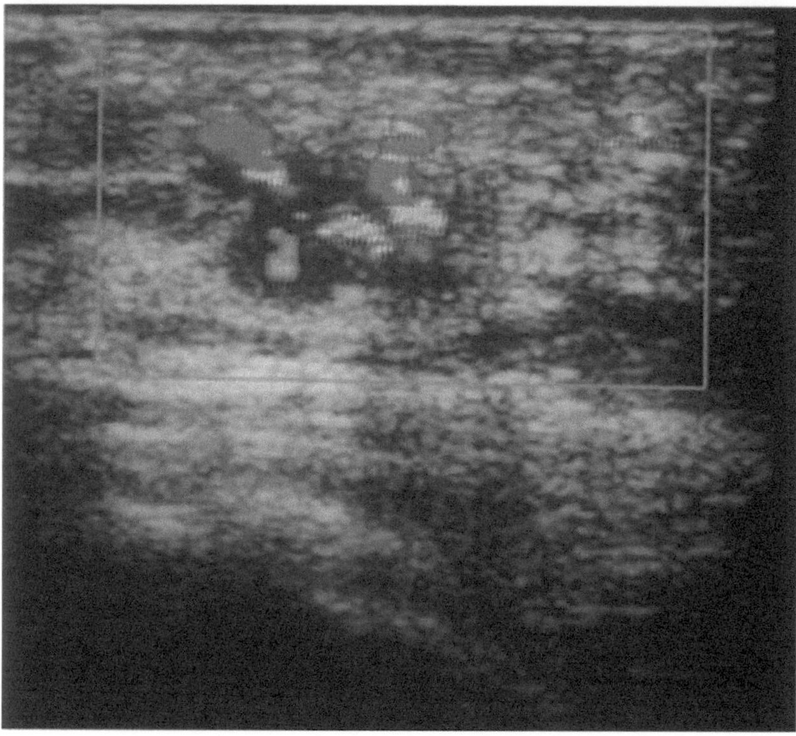

b

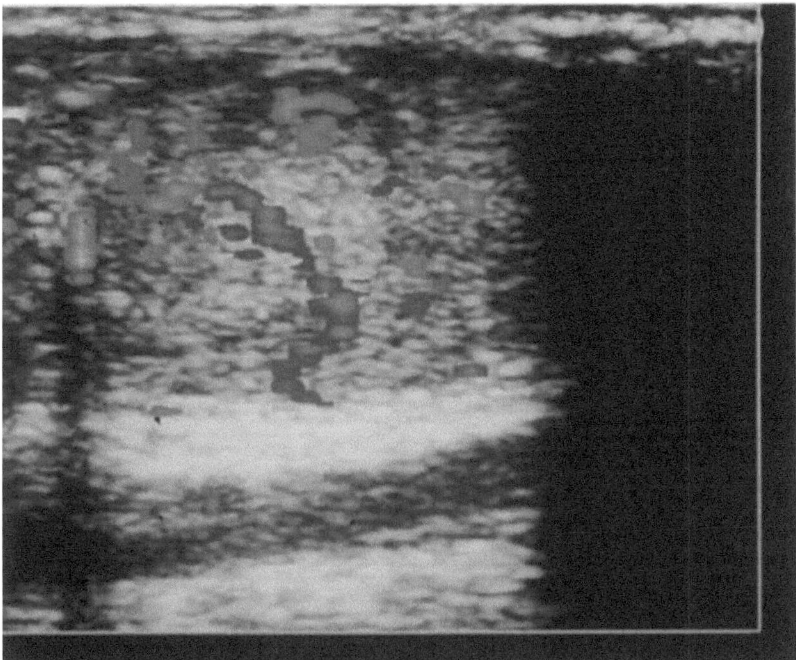

c

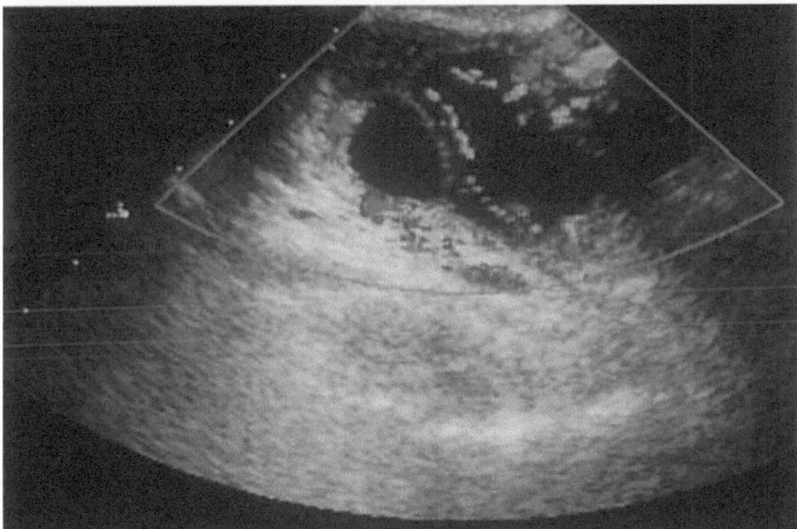

d

Fig. 24.11 a–d. Tumour vascularization on colour Doppler. **a** Carcinoma of the prostate showing large irregular vessels (neovascularization). **b** Carcinoma of the breast. **c** Testicular teratoma. **d** Ovarian carcinoma

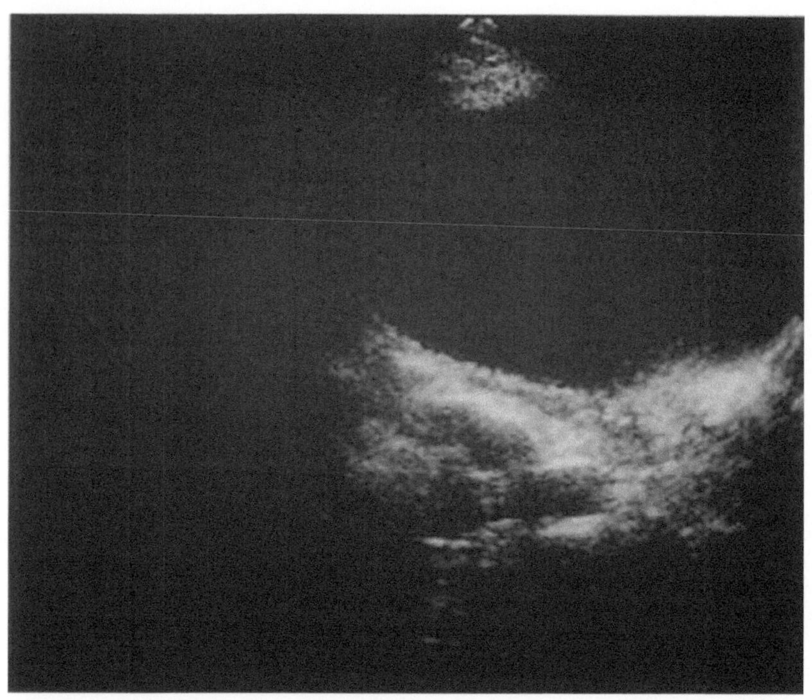

a

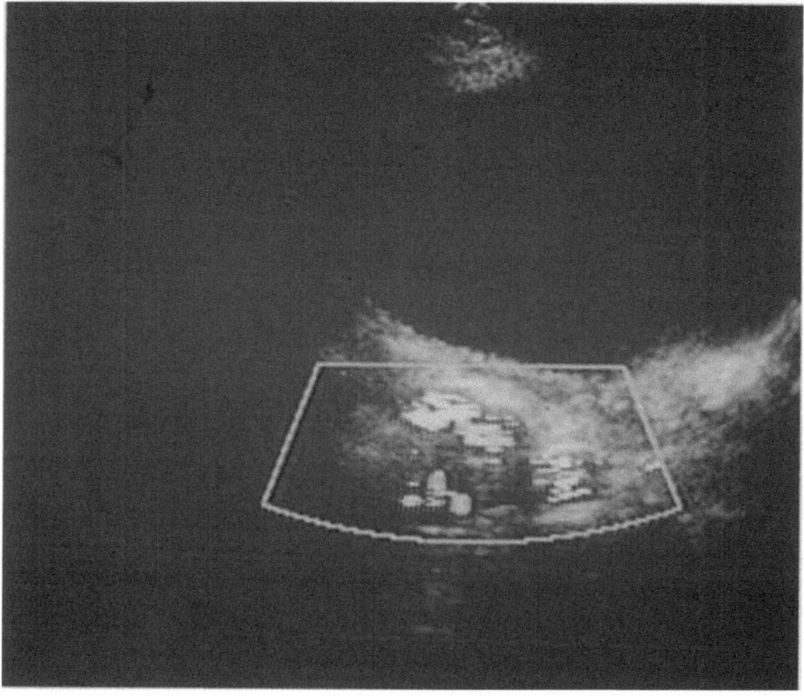

b

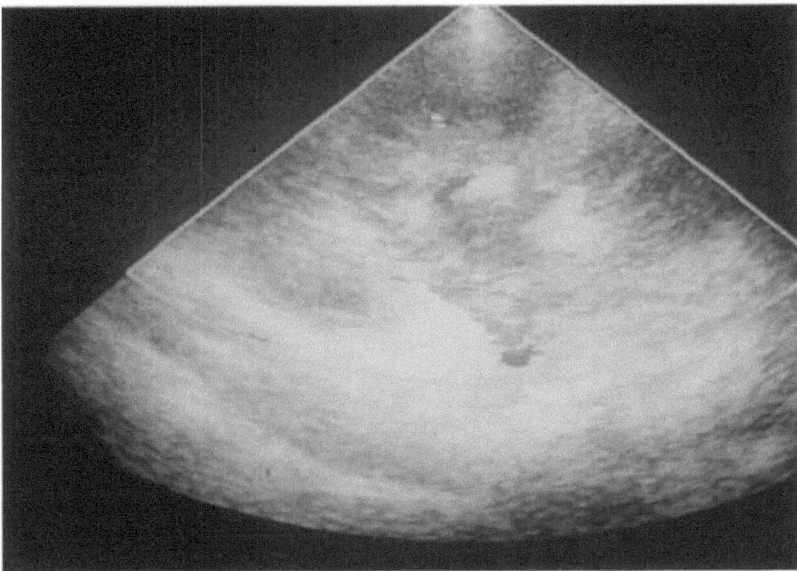

Fig. 24.13. A simple renal cyst shows signals on colour Doppler – intra-cystic renal carcinoma

◀ **Fig. 24.12 a–b.** An adult woman with a history of lymphoma presented with complaint of pelvic discomfort. **a** Transabdominal scan of the pelvis shows an adnexal mass suggestive of recurrence of lymphoma. **b** Colour Doppler shows this to be a tortuous vessel (adnexal varices) and not a nodular mass

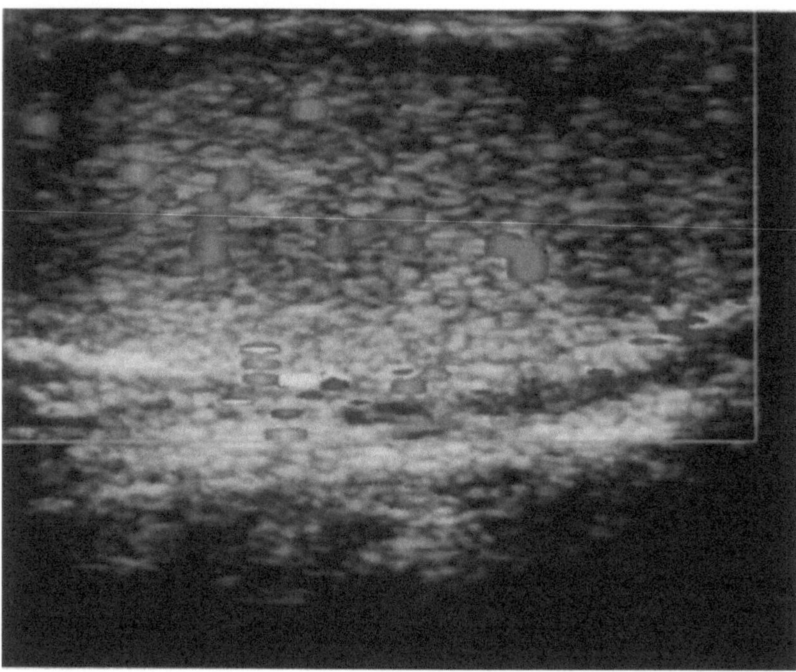

Fig. 24.14. Orchitis. Enlarged hypoechoic testis with increased vascularity. In a normal testis only very few vessels are seen

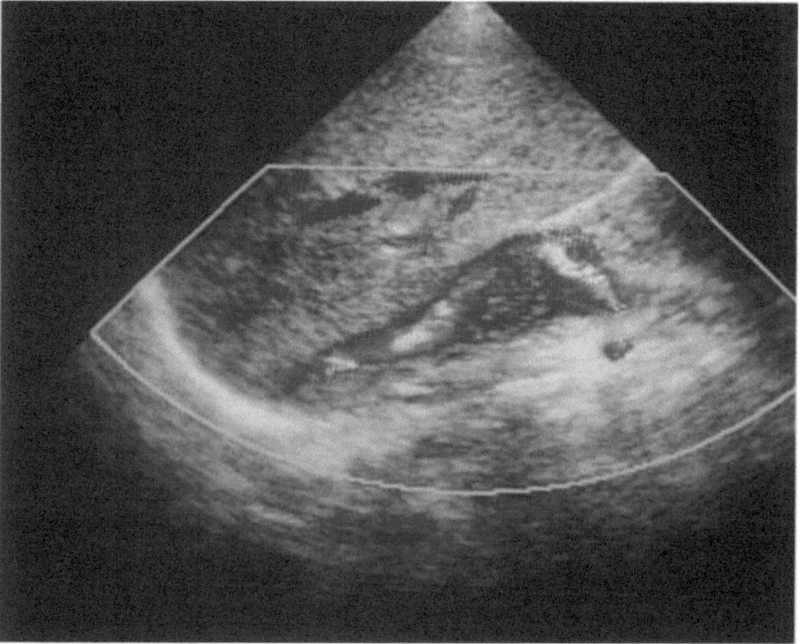

Fig. 24.15. A thrombus in the inferior vena cava extending from a carcinoma of the left kidney. Partial thrombosis was difficult to identify on real-time ultrasound

Subject Index

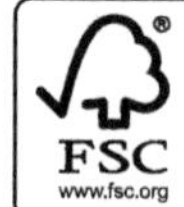 MIX
Papier aus verantwortungsvollen Quellen
Paper from responsible sources
FSC® C105338
FSC
www.fsc.org

If you have any concerns about our products,
you can contact us on
ProductSafety@springernature.com

In case Publisher is established outside the EU,
the EU authorized representative is:
Springer Nature Customer Service Center GmbH
Europaplatz 3, 69115 Heidelberg, Germany

Printed by Libri Plureos GmbH
in Hamburg, Germany